FURTHER STUDIES

for

*H*EALTH

Hilary Thomson

Jean Manuel

Hodder & Stoughton

A MEMBER OF THE HODDER HEADLINE GROUP

Cataloguing in Publication Data is available from The British Library

ISBN 0 340 620552

First published 1996
Impression number   10   9   8   7   6   5   4   3   2   1
Year   2000   1999   1998   1997   1996

Typeset by Wearset, Boldon, Tyne and Wear.
Printed in Great Britain for Hodder & Stoughton Educational, a
division of Hodder Headline Plc, 338 Euston Road, London
NW1 3BH by the Bath Press

FURTHER STUDIES

for

*H*EALTH

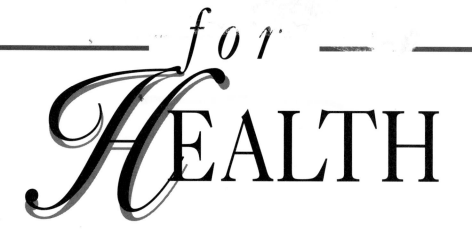

Dedicated to my friend and colleague Jean Manuel,
who sadly died shortly before the publication of this book

CONTENTS

Acknowledgements   ix

1 Chemical science for health care   **1**
Chemical structures in a physiological context   1
Physiological chemical reactions   10
Physical chemistry relevant to physiology   12
Looking again at biological reactions   14
Acids, bases and salts   17
Separation techniques for biological molecules   23
The chemical basis of life   27
Safety in the laboratory   52

2 Environment and health   **58**
Environmental health provision   58
Social and economic influences on the environment   74
The harmful effects of human activity on the environment and health   75
Human activities designed to reduce harm to the environment and health   103

3 Influences on health and disease   **123**
An analysis of research into patterns of disease   123
The purpose of research into patterns of disease   125
Sources of information for determining patterns of disease   127
The examination of specific diseases at a local, national and worldwide level   128
The range of influences on patterns of disease   135
Causes and controlling factors in health and disease   138
Modes of transmission of diseases   158
The control and prevention of disease and illness   160
The role of socioeconomic factors affecting health and disease   171
Processes and responses in disease and illness   179

4 Physical science for health care   **188**
Mechanics in care contexts   188
Electricity, magnetism and their interaction   209
The properties of waves and particles   220
Thermodynamics   232

5 Physiology for health care   **237**
Body systems involved in the transport and elimination of metabolic products   237
The processing and transport of nutrients   254
Sensory and communication systems within the human body   265
The process of seeing   274
The mechanism of hearing   278

Index   **285**

ACKNOWLEDGEMENTS

Many thanks to Nigel Duffin for supplying information for chapter 4.
  Our special thanks go to our families and friends for their support and encouragement.

The publishers would like to thank the following for permission to reproduce copyright material and photographs:

Corbis-Bettmann/UPI, fig 2.5; Sally & Richard Greenhill, figs 2.10, 2.19, 4.40; Sheila Gray/Format, fig 2.12; John Arthur/Impact, fig 2.16; Sam Tanner/Photofusion, fig 4.3; Brenda Prince/Format, fig 4.12; Life Science Images, fig 5.24.

The following figures are reproduced with permission from the Science Photo Library and their photographers:

David Parker, 1.30, 1.31; Will McIntyre, 2.3; Jerome Yeats, 2.15; Omikron, 3.15a; NIBSC, 3.15b; USDA, 3.18; Dr Gary Settles, 3.24; Manfred Kage, 3.25b; Prof P Motta/Dept of Anatomy/University "La Sapienza", Rome, 3.26; BSIP AMAR, 3.27; Prof P Motta, G Macchiarelli, SA Nottola, 3.28; Larry Mulvehill, 4.5; Adam Hart-Davis, 4.31; 4.34; Sinclair Stammers, 4.37; Stammers/Thompson, 4.39; Mehau Kulyk, 4.45; CNRI, figs 5.2b, 5.6 and 5.8c; Alfred Pasieka, 5.8a; Gennard & Grillone, 5.8b; Jan Hinsch, 5.14b; Gene Cox, 5.20b; Patrick Lynch, 5.22; Ralph Eagle, 5.36.

Every effort has been made to trace copyright holders of material reproduced in this book. Any rights not acknowledged here will be acknowledged in subsequent printings if notice is given to the publisher.

CHEMICAL SCIENCE FOR HEALTH CARE

Chemical structures in a physiological context

Chemical structures and reactions in the human body are usually quite complicated. Before studying these in more detail, we must first understand some basic chemistry.

Chemical terms

ELEMENTS

Everything in the universe is made up of *elements*. An element is a substance that cannot be broken down into simpler substances. There are 105 natural elements known so far. The following ones are found in the human body:

- calcium
- carbon
- chlorine
- copper
- fluorine
- hydrogen
- iodine
- iron
- magnesium
- manganese
- molybdenum
- nitrogen
- oxygen
- phosphorus
- potassium
- sodium
- sulphur
- zinc

COMPOUNDS

When bread is well toasted, the surface gets covered with a black solid known as *carbon*. Smoke, containing water vapour and carbon dioxide, rises from the burnt toast.

Bread $\xrightarrow{\text{heat}}$ carbon + carbon + water + toast
dioxide

No matter how the black carbon is treated, it cannot, as an *element*, be changed into anything else. Carbon dioxide and water, on the other hand, *can* be broken down into simpler substances, and so they are *compounds*. Elements are the building blocks of compounds.

Important compounds in the human body are:

- carbohydrates
- lipids
- proteins
- vitamins

ACTIVITY 1

Figure 1.1 shows the apparatus that is required for an experiment to show that the compound water is made up of two elements. When electricity is passed through water containing a little sulphuric acid, the water decomposes into hydrogen and oxygen.

1 Carry out this experiment yourself, if possible.

2 How could you identify that it is hydrogen and oxygen that collect in the two tubes?

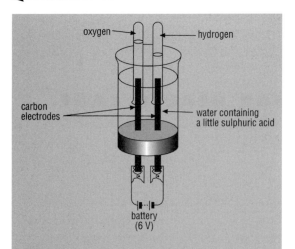

oxygen — hydrogen

carbon electrodes — water containing a little sulphuric acid

battery (6 V)

Figure 1.1 An apparatus for finding the elements of water
Source: Chemistry Counts, G. Hill, Hodder & Stoughton, 1986.

3 Write an equation to show the reaction, first in words and then using chemical formulas. (Read the next section on atoms and molecules before you do this part.)

4 What might the experiment tell us about the proportions of hydrogen and oxygen in water?

ATOMS

The smallest particle of an element is an *atom*. Atoms of the same element are always alike, with the same mass, colour and other properties. Atoms of the various different elements all have their own unique characteristics.

Atoms are represented using *symbols*.

ACTIVITY 2

Find out the symbols for the chemical elements in the human body listed earlier. (For example, the symbol for hydrogen is H, and for Iron it is Fe.)

MOLECULES

Using the symbols for the elements, compounds can be represented as well. Water is represented as H_2O because the smallest particle of water (a molecule) contains two hydrogen atoms and one oxygen atom. Carbon dioxide is written as CO_2: this is one carbon and two oxygen molecules. H_2O and CO_2 are called *formulas*. Formulas show the relative numbers of atoms of each element in the molecules of a compound.

ACTIVITY 3

Take the sugar *sucrose*, i.e. $C_{12}H_{22}O_{11}$, and write a short paragraph about it containing the words 'element', 'atom', 'compound', 'symbol', 'formula' and 'molecule'.

MOLES

It has been found that one atom of carbon is 12 times as heavy as one atom of hydrogen. Therefore, 12 grammes of carbon will have the same number of atoms as 1 gramme of hydrogen. Similarly, one atom of oxygen is 16 times heavier than one atom of hydrogen, so 16 grammes of oxygen will also contain the same number of atoms as 1 gramme of hydrogen and 12 grammes of carbon. These comparisons enable us to work out the *relative atomic mass* (RAM) for each element. The *same* number of atoms, of whatever elements, is assumed when calculating the RAM: 600,000,000,000,000,000,000,000 or 6×10^{23}. This number is called *Avagadro's constant*.

The relative atomic mass in grammes is known as one *mole* of the element. Thus, 12 grammes of carbon equal one mole of carbon; and 16 grammes of oxygen equal one mole of oxygen; and 1 gramme of hydrogen equals one mole of hydrogen.

One mole of an element thus contains 6×10^{23} atoms.

ACTIVITY 4

Notice that:

$$\text{number of moles} = \frac{\text{mass}}{\text{RAM}}$$

and that:

number of atoms present = number of moles $\times 6 \times 10^{23}$

1 How many moles are the following?
- 6 g of hydrogen
- 240 g of carbon
- 6 g of carbon
- 64 g of oxygen

2 How many atoms are there in the following samples?
- 2 g of hydrogen
- 1 g of carbon
- 10 g of carbon
- 8 g of oxygen

3 How many moles are 24×10^{23} hydrogen atoms?

Finding formulas

We have used some formulas already, but how are they obtained? How do scientists know that the formula for water is H_2O?

Experimental results have shown that when water decomposes, 18 g of water give rise to 2 g of hydrogen and 16 g of oxygen. The calculation is then as follows:

$$
\begin{aligned}
18\text{ g of water} \;=\; & 2\text{ g of hydrogen} + 16\text{ g of} \\
& \text{oxygen} \\
=\; & 2\text{ moles of hydrogen} + 1 \\
& \text{mole of oxygen} \\
=\; & 2 \times 6 \times 10^{23}\text{ atoms of} \\
& \text{hydrogen} + 6 \times 10^{23} \\
& \text{atoms of oxygen}
\end{aligned}
$$

Therefore, 2 hydrogen atoms must combine with 1 oxygen atom.

ACTIVITY 5

Find out the formula for magnesium oxide.

The relative atomic mass of magnesium is 24. When magnesium ribbon is heated,

it forms a white powder which is magnesium oxide:

$$\text{magnesium} + \text{oxygen} \rightarrow \text{magnesium oxide}$$

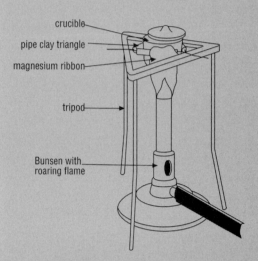

Figure 1.2 An apparatus for finding the formula for magnesium oxide

Heat 0.24 g of magnesium ribbon strongly in a crucible which has been previously weighed together with its lid. (See Figure 1.2 to set up the apparatus). Put a lid on the crucible to stop the magnesium oxide escaping, but leave a small gap so that air can enter. When the magnesium has finished reacting, reweigh the crucible plus lid plus magnesium oxide.

Calculate the amount of oxygen that has combined with the magnesium to form magnesium oxide. Fill in Table 1.1 to give you the formula for magnesium oxide.

Table 1.1 Calculating the formula for magnesium oxide

	Mg	O
Masses reacting	0.24 g	
Mass of 1 mole	24 g	
Moles present	0.01	
Ratio of moles	1	
Ratio of atoms	1	
Formula		

Write a report on your investigation.

Solutes, solvents and solutions

A mixture of (for example) sugar and water forms a *solution*. The substance that dissolves (in this case, the *sugar*) is called the *solute*, and the liquid (in this case, the *water*) in which the solute dissolves is called the *solvent*. In living plants and animals, the solvent is water. Water covers more than 70% of the surface of the earth in oceans, rivers and lakes. It freezes at 0 °C and boils at 100 °C, and so, at most places on the earth, it takes *liquid* form. Water is a very good solvent, dissolving salt, sugar, oxygen and carbon dioxide, and other substances important to life. Table 1.2 shows the solubility of some substances in water at 20 °C. You will notice that some substances are more soluble than others, and that some substances are *insoluble*.

Table 1.2 The solubility of substances in water

Substance	Mass which dissolves in 100 g of water at 20°C
Sand	insoluble
Alcohol	infinite
Salt	36.0 g
Sugar	204.0 g
Oxygen	0.004 g
Carbon dioxide	0.014 g

When the temperature falls below 0 °C, water turns to ice. The ice (unusually) takes up more space than the water that forms it. This makes it less dense than water, and explains why it *floats* on frozen lakes and ponds, allowing fish, plants and other creatures in the water below it to remain alive.

The solubility of a solute in a given solvent (see Table 1.2 again) is defined as the mass of a solute that saturates 100 g of a solvent at a given temperature. Most solids become more soluble in water as the temperature rises. Think of how much easier it is to make a cup of instant coffee with hot water rather than cold, and how much more easily sugar dissolves in hot coffee. Most gases, on the other hand, become less soluble in hot water. This can be important when we remember that fish and other animals depend on dissolved oxygen in seas, rivers and lakes.

You will see from Table 1.2 that carbon dioxide is more soluble than oxygen in water. This is because it reacts with water to form *carbonic acid*, which is a weak acid. This is important in the carriage of carbon dioxide in the blood.

carbon dioxide + water → carbonic acid

ACTIVITY 6

1 Why is water an unusual substance?

2 How does the solubility of solids differ from that of gases?

3 Why is it necessary to give the temperature at which solubility is measured?

4 How would you make sure that a solution is saturated at a particular temperature?

5 Give six examples from the human body where the properties of water are important for physiological processes to take place.

6 Design an experiment to show that water expands when it freezes.

MOLAR SOLUTIONS

Dissolving 1 mole of a substance in sufficient water to make 1 cubic decimetre (i.e. 1 litre) of solution gives a solution of concentration 1 mole per cubic decimetre ($1 \, mol \, dm^{-3}$). This is known as a *molar solution*. The abbreviation for a mole is 'mol'. A solution of sodium chloride of concentration $1 \, mol \, dm^{-3}$ is made by dissolving one mole of sodium chloride, NaCl (58.5 g), in water and making the solution up to a total volume of 1 dm^3. The abbreviation 'M' is often used to indicate this kind of concentration. If the solution had a concentration of 2 mol dm^{-3}, then it would be referred to as '2M' and so on.

ACTIVITY 7

Prepare molar solutions of glucose ($C_6H_{12}O_6$) and potassium nitrate (KNO_3) (1 dm^{-3} of each). How much of each substance should you weigh out? (Relative atomic masses: H = 1, C = 12, N = 14, O = 16, K = 39.)

The atomic structure

All atoms are made up of three basic particles: *protons*, *neutrons* and *electrons*. The *nuclei* (the dense central regions) of atoms contain the protons, which have a positive charge, and

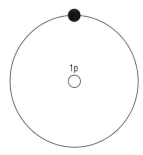

Figure 1.3   A hydrogen atom

the neutrons, which have no charge at all. Moving around the nucleus in orbit are the electrons, which are negatively charged. These electrons are arranged in layers, or 'shells'. The number of protons in an atom is always the same as the number of electrons. We do not usually draw all the protons and neutrons in the nucleus in diagrams of atoms. This would be difficult where atoms have a very large nucleus. For example, uranium has 92 protons and 143 neutrons.

The smallest atom is *hydrogen*, which has one proton in the nucleus, no neutrons and one electron (see Figure 1.3). Carbon, on its part, has six protons, six neutrons and six

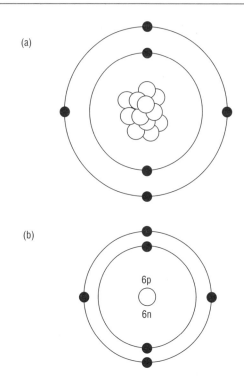

Figure 1.4   A carbon atom

electrons. (Figure 1.4a shows all the protons and neutrons in the nucleus of a carbon atom. Figure 1.4b shows how to simplify the diagram of the carbon atom.) Oxygen has eight protons, eight neutrons and eight electrons (see Figure 1.5).

The first shell of electrons nearest the nucleus can hold up to two electrons. The second shell holds up to eight electrons, the third up to eighteen and the fourth up to thirty-two.

The atomic number and the mass number

The number of protons in the nucleus is called the *atomic number*. The number of

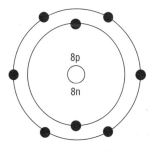

Figure 1.5   An oxygen atom

protons plus the number of neutrons is called the *mass number*.

ACTIVITY 8

1 What is the atomic number and the mass number of hydrogen, carbon and oxygen?

2 Nitrogen has an atomic number of 7 and a mass number of 14. Draw an atom of nitrogen, with its shells of electrons.

There is a convention for writing the chemical symbols for elements together with their mass numbers and atomic numbers, as follows:

mass number
$$^1_1H \text{ and } ^{12}_6C \text{ and } ^{16}_8O$$
atomic number

Look back in this chapter and read the section 'Moles' again. There we saw that one atom of carbon is 12 times as heavy as one atom of hydrogen, and that one atom of oxygen is 16 times as heavy as one atom of hydrogen.

Protons and neutrons each have a relative mass of 1. The mass of an electron is so small that it can be ignored when working out the total mass of the atom.

Isotopes

It has been found that some elements have relative atomic masses (RAMs) which are not whole numbers. We would usually expect whole numbers since the relative atomic mass depends on the numbers of protons and neutrons present, and each of these has a relative mass of 1. However, it turns out that not all atoms of certain elements are exactly the same. An example here is chlorine: the relative atomic mass of chlorine is 35.5. It has been found that there are two different types of chlorine atom, one with a mass number of 35 and one with a mass number of 37:

$^{35}_{17}Cl$ $^{37}_{17}Cl$

There are 17 protons and 17 electrons in both types of chlorine atom, but one has 18 neutrons and the other has 20 neutrons. The two atoms are called *isotopes* of chlorine.

If chlorine contained 100% $^{35}_{17}Cl$ then the relative atomic mass would be 35. If there were a 50:50 mixture of both types of atom, then the relative atomic mass would be 36. Since, however, the RAM is 35.5, we can see that the mixture must be 75% $^{35}_{17}Cl$ and 25% $^{37}_{17}Cl$.

Many elements have relative atomic masses which are *nearly* whole numbers, which means that almost all the atoms are the same with very few isotopes present. Examples are nitrogen, with a RAM of 14.007, and sodium with a RAM of 22.99.

ACTIVITY 9

Almost 100% of naturally occurring hydrogen is ^1_1H. However, there are some hydrogen atoms which have mass numbers of two and three. How many protons, neutrons and electrons do each of the three hydrogen isotopes have?

RADIOACTIVE ISOTOPES

Some isotopes of certain atoms are radioactive. The common form of carbon has a mass number of 12 and an atomic number of 6; this means that it has 6 protons, 6 neutrons and 6 electrons. An isotope of carbon exists, however, which has a mass number of 14 and an atomic number of 6, and thus 6 protons, 8 neutrons and 6 electrons. This type of carbon is described as a *radioactive isotope*. It is not a stable atom and it decays, losing β particles. Experiments have shown that β particles are *electrons*. During the radioactive decay of Carbon-14 ($^{14}_6C$), a neutron in the nucleus of the radioactive atom decays to form an electron and a proton. As well as β particles, *gamma rays* are also given off by radioactive Carbon-14. Both the rays and the β particles can be detected by Geiger–Müller tubes.

In research carried out to discover the sequence of events in metabolic pathways in living organisms, radioactive carbon is often used as a 'tracer', since almost all molecules in cells contain carbon. This type of research is usually done with bacteria, plants or isolated organs since radioactive substances are dangerous: they damage the nucleus in a living cell and prevent it from functioning and dividing correctly.

Forces holding atoms together

We have seen that atoms combine together to form molecules. This chemical bonding results in a more stable electron arrangement in the atoms. When the outermost electron shell is full, the atom is particularly stable. If we are considering the second electron shell, then the most stable configuration is achieved when there are *eight* electrons in this shell: the atom will then be unreactive.

IONIC BONDING

This occurs when atoms exchange electrons with each other to form *ions*. An example is the formation of sodium chloride. Sodium has one electron, in its outer shell, which it is keen to lose. Figure 1.6 shows sodium (Na) combining ionically with chlorine (Cl). The

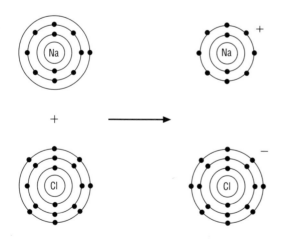

Figure 1.6   Sodium combining ionically with chlorine

sodium atom loses an electron, and the chlorine ion gains it.

The sodium atom is now positively charged since it has lost a negatively charged electron. A positive ion is called a *cation*. The chlorine atom is now negatively charged since it has *gained* an electron. A negative ion is called an *anion*. *Ionic bonds* result from the *attraction* between these two oppositely charged ions.

There are many ions in body fluids in the human body. Sodium chloride is found in blood plasma.

COVALENT BONDING

A *covalent bond* is formed by the sharing of a pair of electrons between two atoms. Figure 1.7 shows covalent bonding in water.

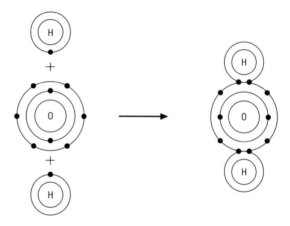

Figure 1.7   Covalent bonding in water

Hydrogen atoms have only one atom in the first electron shell. If there are two, then the atom becomes more stable. Oxygen atoms have six electrons in the second shell; if there are eight, then the atom becomes more stable. So if one oxygen atom combines with two hydrogen atoms, the shells of both atoms are filled through the sharing of electrons, and a stable water molecule is formed.

Biological molecules all contain carbon. Molecules containing carbon are called *organic molecules*. Carbon atoms form covalent bonds with hydrogen, and the simplest organic compound is *methane*.

The carbon atom has four electrons in its second (outermost) shell, and therefore has capacity for four more electrons. Hydrogen

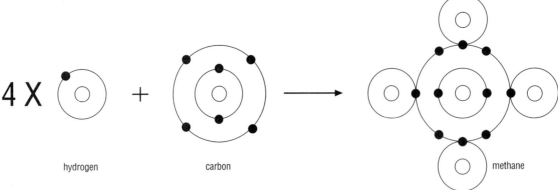

hydrogen   carbon   methane

Figure 1.8   Covalent bonding in methane

has only one electron, but it can share one more electron in this shell – as we have seen in the structure of water. Figure 1.8 shows covalent bonding between one carbon atom and four hydrogen atoms to form methane.

The covalent bonds between carbon and hydrogen can also be illustrated by lines in a two-dimensional representation known as a *structural formula*. Figure 1.9 shows the structural formula for methane. In a methane molecule, the four covalent bonds are arranged symmetrically as if within a tetrahedron (see Figure 1.10).

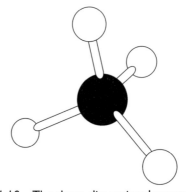

Figure 1.10   The three-dimensional structure of methane

other atoms (see Figure 1.11), including oxygen and nitrogen, thus forming the bulk of the compounds that make up living cells, including carbohydrates, lipids, proteins and nucleic acids
- Carbon can also form double bonds both with itself and with oxygen and nitrogen (see Figure 1.11)

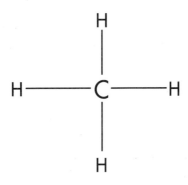

Figure 1.9   The structural formula for methane

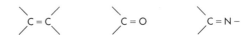

Figure 1.11   Varieties of carbon bond

IMPORTANT CHEMICAL PROPERTIES OF CARBON

- Carbon has the unusual ability to form covalent bonds with *itself*, which allows the formation of multiple chains and rings of carbon atoms
- Carbon can also form covalent bonds with

OTHER MOLECULES INVOLVING COVALENT BONDING

- hydrogen (H_2)
- oxygen (O_2)
- nitrogen (N_2)
- carbon dioxide (CO_2)

(all gases).

ISOMERS

Carbon can form a very large number of compounds, and it is possible for the same group of atoms to be joined up in a number of different ways. Take the formula C_4H_{10}. Two chemicals share this chemical formula but have different *structural* formulas, namely *butane* and *methylpropane* (see Figure 1.12).

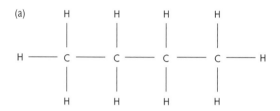

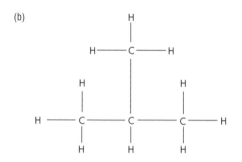

Figure 1.12 The structural formulas for (a) butane and (b) methylpropane

Butane and methylpropane are *isomers* of each other.

The formula $C_6H_{12}O_6$ normally refers to glucose. *Fructose* and *mannose*, two other sugars, have the same chemical formula, but their atoms are arranged differently. These three sugars thus have different structural formulas but are again all isomers of each other.

HYDROGEN BONDS

A water molecule – as already shown on p. 7 above – is formed when two hydrogen atoms combine with an oxygen atom by the sharing of electrons in covalent bonds. The resulting molecule is stable and relatively unreactive. Overall, this molecule is also electrically neutral, but in both the oxygen–hydrogen bonds, the oxygen nucleus draws electrons *away* from the hydrogen

nucleus. Thus, there is a net negative charge on the oxygen atom and a net positive charge on the hydrogen atoms. A molecule – such as the water molecule – that carries an unequal distribution of electrical charge is called a *polar molecule*.

Because of this charge separation in an overall neutral molecule, water molecules form relatively weak bonds called *hydrogen bonds* with other water molecules. This is illustrated in Figure 1.13. Hydrogen bonds form when there is an attraction between the positively charged region of one molecule and the negatively charged region of a neighbouring molecule. They are very important in maintaining the arrangements of polypeptide chains in the three-dimensional structures of proteins which are described later in this chapter.

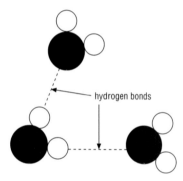

Figure 1.13 A water molecule and the hydrogen bonds that it forms with other water molecules

VALENCY

The valency of an atom is a measure of its *combining power*. We have seen that the carbon atom has four electrons in its outer shell, and that it is able to combine with four hydrogen atoms. The valency of carbon is thus 4; and the valence of hydrogen – which has only one electron – is 1. Oxygen has the ability to combine with two hydrogen atoms to make water, so its valency is 2. Nitrogen has the ability to combine with three hydrogen atoms to make ammonia (NH_3), so its valency is 3.

If we look at atoms which form ionic bonds, like sodium and chlorine, we need to look at the number of charges on the ions to determine the valency. Sodium forms ions with *one* positive charge: Na^+. Chlorine forms ions with *one* negative charge: Cl^-. The valency of both sodium and chlorine is 1.

ACTIVITY 10

Earlier in this chapter, you were asked to list chemical elements found in the human body, and to find out their chemical symbols. Now go back to this list and note the valency of the element by looking at each symbol. Some elements have more than one valency. Try to explain why this is so.

PHYSIOLOGICAL CHEMICAL REACTIONS

Chemical equations

In a chemical reaction, the reacting substances (*reactants*) are converted into new substances (*products*). An equation summarises the chemical changes involved here, with chemical formulas used rather than chemical names. The equation indicates the numbers of moles of reactants and products, and information is also often given about the physical state of each reactant and product, by adding 'g' (gas), 'l' (liquid), 's' (solid) or 'aq' (aqueous, meaning in dilute solution in water) to the formula.

Constructing a chemical equation involves four steps:

1 The word equation is written. For example:

hydrogen + oxygen → water

2 The words are replaced by the formulas of the substances involved:

$H_2 + O_2 \rightarrow H_2O$

3 The equation is balanced: the numbers of atoms on both sides of the equation must be equal.

$2H_2 + O_2 \rightarrow 2H_2O$

4 The physical states may then be added:

$2H_2 (g) + O_2 (g) \rightarrow 2H_2O (l)$

Metabolic reactions

The totality of all the chemical reactions in a living organism is called *metabolism*. Those reactions that are involved in making substances and building up molecules, some of which are very large, are called *anabolism*: simple chemicals are combined to make larger molecules, some of which are stored as energy sources for later use. Examples of anabolism include protein synthesis from amino acids and starch synthesis from glucose. Where larger molecules are broken down to release smaller ones, the processes are collectively known as *catabolism*. Examples include the breakdown of glucose to release energy in respiration and the production of urea from unwanted amino acids in excretion.

The reactions of metabolism are controlled by the organism through enzyme activity. The cell nucleus controls which enzymes are present in the cell. Consequently, the nucleus indirectly controls metabolism.

Oxidation and reduction

Many reactions which occur in everyday life involve substances combining with oxygen to form *oxides*. Burning, respiration and rusting are three important examples.

In burning, fuels containing carbon and hydrogen react with oxygen to form carbon dioxide and water:

fuel + oxygen → carbon dioxide + water

During respiration, glucose, which contains carbon and hydrogen, reacts with oxygen to form carbon dioxide and water:

glucose + oxygen → carbon dioxide + water

During rusting, iron reacts with oxygen and water to form hydrated iron oxide:

iron + oxygen + water → hydrated iron oxide

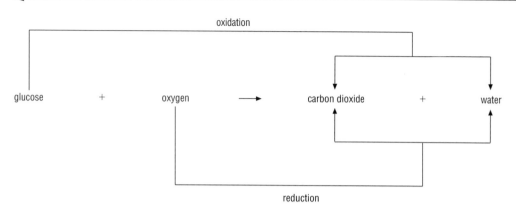

Figure 1.14 Oxidation and reduction in aerobic cellular respiration

Oxidation is thus the term used for the reaction which occurs when substances combine with oxygen. If one substance combines with oxygen, another substance, possibly the oxygen itself, must *lose* oxygen. The substance that loses oxygen in chemical reactions is *reduced*, and the loss process is called *reduction*.

Oxidation and reduction always happen together, and the combined process is called *redox*.

ACTIVITY 11

Look at Figure 1.14. This shows a word equation. Replace the words with the formulas of the substances involved. Then balance the equation – remember that the numbers of atoms on both sides of the equation must be equal. Finally, add the physical state of all the molecules.

Condensation and hydrolysis reactions

These reactions are very common in metabolism. When two glucose molecules react together to form maltose, with the elimination of water, this is called a *condensation* reaction:

glucose + glucose → maltose + water

During digestion, maltose is broken down by a digestive enzyme, which enables water to be added, to release two glucose molecules. This reaction is an example of *hydrolysis*:

maltose + water → glucose + glucose

ACTIVITY 12

Replace the word equations for the condensation reaction of glucose to form maltose and the reverse hydrolysis of maltose to form glucose with balanced equations using the formulae for all the substances involved. The formula for glucose is $C_6H_{12}O_6$.

ASSESSMENT OPPORTUNITY

1 Produce a report on two important chemical reactions taking place in the physiology of the human body which includes:
   - the use of chemical terms to describe the reactions
   - an identification of the name, symbol and valency of the common chemical elements in the human body
   - a description of the atomic structure of carbon, hydrogen and oxygen
   - an explanation of the forces holding atoms together
   - chemical equations related to two physiological chemical reactions

- an explanation of the following chemical terms:

  (a) element   (b) compound

  (c) atom   (d) molecule

  (e) ion   (f) isotope

  (g) isomer   (h) mole

  (i) molar solution   (j) solvent

  (k) solute   (l) reactants

  (m) products   (n) atomic

  (o) atomic mass   number

2 Make notes on the other types of chemical reaction not covered by your main report.

PHYSICAL CHEMISTRY RELEVANT TO PHYSIOLOGY

States of matter: solids, liquids and gases

Chemical substances are sometimes called 'matter'. The theory that matter is made up of moving particles, which are atoms or molecules, is called the *kinetic theory*. The main points of this theory are as follows:

1 All matter is made up of tiny, invisible moving particles.
2 Particles of different substances have different sizes.
3 As the temperature rises, the particles move faster.
4 In a solid, the particles are very close together and can only vibrate about fixed positions.
5 In a liquid, the particles are a little further apart and have more energy so that they can move round each other.
6 In a gas, the particles are far apart and move rapidly and randomly in all the space they can find.

ACTIVITY 13

Studying particles in motion:

1 *Diffusion.* Set up two gas jars. Place some copper sulphate crystals in the bottom of one and carefully fill it with water. Place some liquid bromine in the bottom of the other gas jar. Make some observations. You will have to leave the copper-sulphate jar for a week, but you can see what happens to the bromine in an hour or two.

Write a report on your findings. What does this experiment tell us about the movement of particles? List three important processes in the human body where diffusion is very important.

2 *Brownian motion.* The movement of tiny particles in a gas or liquid is called Brownian motion.

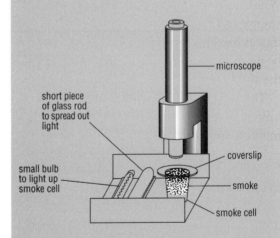

Figure 1.15 A microscope set up to show Brownian motion

Set up a microscope as shown in Figure 1.15. Inject some smoke from a piece of smouldering string into the smoke cell using a test pipette. Observe, through the microscope, the movement of the smoke particles. The air particles are too small to be seen, but they move very fast and hit the smoke particles at random.

Changes of state

Solids, liquids and gases are sometimes called the *three states of matter*. The kinetic theory can be used to explain how a substance changes from one state into another. These changes are usually caused by heating or cooling a substance.

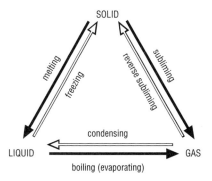

Figure 1.16 Changes of state in matter

A summary of the different changes of state is shown in Figure 1.16.

MELTING AND FREEZING

When a solid is heated, the particles gain energy and vibrate faster and faster. Eventually, they break free from their fixed position and begin to move round each other. As a result, the solid melts to form a liquid.

The temperature at which the solid melts is called the *melting point*. Metals have very high melting points.

EVAPORATING AND BOILING

When a liquid is heated, the particles gain energy and move around each other faster and faster. Some particles near the surface of the liquid have enough energy to escape from those around them into the air, and some of the liquid thus evaporates to form a gas.

Eventually, a temperature is reached at which the particles are trying to escape from the liquid so rapidly that bubbles of gas start to form inside the liquid. The temperature at which this evaporation begins to occur in the bulk of the liquid is called the *boiling point*. Liquids with high boiling points have stronger forces between the particles than liquids with low boiling points.

ACTIVITY 14

1 What happens to particles of a liquid as it cools down and then freezes?

2 Use the kinetic theory to explain why
   - gases exert a pressure on the walls of their container
   - solids have a fixed size and a fixed shape
   - liquids have a fixed size but not a fixed shape
   - solid blocks of air freshener can disappear without leaving any solid

3 Table 1.3 shows the melting points and boiling points of substances W, X, Y and Z.

Table 1.3 The melting and boiling points of four substances

Substance	Melting point (°C)	Boiling point (°C)
W	1,083	2,600
X	−7	58
Y	−101	−35
Z	27	98

(a) Which substance is a liquid at room temperature?
(b) Which substance is a gas at room temperature?
(c) Which substance is a metal?
(d) Which substance cannot be a metal?
The substances here are bromine, chlorine, copper and iodine. Which is which?

THE EVAPORATION AND CONDENSATION OF WATER

The molecules in liquid water are held quite close together by *intermolecular forces*. These forces are absent in water vapour, where molecules are free to separate and take up far more volume.

When water evaporates, changing from

liquid to vapour, the intermolecular attractions are overcome. This process uses energy, and the amount of energy used is called the *molar latent heat of vaporisation* (or the *enthalpy change of vaporisation*). Its symbol is: ΔH_{Vap}. In the reverse process, *condensation*, molecules come together again, intermolecular attractions re-form and an equal quantity of energy is released.

The importance of these processes to life

- 17% of the sun's energy received at the tropics is transported by water vapour to colder parts of the earth
- When rain is formed by the condensation of water vapour, energy is released, and this warms the land
- Humans rely on the evaporation of water to cool the body when we sweat. The heat needed to cause water vapour to form comes from the body, which is thus cooled down

LOOKING AGAIN AT BIOLOGICAL REACTIONS

Oxidation and reduction

Earlier in this chapter, we saw that oxidation and reduction always happen together. To recap, we defined oxidation as the term for the reaction that occurs when a substance combines with oxygen. And if oxygen is gained by one substance, then it must be *lost* from another. The substance losing oxygen is then described as being *reduced*. Together, these reactions are described as *redox* reactions.

There are, however, ways of defining oxidation and reduction in more detail.

1 Something is *oxidised* if
   - it gains oxygen
   - it loses electrons
   - it loses hydrogen
2 Something is *reduced* if
   - it loses oxygen
   - it gains electrons
   - it gains hydrogen

An oxidising agent *removes electrons from something else*. A reducing agent *gives electrons to something else*.

Aerobic respiration is represented by the equation:

$$C_6H_{12}O_6 + 6O_2 \rightarrow 6CO_2 + 6H_2O$$

Glucose is oxidised, and oxygen is the oxidising agent. The latter itself becomes reduced to form water.

ACTIVITY 15

Look at Figure 1.17. Earlier in your course (when you studied the physical aspects of health and social well-being), you learned about cellular respiration, which includes both aerobic and anaerobic respiration.

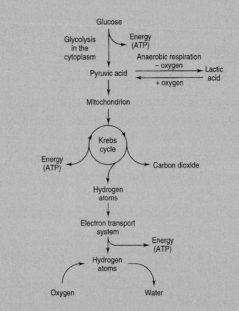

Figure 1.17 **Stages in cellular respiration**

Revise this topic by writing a brief account of the stages of respiration shown in the present figure. Use the following paragraph headings:
- glycolysis and anaerobic respiration
- the Krebs cycle (the tri-carboxylic acid cycle)
- the electron transfer system

Is this an anabolic or catabolic series of reactions?

There are about 40 different reactions involved in the three stages of cellular respiration listed in the above Activity. We will now look in more detail at some of these stages to illustrate the particular features of *redox* reactions.

1 *Glycolysis and the Krebs cycle.* You will see that hydrogen atoms are released during the first two stages, glycolysis and the Krebs cycle. The hydrogen atoms are progressively 'stripped off' the carbon atoms of the glucose molecules, leaving carbon dioxide. The glucose molecules have been gradually *oxidised* in this series of reactions since they have *lost* hydrogen atoms.

The released hydrogen atoms are carried away by special carriers, the main one being *nicotinamide adenine dinucleotide* (NAD). These carriers are therefore *reduced* since they gain hydrogen atoms whilst glucose is oxidised:

Glucose + NAD → carbon dioxide + reduced NAD

2 *The electron transfer system.* The reduced carriers take the hydrogen atoms to the electron transfer system (see Figure 1.18). Here, the hydrogen atoms separate into protons and electrons. The protons go into solution and the electrons pass to a series of protein molecules called *cytochromes*. As each cytochrome gains an electron, it is reduced, and as it loses an electron it is oxidised. The electrons then pass to an enzyme called *cytochrome oxidase* which transfers the electrons to oxygen molecules. Then, the protons join to make water. You can see that oxygen is only reduced at the very last stage of cellular respiration.

The purpose of the electron transfer system is to release energy in a controlled way so that *adenosine triphosphate* (ATP) can be made. This carries the energy from respiration to the metabolic activities that need it. Three energy-carrying ATP molecules are made for each H_2.

3 *Anaerobic respiration.* You will see in Figure 1.17 that in the last stage of glycolysis, pyruvic acid does not enter the Krebs cycle if oxygen is absent, but instead forms *lactic acid*. During strenuous exercise, the circulatory system may not be able to supply the muscle with oxygen fast enough. Lactic acid accumulates, and in time can cause cramp and so prevent the muscle from operating. Lactic-acid formation is a *redox* reaction. This reaction is reversible, so that when the muscle stops working and oxygen supplies return to normal, the lactic acid forms pyruvic acid again, and this continues on the respiration pathway.

To make lactic acid, hydrogen atoms are required, and these are supplied by the hydrogen carrier NAD. (Notice, in Figure 1.19, where the hydrogen atoms have joined with the pyruvic acid, which is *reduced* to make lactic acid.)

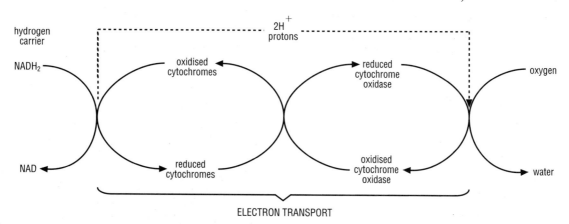

Figure 1.18 **The electron transfer system**

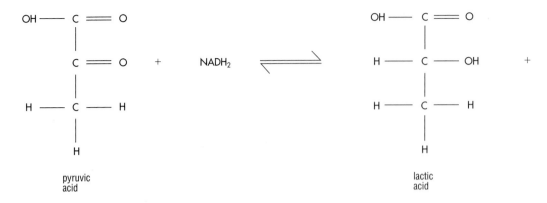

pyruvic
acid

lactic
acid

Figure 1.19 Lactic-acid formation

The reversibility of reactions

You will notice that lactic-acid formation from pyruvic acid is a reversible reaction. This is because the energy change involved is very small, and because the product, lactic acid, is not removed from where it is formed. Aerobic cellular respiration, on the other hand, is not reversible because there is a relatively large energy difference between the substrate, glucose, and the products, carbon dioxide and water. Another product, adenosine triphosphate (ATP), carries energy away from the site of production to cellular reactions.

Figure 1.20 shows that 2,900 kJ mol energy is released from glucose in a controlled way in a step-by-step series of reactions. About 50% is transferred to ATP, and the rest is released as heat.

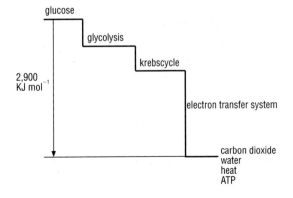

Figure 1.20 Energy release in aerobic cellular respiration

Condensation and hydrolysis

Earlier on in this chapter, we looked at the formation of the disaccharide maltose from two glucose molecules as an example of a condensation reaction. Here, water is eliminated in the formation of the *glycosidic bond* which joins the glucose molecules:

$$C_6H_{12}O_6 + C_6H_{12}O_6 \rightarrow CH_{22}O_{11} + H_2O$$

Condensation reactions involving the elimination of water also occur in the formation of

- starch from glucose
- proteins from amino acids
- lipids from fatty acids and glycerol

ATP from respiration is used to make the bonds in the formation of the large molecules.

These are all *anabolic* reactions because they involve building up larger molecules from smaller ones. Hydrolysis reactions, which involve the breaking of bonds through a reaction to water, are *catabolic* reactions. Energy is released during this reaction. Enzymes which *catalyse* (i.e. speed up) hydrolysis reactions will be considered later on in this chapter.

At first glance, it looks as if condensation and hydrolysis reactions are simple reverse processes. However, different enzymes are involved, and condensation reactions need an energy input from ATP to make the new bonds. So although the processes *are* reversible, each pathway involves its own specific enzymes.

ACTIVITY 16

1 Why is hydrolysis so important in digestion?

2 Find out about how proteins, starch and other carbohydrates, and lipids are digested in the alimentary canal.

3 List two other hydrolytic processes that are important in metabolism, and explain why the reaction is important.

4 The synthesis of glycogen in the liver is an important condensation reaction. Explain how this is carried out. Look particularly at how the energy is supplied to make the new glycosidic bonds.

5 The hydrolysis of glycogen is also important. Explain using a diagram how the balance between condensation and hydrolysis is achieved. Why is this process so important?

ACIDS, BASES AND SALTS

Acids

We can think of an acid as a compound which breaks down (dissociates) in water to liberate hydrogen ions. Substances which we call acids do not behave as acids in the absence of water. Water reacts with substances to produce the H^+ (aq) ions which cause acid properties. And acids are thus defined as substances which can *give* (i.e. *donate*) these H^+ ions.

The stronger the acid, the more hydrogen ions it liberates per mole. Inorganic acids, such as the hydrochloric, nitric and sulphuric acids, are strong acids because a large degree

of dissociation occurs in an aqueous solution in order to form ions (in a process called *ionisation*). For hydrochloric acid:

$$HCl\ (aq) \rightarrow H^+\ (aq) + Cl^-\ (aq)$$

For sulphuric acid:

$$H_2SO_4\ (aq) \rightarrow 2H^+\ (aq) + SO_4^{2-}\ (aq)$$

For nitric acid:

$$HNO_3\ (aq) \rightarrow H^+\ (aq) + NO_3^-\ (aq)$$

The balance (equilibrium) between dissociated and undissociated molecules lies far to the right, so we draw in just one arrow above to show this.

Acids like sulphuric acid – H_2SO_4 – react with metals to forms salts and hydrogen:

$$Mg + H_2SO_4 \rightarrow MgSO_4 + H_2$$

They also react with metal oxides to form salts and water:

$$CuO + H_2SO_4 \rightarrow CuSO_4 + H_2O$$

Carbonic acid (H_2CO_3) forms when carbon dioxide dissolves in water (HCO_3^- are the hydrogen carbonate ions):

$$CO_2 + H_2O \rightleftharpoons H_2CO_3 \rightleftharpoons H^+ + HCO_3^-$$

Carbonic acid is quite a weak acid as not all its molecules dissociate. (See Figure 1.21 and the discussion on the pH scale on pp. 18–19.) This latter reaction is of physiological importance since carbon dioxide is produced in respiration and has to be carried in the blood plasma from the site of production to the lungs for excretion.

The more usual acids found in living systems are *organic acids*. These are also weak acids since relatively few of their molecules are dissociated in solution.

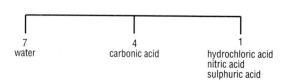

Figure 1.21 **The pH scale for water and various acids**

TWO OTHER PROPERTIES OF ACIDS

- They give characteristic colours with *indicators*: they give a red colour with litmus and an orange or red colour (depending on how acid they are) with universal indicator
- They conduct electricity, and are decomposed by it. Hydrogen is produced at the cathode during electrolysis

Bases and alkalis

Bases are chemical opposites to acids: bases *take* in H ions whereas acids *donate* them. Bases can neutralise acids by combining with the H^+ ions. Bases that are soluble in water are called *alkalis*.

Sodium, potassium and zinc hydroxides are examples of strong bases since they are fully ionised in solutions. The following reaction shows how zinc hydroxide ($Zn(OH)_2$) neutralises sulphuric acid (H_2SO_4):

$$Zn(OH)_2 \text{ (s)} + H_2SO_4 \text{ (aq)} \rightarrow ZnSO_4 \text{(aq)} + 2 H_2O \text{ (l)}$$

The OH ions from the zinc hydroxide combine with the hydrogen ions from the acid to form water ($2H_2O$) and *zinc sulphate* ($ZnSO_4$).

Ammonia (NH_3) is only partially ionised in solution and is thus a weak base:

$$NH_3 \text{ (aq)} + H_2O \rightleftharpoons NH_4OH \rightleftharpoons NH_4^+ \text{ (aq)} + OH^- \text{ (aq)}$$

Ammonia is produced in the breakdown of amino acids in the liver prior to excretion processes in the kidneys.

As well as hydroxides, *metal oxides* also are bases. These neutralise acids in a similar way. This example involves zinc oxide – ZnO:

$$ZnO \text{ (s)} + H_2SO_4 \text{ (aq)} \rightarrow ZnSO_4 \text{ (aq)} + H_2O \text{ (l)}$$

Salts

Salts are formed when acids react with metals or bases. Most salts contain a positive metal ion and a negative non-metal or *radical* ion.

Radicals are groups of atoms like NO_3^- and CO_3^{2-}.

Sodium chloride is the best-known salt.

PROPERTIES OF SALTS

- They have high melting points and boiling points
- They are electrolytes – they dissociate into ions in solution
- They are often soluble in water

The ionisation of water

We have seen that acids, bases and salts dissociate to form ions to varying degrees when they are in an aqueous (water) solution. This is called ionisation. We have also seen that water itself can form ions. In pure water, very few molecules dissociate to form hydrogen ions (H^+) and *hydroxyl ions* (OH^-):

$$H_2O \rightleftharpoons H^+ + OH^-$$

The hydrogen and hydroxyl-ion concentration in pure water is 0.0000001 (or 10^{-7}) moles dm^{-3}.

The pH scale

The pH (potential of hydrogen) scale is a measure of the degree of acidity or alkalinity of a solution. Pure water has a pH of 7. Solutions with a pH of less than 7 are acidic. Solutions with a pH of more than 7 are alkaline. The pH scale represents the concentration of H^+ ions in a solution on a *logarithmic* scale. This means that a *tenfold* change in concentration is needed to produce a pH change of 1. Figure 1.22 gives the hydrogen ion concentrations corresponding to some pH numbers. At pH 7, the concentration of hydrogen ions (represented symbolically by $[H^+]$) is equal to the concentration of hydroxyl ions ($[OH^-]$), and the solution is therefore *neutral*.

The pH value of a liquid is the logarithm to the base 10 of the reciprocal of the hydrogen ion concentration expressed in moles per dm^{-3}. In pure water or a neutral solution:

$$[H^+] = [OH^-] = 10^{-7} \text{ mol dm}^{-3}$$

Therefore:

$$pH = \log \frac{1}{[H^+]} = \log \frac{1}{10^{-7}} = 7$$

ACTIVITY 17

An experiment to find out how fast carbon dioxide escapes from a solution

A pH reading is determined experimentally using either coloured indicator papers or an electronic pH meter equipped with a probe that is sensitive to hydrogen ions.

You will remember that carbon dioxide dissolves in water to form carbonic acid which is a weak acid. This dissociates to form hydrogen carbonate ions and hydrogen ions. (Look back to p. 17 to remind yourself of the equation involved.) A saturated solution of carbon dioxide at room temperature and pressure has a pH of 4. If the concentration of H^+ ions in a solution is halved, the pH only changes by 0.3. This means that the pH changes to be observed are only very small.

Water has a pH of 7.

Requirements

- a solution of CO_2 in water (e.g. soda water)
- a pH meter and glass electrode (or narrow-range pH paper)
- buffer solutions to calibrate the pH meter
- a thermometer
- a glass rod
- a stopwatch
- small beakers

1 Place some of your CO_2 solution in a small beaker, and measure the initial pH.

2 When dissolved CO_2 escapes from a solution and becomes gaseous, it can only do so at the interface between the solution and the atmosphere. If the solution is left undisturbed, then the CO_2 molecules take time to diffuse to the surface of the liquid. Systematic stirring, or bubbling air through the solution, is therefore important to help this diffusion process. Stir, or bubble air through, the solution for a timed period and then measure the pH again. Do this several times.

3 Write a report on your findings, with an accurate method and results table. Record your results on a graph.

4 Calculate the concentration of hydrogen ions in mol dm^{-3} for each of your readings, and plot a second graph.

5 Provide a conclusion and full discussion. Evaluate your experiment.

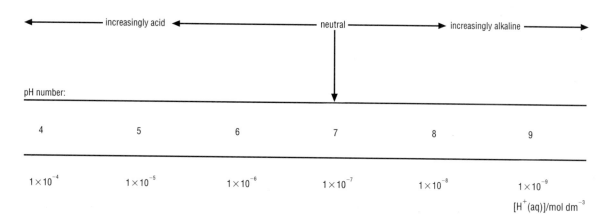

Figure 1.22 The pH scale

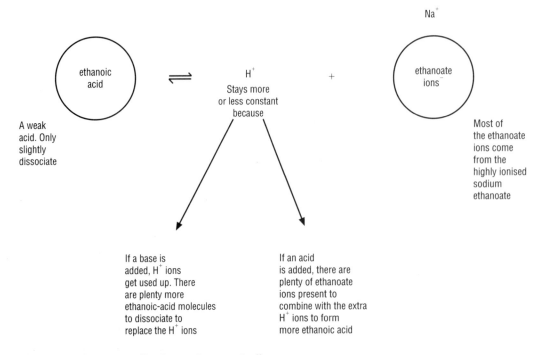

Figure 1.23   The ethanoic acid/sodium ethanoate buffer system

THE BIOLOGICAL IMPORTANCE OF pH

The pH of the external environment is one of the most important ecological factors. The availability of mineral ions for uptake by plants is affected by the pH of the soil. The productivity of crops is therefore dependent on this factor.

Slight changes in the pH of the internal environment of the human body can adversely affect physiological and metabolic reactions. We have seen that acids and bases are involved in cell reactions.

Earlier in this chapter, we saw that carboxylic acids are part of the Krebs cycle of cellular respiration, and that ammonia, a base, forms as a product of amino-acid breakdown in the liver. Carbon dioxide forms all the time as a waste product of respiration – it dissolves to become carbonic acid, a weak acid, in the blood plasma.

The shapes of protein molecules and the functioning of enzymes are greatly affected by pH change. This is discussed in more detail later on in this chapter.

Here are the pH values of some physiological fluids:
- Blood   7.40
- Milk, urine   6.50
- Gastric fluid 1.75

BUFFERS

In a *buffer* solution, the pH does not change significantly when a small amount of acid or base is added to it. Some chemical buffers contain a weak acid together with a strongly ionised soluble salt of the same acid. An example is a buffer composed of ethanoic acid, which is slightly ionised and is therefore a weak acid, and sodium ethanoate, a salt which is strongly ionised in solution. Figure 1.23 shows how the ethanoic acid/sodium ethanoate buffer system works.

The maintenance of pH in the human body is often called the *acid/base balance*. The pH of human blood is maintained between 7.35 and 7.45 in arteries and 7.30 and 7.41 in veins. Any significant change in pH outside these narrow ranges causes disturbances in blood gas carriage. *Acidaemia* is the name given to the condition where the blood pH falls *below* normal, and *alkalaemia* is where the blood pH rises *above* normal. Although a more or less constant blood pH is achieved, concentrations of carbon dioxide, and hence carbonic acid, vary greatly. The buffer in blood consists of two main factors, the hydrogen carbonate ions and proteins – especially haemoglobin. The property of hydrogen carbonate ions acting as a buffer depends on the fact that the equilibrium of the following reaction lies well to the left:

$$H_2O + CO_2 \rightleftharpoons H_2CO_3 \rightleftharpoons H^+ + HCO_3^-$$

Additional hydrogen ions added will be 'mopped up' by more carbonic acid forming. The buffering properties of blood proteins, including the plasma proteins as well as the above-mentioned haemoglobin, are also very important in maintaining a constant internal pH.

Proteins are made up of amino acids with the general formula as shown in Figure 1.24: R is any one of a variety of chemical structures, and the —NH_2 and —COOH groups shown in the formula are part of the

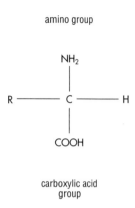

Figure 1.24 The general formula for an amino acid

peptide links which join amino acids to make a protein (see Figure 1.24). In some amino acids, R contains extra amino or carboxylic acid groups, and these then form *charged groups* in the protein molecule.

The negatively charged carboxyl groups can take up additional hydrogen ions, and the positively charged amino groups can take up additional hydroxyl ions. This is how proteins act as buffers – see Figure 1.25. Having said that, the *final* control of pH will, however, occur when carbon dioxide is released in the lungs.

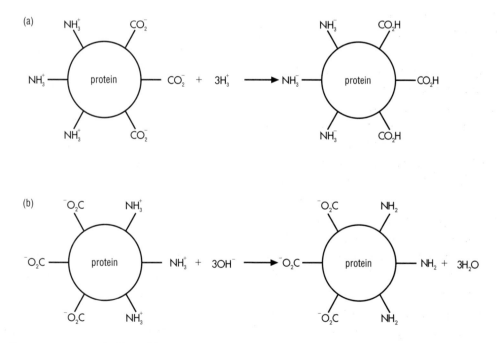

Figure 1.25 Proteins acting as buffers: (a) protein acting as a base combining with hydrogen ions; (b) protein acting as an acid combining with hydroxyl ions

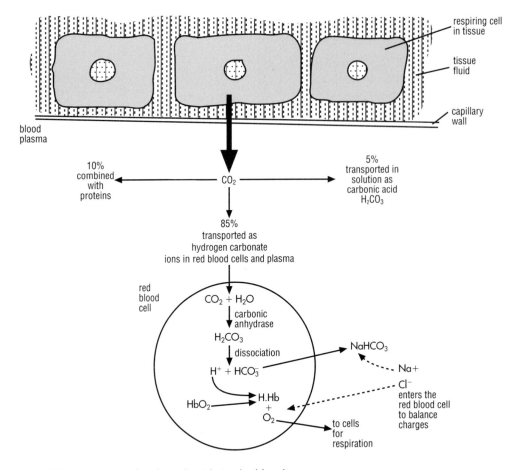

Figure 1.26   The transport of carbon dioxide in the blood

ACTIVITY 18

1 Look at Figure 1.26, which diagramatically shows how carbon dioxide is carried in the blood. *Carbonic anhydrase* is an enzyme found in red blood cells which catalyses the formation of carbonic acid from carbon dioxide and water. Write a description of the sequence of events involved here, emphasising the stage where haemoglobin (Hb) acts as a buffer by absorbing H^+ ions and thus preventing the blood from becoming acid.

2 This whole process is called the 'chloride shift'. Explain why.

THE ROLE OF THE KIDNEYS IN pH REGULATION

Buffers are limited in the extent to which they can cope with excess hydrogen ions in the body. We have seen that the lungs play an important role in the final regulation of pH by eliminating carbon dioxide from the body. However, the kidneys also play a vital role in regulating acid levels.

As well as the acids produced by the body itself, *food intake* will also contribute to acid levels. Acid excretion takes place in the distal convoluted tubule of the nephrons of the kidney. Carbonic acid is produced in the tubule and carbonic anhydrase causes a rapid dissociation into hydrogen and hydrogen carbonate ions. The hydrogen ions are then actively secreted into the tubule, where they react with *disodium hydrogen phosphate* in the filtrate. The hydrogen replaces some of the sodium, producing *sodium dihydrogen phosphate*. The sodium ions are then actively reabsorbed back into the blood.

This system has two advantages:

1 sodium is not lost to the body
2 hydrogen ions are buffered in the urine.

This system is shown in Figure 1.27a.

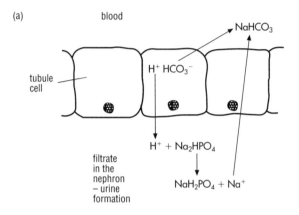

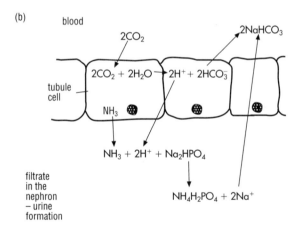

Figure 1.27 The regulation of pH in the kidney

There is a second system which comes into play if the pH of the blood is very high. The resulting low pH in the filtrate stimulates the tubule cells to release ammonia, which then completely replaces sodium ions from disodium hydrogen phosphate. This system is shown in Figure 1.27b.

SEPARATION TECHNIQUES FOR BIOLOGICAL MOLECULES

One problem facing scientists studying biological molecules is how to separate them from each other, since every cell is made up of millions of different molecules. The reasons for isolating molecules are:
• to analyse them
• to measure amounts of molecules present
• to obtain large amounts for further study or commercial production

Chromatography

This is one of the most commonly used techniques for separating molecules. It involves two phases:

1 the *stationary* phase, which is the chromatographic material – this can be paper or silica gel
2 the *mobile* phase, which can be a liquid or a gas.

The mobile phase moves through the stationary phase, carrying with it the molecules to be separated. How much these will separate will depend on how much they interact with the stationary phase. If they link strongly to it, they will be left behind as the mobile phase moves along the stationary phase.

If a mixture of unknown substances is separated by chromatography, we then need to identify them. Sometimes they are already coloured, so it is easy to see where they are on a *chromatogram* (a strip of material containing constituents of a mixture separated by chromatography). If the substances are not coloured, then they have to be treated with a dye so that they can be located.

We can compare the position of an unknown substance on the chromatogram with known ones to try to identify it. To help us do this, we calculate the Rf ('ratio of fronts') value:

$$Rf = \frac{\text{distance travelled by substance}}{\text{distance travelled by solvent}}$$

We measure from the point of original application of the mixture of substances. Each substance has an Rf value for a particular solvent.

ACTIVITY 19

The chromatography of leaf pigments.

Grind up some nettle leaves in propanone. Filter this through muslin into a small beaker. Cut a strip of chromatography or filter paper long enough to fit into a boiling tube and narrow enough not to touch the sides. Draw a line 30 mm from one end of the paper. Place a drop of the pigment on the middle of this line and let it dry. Do this several times to get a concentrated spot. Suspend the paper in a boiling tube containing some solvent (see Figure 1.28).

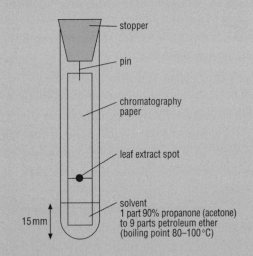

Figure 1.28 The chromatographic separation of leaf pigments

Watch the solvent rise and reach the leaf-extract spot. It will then carry pigments up the paper. Stop the experiment when the solvent has not quite reached the top – this will be within half an hour. Mark the point reached by the solvent. (A thin layer of silica gel on a backing could be used instead of paper.)

Calculate your Rf values for all the separated pigments. Compare these with the values in Table 1.4 and identify the pigments present.

Table 1.4 Colours and Rf values for leaf pigments separated in propanone/ether solvent

Pigment	Colour	Rf
Carotene	Yellow	0.95
Phaeophytin	Yellow-grey	0.83
Xanthophyll	Yellow-brown	0.71
Chlorophyll a	Blue-green	0.65
Chlorophyll b	Green	0.45

Electrophoresis

Electrophoresis is a process used to separate *charged* molecules such as proteins, peptides and nucleic acids. Separation of proteins are normally carried out using a *polyacrylamide gel* (PAG). This method relies not only on the charge but also on the *molecular mass*, and only very small quantities of proteins are required. These are first treated with a detergent, called SDS, which 'unwinds' the protein molecules. One SDS molecule then attaches itself to each peptide bond. (These bonds join the amino acids together to form the protein.) The SDS molecules are negatively charged, so at the end of the initial treatment the proteins too are negatively charged.

All the SDS-treated protein molecules move towards the anode, but the smaller ones move faster.

Electrophoresis patterns of proteins can be used to help diagnose certain diseases.

ACTIVITY 20

People with sickle-cell anaemia have an abnormal form of haemoglobin (Hb S) in their red blood cells. A difference between Hb S and normal haemoglobin (Hb A) can be detected by electrophoresis and chromatography. Figure 1.29 outlines these processes.

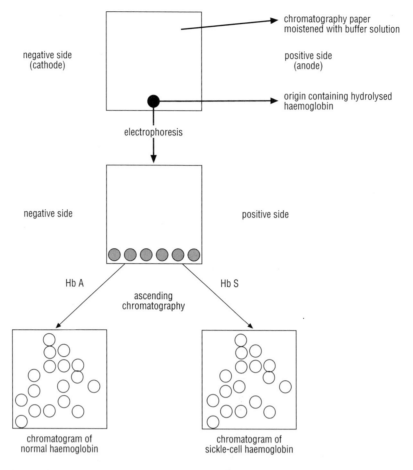

Figure 1.29 Using electrophoresis and chromatography to distinguish between normal and abnormal forms of haemoglobin

1 Before electrophoresis, the haemoglobin was hydrolysed to a mixture of 17 peptides. Suggest how this could have been done.

2 Describe the results after electrophoresis. What property of the different peptides results in their separation by electrophoresis?

3 Use information in Figure 1.29 to suggest how Hb S differs from Hb A.

THE ELECTROPHORESIS OF DNA

DNA (*deoxyribonucleic acid*) is part of all chromosomes. DNA can be extracted from very small samples of tissue and treated so that it can be separated into its fragments by electrophoresis. The DNA sample is negatively charged so that it moves towards the anode when an electric current is passed through a DNA solution in buffer.

The fragments separate according to their size and charge, and can then be stained. Each individual has a unique DNA complement, and the personal electrophoresis pattern is called a *DNA fingerprint* (see Figure 1.30).

USES OF DNA FINGERPRINTING

• Establishing family relationships. We inherit half our DNA from our father and half from our mother. The DNA fingerprint bands of a child must therefore match with those in the parents' DNA fingerprints (see Figure 1.31).

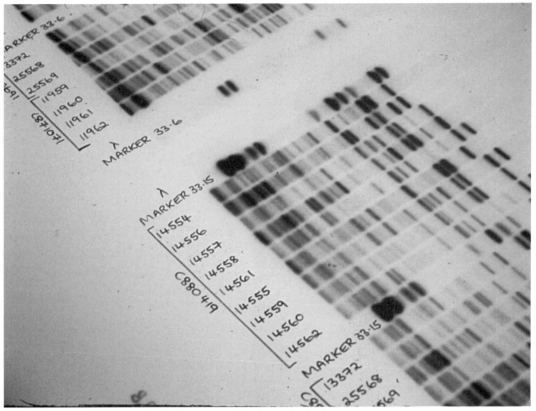

Figure 1.30 A photograph of DNA fingerprints for five individuals

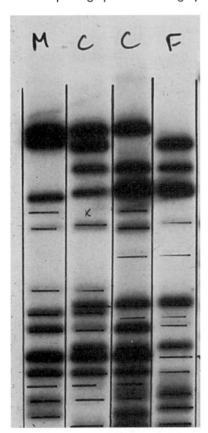

Figure 1.31 An analysis of DNA fingerprints in paternity testing

- Testacy cases can be solved using this technique. DNA fingerprints will show whether 'long-lost' claimants are really part of the family
- Forensic science investigations can use DNA fingerprinting when a biological specimen is left at the scene of the crime. The offender can be identified with certainty
- The confirmation of animal pedigrees
- Monitoring bone-marrow transplants. DNA fingerprinting can be used to detect whether a transplanted marrow is being rejected
- The detection of inherited diseases. Work is currently being done to identify members of families who may have inherited certain diseases but who do not show any symptoms yet. *Neurofibromatosis* (a type of cancer) and Huntington's chorea are examples

ACTIVITY 21

Discussion points

1 A *vasectomy* is a minor operation to cut the *vas deferens* leading from each testicle and is used as a method of birth control. Rapists who have had a vasectomy are less likely to be identified using the DNA fingerprinting technique – research this area and explain why.

2 Is DNA fingerprinting for forensic science an important development? What advantages does it have over previous methods of detection?

3 Explain how a series of DNA fingerprints would show the success or otherwise of a bone-marrow transplant.

4 Is there any point in having a test for certain fatal genetic conditions if there is no possible cure?

5 If everyone was required by law to supply a genetic fingerprint for storage in a national police computer, would our lives be better and the world a safer place?

Source: SATIS 16–19 Unit 6

ASSESSMENT OPPORTUNITY

Make records of investigations into those areas of physical chemistry that are relevant to physiology. These records must include:
- an explanation of one change of state of matter into another
- a summary of different types of chemical reaction, with one physiological example of each
- a description of acid, base and salts
- an explanation of two buffer systems, one in blood and one in urine

formation, with pH notation and the relationship to hydrogen ion concentration explained
- an explanation of the separation of different substances using chromatography or electrolysis
- an explanation of how electrolysis and electrophoresis are applied to health care

THE CHEMICAL BASIS OF LIFE

Water

Earlier in this chapter, we looked at various properties of water. (You will find information about water in the sections above on elements and compounds, the atomic structure of molecules, bonding and the properties of solvents.) Water can exist as a vapour, a liquid or a solid, and these aspects were considered in the discussions on changes of state. Water can also react in cells in both hydrolysis and condensation.

ACTIVITY 22

1 What elements are in water, and how can you show this?

2 What is the structure of the atoms in water, and how are these atoms joined together to make water?

3 Discuss the two types of bonding shown by water.

4 Why is water described as a polar molecule?

5 Water is a good solvent. List four substances important to life that dissolve easily in water.

6 What is the molar latent heat of vaporisation, and why is this important in human physiology?

7 Water can be a reactant in physiological reactions. Name two types of reaction that it is involved in, and give an example of each.

8 Water is weakly ionised, and has a pH of 7. What does this mean, and how are these two properties linked?

9 To what extent are the properties of water reflected in the human blood?

WATER AS A SOLVENT

Water can dissolve more substances than virtually any other liquid. It is such an excellent solvent because it is a *polar molecule*. Other substances that are *polar* or *ionic* will dissolve in water. Sodium chloride (a common salt) is made up of positive sodium ions strongly attracted to negative chloride ions.

Usually, it would take a large amount of energy to break this strong ionic bond, but when salt is dissolved in water, the negative oxygen atoms cluster round the sodium ions and the positive hydrogen ions are attracted to the chloride ions. The attraction between the sodium and chloride ions is weakened, and the ions separate. See Figure 1.32.

Many biological molecules are joined together by covalent bonds, and these too will dissolve in water so long as they have polar

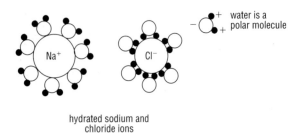

hydrated sodium and chloride ions

Figure 1.32 Sodium and chloride ions separated in water

groups within them. *Carbohydrates* have many hydroxyl groups (—OH) which are polar. These form hydrogen bonds with water, so separating the carbohydrate molecules from each other and allowing them to dissolve easily.

It is not surprising that about 90% of *cytoplasm* – the protoplasm of a cell contained within the cell membrane but excluding the nucleus – is water.

ACTIVITY 23

The solubility of gases in water
Look at Table 1.5.

Table 1.5   Gas solubility

	Oxygen	Nitrogen	Carbon dioxide
Air	20.95	78.00	0.03
Water	0.79	1.20	0.03

1 Which are the most and which are the least soluble gases?

2 What are the implications of these solubilities, for living organisms?

3 What is surprising about the solubility of oxygen?

4 How does the human body cope with this feature of oxygen?

WATER AS A TEMPERATURE STABILISER

Water has a very high *specific heat capacity*, which is the amount of heat required to raise the temperature of 1 gramme of a substance by 1 °C. This value for water (between 0 °C and 50 °C) is $4.2 \, J \, g^{-1}$, which is much higher than that for compounds of a similar molar mass. This means that it takes quite a large amount of energy to raise the temperature of water; and once it is warm, it cools down *slowly*.

Water can therefore act as a *thermal buffer* in the body to prevent it from undergoing rapid changes of temperature as the air temperature changes. And in the environment also, it means that large bodies of water like oceans and lakes tend to have a steady temperature suitable for cold-blooded animals such as fish.

WATER AS A LUBRICANT

In some cases, water acts as a lubricant, for example in the alveoli of the lungs where a secretion lubricates and maintains the suppleness of the elastic air sacs.

Often, lubricants in the body contain *colloids*. Particles smaller than 10^{-3} cm in diameter form true solutions in water.

Particles which are larger, up to 10^{-5} cm, do not form true solutions but instead attract water to form a *colloidal state*. In colloids, water acts as a dispersion medium. The particles involved here are known as the *disperse phase* and are permanently suspended. Large *carbohydrate* and *protein* molecules form colloids in the body. Cytoplasm and blood plasma are both colloids.

Colloids are more *viscous* than true solutions. Viscosity is a measure of how easily molecules can slide over each other. If the molecules can do this very readily, like water, then the liquid is described as having a low viscosity, and it flows easily. More viscous liquids are 'thick and sticky'.

Colloids have ideal properties for biological lubricants. Two examples of such lubricants are:

1 *Synovial fluid.* This colloid contains large molecules of a polysaccharide containing nitrogen, loosely linked to protein, which bind to large numbers of water molecules to make a jelly-like substance.
2 *Mucus.* This contains polysaccharides linked more strongly to proteins to form a substance known as a *proteoglycan*. Mucus is found in the following places:
   • the alimentary canal
   • tears in the eyes
   • the respiratory system

ACTIVITY 24

1 Find out about the production and functions of lubricants in the alimentary canal, the eye, the respiratory system and joints.

2 Are there any other examples of lubrication in the human body? Find out about these as well.

Oxygen and carbon dioxide

Both oxygen and carbon dioxide are gases with atoms joined by covalent bonds.

ACTIVITY 25

Revise the sections on atomic structure and covalent bonding earlier in this chapter (see pp. 5, 7 and 8), and then explain the atomic structures of these two gases.

COMBUSTION

All elements burn better in oxygen than in air. This burning process is called *combustion*, and the substances produced are *oxides*. Metals like sodium, magnesium, iron and copper form basic oxides. Sodium and magnesium oxides are soluble in water, forming alkaline solutions with a pH greater than 7. These oxides are called *alkaline oxides*. When non-metals are burnt with oxygen, they form oxides as well, but these dissolve in water to produce acidic solutions with a pH of less than 7. Carbon dioxide is one example of such an *acidic oxide*. It is formed when carbon is burnt with oxygen. Carbon dioxide is also formed when fossil fuels, mainly compounds of carbon and hydrogen, are burnt in oxygen.

Carbon dioxide does not burn itself, and substances will not burn in it. It is used in fire extinguishers because, being heavier than air, it covers the fire and prevents oxygen from reaching it. The fire 'goes out' because carbon dioxide does not support burning.

SOLUBILITY IN WATER

We have already looked at the properties of water as a solvent. Table 1.5 showed us that in 100 cm^3 of air there is approximately 21 cm^3 of oxygen and 0.03 cm^3 of carbon dioxide. If water is placed in contact with air, 100 cm^3 of water takes up only 0.79 cm^3 of oxygen but is able to dissolve 0.03 cm^3 of carbon dioxide – which is the same amount as is in the air. We can see that carbon dioxide is far more soluble in water than is oxygen, since water absorbs only about 4% of the oxygen present in the air.

THE TRANSPORT OF GASES IN THE BLOOD

Earlier in this chapter, we considered how carbon dioxide is carried in the blood, and how haemoglobin acts as a buffer to prevent changes of pH while the carbon dioxide is being carried to the lungs for expulsion (see Figure 1.26, p. 22). The transport of *oxygen* requires a special mechanism because of its relative insolubility. Haemoglobin (Hb), the red pigment in red blood cells, combines reversibly with oxygen to form *oxyhaemoglobin* (HbO_8). There are 280 million molecules of haemoglobin in one red blood cell.

$$Hb + 4O_2 \underset{\text{tissues}}{\overset{\text{lungs}}{\rightleftharpoons}} HbO_8$$

At body temperature, only about 0.3 cm^3 of oxygen can dissolve in 100 cm^3 of plasma, but the total oxygen-transporting facility of blood is about 20 cm^3 per 100 cm^3 of blood. Thus, about 98% of oxygen is carried by haemoglobin.

HAEMOGLOBIN

Haemoglobin is a large globular protein consisting of four sub-units: namely polypeptide molecules, each containing about 140 amino acids plus one haem group. Each of these haem groups is a molecule, containing carbon, hydrogen and nitrogen, called a *porphyrin*, with an iron(II) (the small-capital 'I's indicate the *oxidation state*) atom in

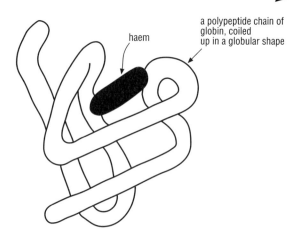

Figure 1.33   A sub-unit of haemoglobin in detail

the middle. Figure 1.33 shows the structure of a sub-unit of haemoglobin.

The haem groups are responsible for the red colour of the haemoglobin, and provide the iron(II) sites where oxygen can be loosely attached without any oxidation taking place.

THE FORMATION OF OXYHAEMOGLOBIN

In a mixture of gases, each component exerts a pressure in proportion to its molar percentage in the mixture. We usually refer to this as the *partial pressure* (p) of a gas, rather than its percentage concentration, and it is measured in *pascals* (Pa). Table 1.6 shows the partial pressures of gases in air.

The affinity of haemoglobin for oxygen can be measured experimentally by measuring the amount of oxyhaemoglobin formed with increasing partial pressures of oxygen. The result is called an *oxygen dissociation curve*. The partial pressure of oxygen in the alveoli of human lungs is about 13.0 kPa, and in the

Table 1.6   The volume of some common gases in 100 cm^3 of air or water (the latter at 10 °C and in direct contact wth air)

Gas	% composition	Partial pressure (kPa)
Carbon dioxide	0.03 approximately	negligible
Nitrogen	79.0	80.0
Oxygen	21.0	21.3

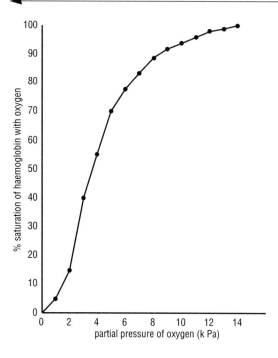

Figure 1.34 The oxygen dissociation curve for human haemoglobin at body temperature

tissues it is much lower (0.0–4.0 kPa). If you now look at Figure 1.34, you will see that the haemoglobin in the capillaries in the alveoli will be almost completely saturated with oxygen, whilst at the tissues it will be almost completely dissociated and will release the oxygen for cellular respiration.

ACTIVITY 26

1 What change in percentage saturation will occur if the oxygen partial pressure drops from 6.2 to 2.5 kPa? Will oxygen be released or taken up?

2 List four properties of haemoglobin which make it efficient in its role as a transporter of oxygen.

3 Find out why smoking cigarettes can damage an athlete's performance. What happens to the haemoglobin?

4 Find out about myoglobin, which is found in muscles. How is it similar to haemoglobin, and what is its function?

THE EFFECT OF CARBON DIOXIDE

The partial pressure of carbon dioxide in blood arriving at respiring tissues is about 5.3 kPa, and this increases to 6.00 kPa as the blood flows through the capillaries in the tissues.

ACTIVITY 27

Plot the data in Table 1.7 which shows the effect of increasing the partial pressure of carbon dioxide on the saturation of haemoglobin with oxygen, at different partial pressures of oxygen.

Table 1.7 Partial pressures of gases in air (dry air at sea level)

Partial pressure of oxygen (kPa)	Saturation of haemoglobin with oxygen (%)	
	Partial pressure of carbon dioxide at 5.3 kPa	Partial pressure of carbon dioxide at 9.3 kPa
0	0	0
2	20	10
4	55	35
6	77	63
8	87	78
10	95	89
12	98	98
14	100	100

1 Does an increase in carbon dioxide partial pressure increase or decrease the affinity that haemoglobin has for oxygen?

2 Is this effect helpful or unhelpful when the oxyhaemoglobin is in the process of dissociating to release oxygen at the tissues because of the low partial pressure of oxygen there?

3 Look again at Figure 1.26. Can you see an effect that carbon dioxide has on the haemoglobin?

4 When haemoglobin is acting as a buffer, does it increase or decrease its affinity for oxygen?

Carbohydrates

Carbohydrates are made up of carbon, hydrogen and oxygen. The simplest units are called *monosaccharides* and have the general formula $C_nH_{2n}O_n$. Monosaccharides can be built up into *disaccharides* and *polysaccharides* in condensation reactions involving the elimination of water. These all yield monosaccharides again upon hydrolysis.

THE IMPORTANCE OF CARBOHYDRATES

- Carbohydrates are produced using energy from the sun during photosynthesis, and are the main energy source for all living organisms, reaching them through food chains
- Energy is released from carbohydrates in cellular respiration, and is transferred to adenosine triphosphate molecules to provide energy for metabolic reactions
- Energy is stored in the form of carbohydrates in plants and animals
- Carbohydrates can be used to make other molecules, for example lipids, which also contain carbon, hydrogen and oxygen. With the addition of amino groups, amino acids and other molecules containing nitrogen can also be made from substances derived from carbohydrates
- Cellulose, found in the structure of plant cell walls, is a carbohydrate, as is the material forming the exoskeletons of insects and other arthropods
- Mucus and other lubricants contain carbohydrates linked to proteins, sometimes in structures called *proteoglycans*

ACTIVITY 28

1 Find out about the carbon cycle. Explain the role of carbohydrates in the transfer of energy.

2 Find out the amount of energy stored in 1 gramme of glucose. Compare this with that stored in 1 gramme of fat. Why are carbohydrates used more readily in respiration?

3 Revise cellular respiration, and note how energy is gradually released in the breakdown of glucose.

4 How and where is energy stored in plants? Why is this called an 'unlimited' energy store?

5 How and where is energy stored in carbohydrates in the human body? Why is this called a 'limited' energy store?

6 What other uses do we make of carbohydrates in our daily life?

STRUCTURES OF CARBOHYDRATES

Monosaccharides

These form the basic unit of all carbohydrates. Monosaccharides are classified according to the number of carbon atoms they contain:

- Trioses $C_3H_6O_3$
- Tetroses $C_4H_8O_4$
- Pentoses $C_5H_{10}O_5$
- Hexoses $C_6H_{12}O_6$
- Heptuloses $C_7H_{14}O_7$

Pentoses (part of the structure of nucleic acids) and hexoses are the most common monosaccharides in living organisms.

Although we can show monosaccharides as straight chain molecules, in solution they are mostly joined up to form rings – see Figure 1.35.

All monosaccharides are described as *reducing sugars*. A test for reducing sugars is to heat the solution with *Benedict's solution*. This blue solution contains an alkaline solution of copper (II) sulphate ($CuSO_4$). The aldehyde group (on carbon 1) or keto group (on carbon 2) of the monosaccharide is able to reduce Cu^{2+} to Cu^+, itself being oxidised to a carboxyl (—COOH) group. A red precipitate

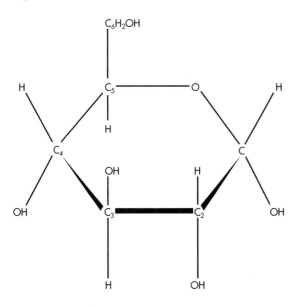

Figure 1.35 The ring structure of glucose

of copper(I) oxide is formed. Reducing sugars form a *red/orange precipitate* when heated with Benedict's solution.

Disaccharides

These are formed in a condensation reaction when two monosaccharides join with the elimination of water. The condensation of two glucose molecules to make maltose is shown as:

$$C_6H_{12}O_6 + C_6H_{12}O_6 \rightarrow C_{12}H_{22}O_{11} + H_2O$$

Figures 1.36 and 1.37a show the same formation.

Another important disaccharide is *sucrose*, commonly called just 'sugar', made from the condensation of one glucose molecule and one fructose molecule – see Figure 1.37b.

A third important disaccharide is *lactose*, or milk sugar, made of one molecule of glucose and one molecule of *galactose*. Galactose is another isomer of glucose.

These three disaccharides all have the formula $C_{12}H_{22}O_{11}$.

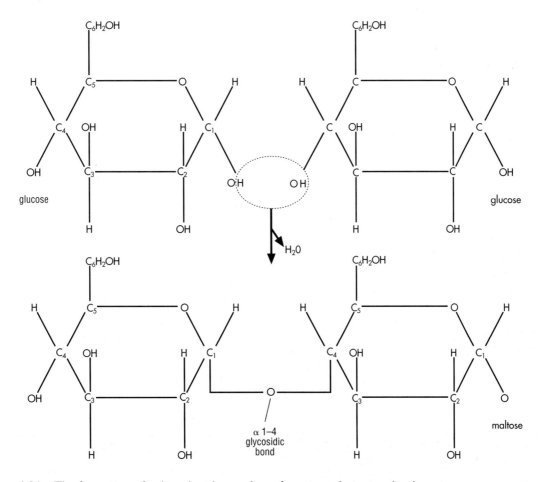

Figure 1.36 The formation of a disaccharide – maltose from two glucose molecules

ACTIVITY 29

1 Build a glucose molecule using chemical molecular modelling beads. Carbon atoms are black, oxygen atoms are red and hydrogen atoms are white. Refer to Figure 1.35 for the structure of glucose. Then link two of the model glucose molecules with a α 1–4 glycosidic bond by removing a water molecule, to form maltose. Refer to Figure 1.36.

2 List three differences between the maltose and sucrose molecules.

3 List two specific functions of disaccharides in living organisms.

4 Look at Figure 1.37. Do you think that disaccharides can be reducing sugars? Before you answer this, you need to know that only 'free' aldehyde and keto groups in disaccharides react with Benedict's solution. If the carbon atom bearing the aldehyde or keto group is part of a glycosidic link, then the sugar is not a reducing sugar and will therefore not react with Benedict's solution.

   You will be able to test your theory in an experiment in Activity 32.

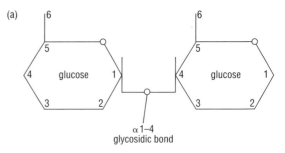

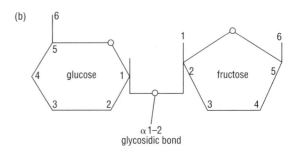

Figure 1.37 Simplified ring structures for (a) maltose and (b) sucrose

Polysaccharides

Polysaccharides are *macromolecules* made up of many condensed monosaccharides joined by glycosidic bonds. Energy is required in their synthesis. Molecules that have many repeating units are known as *polymers*. The repeating units are themselves called *residues* or *monomers*. Usually, only *one* type of sugar monomer is involved in the making of a polymer.

1 *Starch and glycogen*. Starch is an important energy-storage molecule in plants, and it consists of a mixture of two types of polysaccharide, *amylose* and *amylopectin* – see Figure 1.38. Amylose usually makes up about 30% of the starch, and is an unbranched chain containing 200–1,500 molecules of glucose linked together by α 1–4 glycosidic bonds. Amylopectin makes up the rest of the starch, and is a branched chain containing 2,000 to 200,000 molecules of glucose. The straight chain part is the same as amylose, but there are α 1–6 branching points occurring about every 20 glucose residues. Both these molecules are wound up to form a *helix*, which is a spiral structure.

   Glycogen has a very similar structure to amylopectin, but is larger and more highly branched. It is found in the liver, muscles and (in a small amount) the brain. Glycogen granules can be seen in the cells in a section of liver viewed through a microscope.

   Starch and glycogen are only sparingly soluble in water but can be easily hydrolysed by enzymes in the human body.

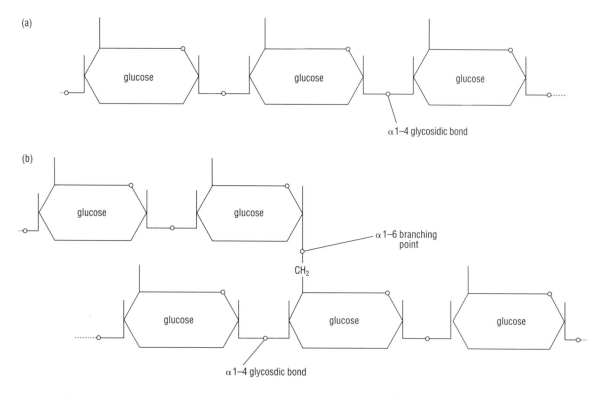

(a)

glucose

glucose

glucose

α1–4 glycosidic bond

(b)

glucose

glucose

α 1–6 branching point

CH₂

glucose

glucose

glucose

α1–4 glycosdic bond

Figure 1.38 Starch: (a) amylose , (b) amylopectin

ACTIVITY 30

1 Look at starch grains of wheat, potato, maize and rice under the microscope, and make sketches to compare them. The concentric rings that you see are alternate layers of amylose and amylopectin.

2 You will have briefly touched on glycogen storage in an earlier exercise in this chapter (see p. 32). Now explain how sugar in the blood is maintained at a constant level by the condensation of glucose molecules to make glycogen in the liver, and by the subsequent hydrolysis of this glycogen. Discuss the role of insulin.

2 *Cellulose*. This is a straight-chain polysaccharide (see Figure 1.39) consisting of 2,000–3,000 glucose molecules. It differs from starch and glycogen in that the bonds that join the glucose molecules are β 1–4 glycosidic bonds. *Microfibrils* of up to 2,000 cellulose chains held together by hydrogen bonds form to make very strong structures, found tightly packed in plant cell walls, which contribute to mechanical support in plants.

Cellulose can only be hydrolysed with difficulty. Herbivorous mammals have symbiotic bacteria in their guts which can digest cellulose, by producing the enzyme *cellulase*, so that the glucose becomes available for absorption and use in the body. Humans, on the other hand, cannot digest cellulose. Together with *hemicelluloses*,

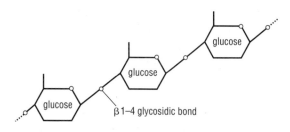

glucose

glucose

glucose

β1–4 glycosidic bond

Figure 1.39 Cellulose – a structural polysaccharide

lignin and *pectins*, cellulose acts as 'roughage' or 'fibre' in the diet which adds bulk to the gut contents in the colon by retaining water. This stimulates movement by *peristaltic* activity leading to defecation. Roughage in the diet helps prevent intestinal disorders.

3 *Pectins and hemicelluloses.* These are other polysaccharides found in plant cell walls. Pectins consist mainly of galactose, and hemicelluloses contain pentose sugars.

4 *Inulin.* This is a fructose polymer found in some plants as an alternative to starch.

5 *Chitin.* This is quite similar to cellulose, but contains nitrogen. Chitin macromolecules are found in long, straight, parallel chains in the cell walls of fungi and the exoskeletons of arthropods.

6 *Mucus.* Mucus contains polysaccharides linked to proteins – structures which are called *proteoglycans*. These form lubricants, and have been mentioned before in this chapter (see p. 29).

ACTIVITY 31

Carbohydrate identification

1 Prepare four test tubes and label one for each of fructose, glucose, starch and sucrose. Add 2 cm^3 of each solution. Then add 1 cm^3 of Benedict's solution to each, and boil in a boiling-water bath. Carry out a control. Record your observations.

Prepare another set of test tubes with the same solutions. Add a drop of iodine to each. Carry out a control. Record your observations.

List your conclusions from this experiment.

2 Boiling disaccharides and polysaccharides with HCl causes hydrolysis of the molecules. Take four test tubes and place 2 cm^3 of the disaccharide into two tubes and 2 cm^3 of the polysaccharide into the other two tubes. Add 2 cm^3 of 2M HCl. Boil for 30 minutes. Neutralise with sodium hydroxide (use pH paper). Then carry out Benedict's test and the iodine test on each. Carry out controls. Record your observations and conclusions.

3 Design and carry out an experiment to discover the contents of two unknown solutions, X and Y, which contain various mixtures of the above carbohydrates.

Lipids

Lipids contain carbon, hydrogen and oxygen, as do carbohydrates, but in lipids the proportion of oxygen is much less. Lipids are insoluble in water, but do dissolve in organic solvents such as ether and ethanol.

There are four groups of lipids:

1 true fats – animal fats and plant oils
2 phospholipids
3 waxes
4 steroids.

Lipids contain *fatty acids* which are usually combined with other molecules. Fatty acids consist of long-chain hydrocarbons in which only carbon and hydrogen are present and which are *non-polar*, which means that they are *not charged*. It is this latter property which makes fatty acids insoluble in water. There is also one terminal carboxylic acid group.

In some fatty acids, there are double bonds between one or more of the carbon atoms in the hydrocarbon chain. If there are no double bonds, the fatty acid is described as *saturated*, and if double bonds *are* present then the fatty acid is *unsaturated*. *Monounsaturated* means that there is only one double bond in the fatty acid. *Polyunsaturated* means that there is more than one double bond in the fatty acid.

You will see in Figure 1.40 that there are

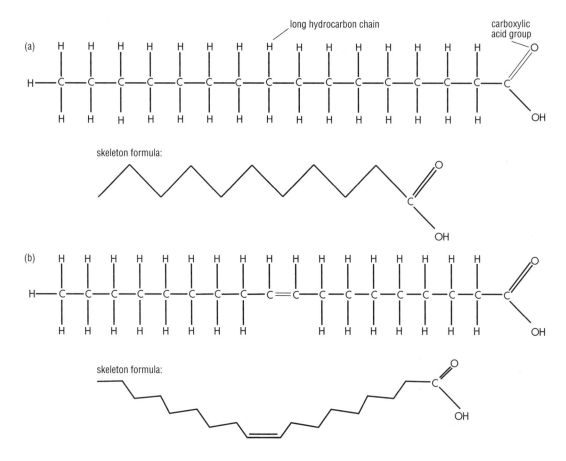

Figure 1.40 The structures and skeleton formulas for two fatty acids: (a) palmitic acid ($C_{15}H_{31}COOH$) – saturated; (b) oleic acid ($C_{17}H_{33}COOH$) – unsaturated

'shorthand' ways of illustrating fatty acids called *skeleton formulas*.

Table 1.8 shows a series of commonly occurring fatty acids.

ACTIVITY 32

1 Look at Table 1.8. List the saturated and unsaturated fatty acids.

2 How do the melting points of saturated and unsaturated fatty acids differ? How would this affect their physical state at room temperature?

Table 1.8 Fatty acids

Name	Formula	Number of double bonds	Melting point (°C)
Lauric acid	$C_{11}H_{23}COOH$	0	44.2
Myristic acid	$C_{13}H_{27}COOH$	0	53.9
Palmitic acid	$C_{15}H_{31}COOH$	0	63.1
Palmitoleic acid	$C_{15}H_{29}COOH$	1	−0.5
Stearic acid	$C_{17}H_{35}COOH$	0	69.6
Oleic acid	$C_{17}H_{33}COOH$	1	13.4
Linoleic acid	$C_{17}H_{31}COOH$	2	−5.0
Linolenic acid	$C_{17}H_{29}COOH$	3	0.11
Arachidic acid	$C_{19}H_{39}COOH$	0	76.5
Arachidonic acid	$C_{19}H_{31}COOH$	4	−49.5

TRUE FATS – ANIMAL FATS AND PLANT OILS

These are composed of a glycerol molecule combined with three fatty acids, which may all be different. This molecule is called a *triglyceride*. Triglycerides are formed in a condensation reaction, with the elimination of three molecules of water for each reaction. Energy is required for this.

True fats are synthesised in the adipose cells of fat tissue in the human body. Animal fats contain mostly saturated fatty acids. True fats in plants are liquid at temperate temperatures since they contain more unsaturated fatty acids. These latter fats are called *oils*.

ACTIVITY 33

1 Find out about adipose tissue and write a short report on its distribution and role in the body. Comment on its functions using three headings:
 • energy store
 • insulation
 • protection

2 The amount of energy in one gramme of fat is higher than that in one gramme of carbohydrate:
 • carbohydrate 16 kJ g
 • fat 37 kJ g
 yet carbohydrates rather than fats provide the immediate substrates for cellular respiration. Suggest a reason for this.

3 Plant oils are often found in seeds. Why should oil be a more efficient energy store than carbohydrates for some seeds?

4 Test a range of foodstuffs for the presence of fats and oils by shaking them in absolute ethanol for a minute. Then, pour the ethanol into a test tube of water, leaving the foodstuff behind. A cloudy white emulsion will indicate a lipid.

5 Test liquid or homogenised foods for lipids by boiling for a few minutes. If lipids are present, they will rise to the surface. Add Sudan(III), shake and allow the oil to settle. Oils, if present, will now be stained red.

Fats in the diet – essential fatty acids and fat-soluble vitamins

Fats in the diet provide an energy source, and also contain essential fatty acids and fat-soluble vitamins. Most of the fatty acids required for the synthesis of body fats can be made from molecules derived from carbohydrate. Glycerol comes from this source as well. There are some fatty acids, known as *essential fatty acids*, that we need but cannot make for ourselves, so these have to be included in the diet. *Arachidonic acid* is an example.

The fat-soluble vitamins are A, D, E and K. Since these are soluble in lipids, they can be stored in the body to a greater extent than the water-soluble vitamins. Fat-soluble vitamins are found in fatty tissues, and vitamin A can be stored in quite large amounts in the liver.

PHOSPHOLIPIDS

If one of the fatty acids in a triglyceride is replaced by a phosphate group, the molecule is called a *phospholipid* – see Figure 1.41. The phosphate group is *polar*. It is ionised and negatively charged, so it is soluble in water or *hydrophilic* ('water-loving'). However, the long-chain fatty acids in the rest of the molecule are *non-polar* and insoluble in water or *hydrophobic* ('water-hating').

Phospholipids are very important in the structure of cell membranes.

WAXES

Waxes contain fatty acids that are joined not to glycerol (as in true fats and phospholipids) but instead to *complex alcohols*. In plants, waxes occur in the cuticle covering the epidermis of leaves, stems, fruits and seeds. In human skin, sebaceous glands produce *sebum* which contains waxes. This keeps the epidermis supple, reduces evaporation and can inhibit the growth of some bacteria.

STEROIDS

Steroids have little in common with the

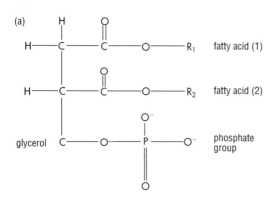

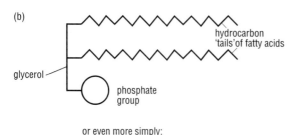

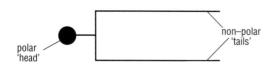

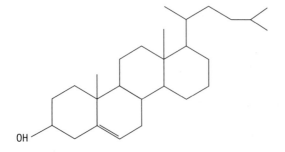

Figure 1.41 A phospholipid: (a) the chemical structure, (b) the skeleton structure

structure of other lipids except that they have carbon and hydrogen in their molecules, with a small amount of oxygen. Steroids consist of four carbon rings – see Figure 1.42.

Cholesterol in the blood and saturated fats

Cholesterol is a steroid itself and is required in the body for making other steroids including:

- the hormones of the adrenal glands
- sex hormones in the ovaries and testes
- steroids in cell membranes linked to the hydrocarbon tails of the phospholipids
- bile salts

Figure 1.42 A steroid molecule

The cholesterol that we need is either absorbed in the diet or synthesised in the liver if the dietary intake is inadequate.

Low density lipoproteins (LDLs) are involved in carrying cholesterol in the bloodstream. The composition of LDLs is only 25% protein. The rest is largely cholesterol, with some triglycerides and phospholipids. LDLs are carried around the body attached to soluble protein because of the insoluble nature of lipid molecules.

High cholesterol levels in the blood have received much attention recently because of the suspected link between high blood-cholesterol levels and certain types of heart disease – including *atherosclerosis*, where cholesterol and other fatty substances are deposited in the walls of the arteries, including the coronary arteries, causing a narrowing of the *lumen*. Excess cholesterol is difficult to transport in the blood since the LDLs can carry only a certain amount. And although the excess is taken to the liver by other proteins and secreted in the bile, it is quite difficult for the body to get rid of cholesterol since it can be *reabsorbed* later on in the intestine.

Although the evidence is still quite controversial, it is seen as important to have a low blood-cholesterol level. Cholesterol is found in animal fats, and saturated fatty acids are more readily converted into cholesterol, so dieticians recommend a lowered intake of foods containing animal fats, like butter, dairy products, eggs and red meat. In addition, we should increase the use of margarines and other products based on unsaturated oils which are derived from plant sources like sunflower seeds, corn and olives. Finally, lowering the body fat level also helps: when less fat has to be transported round the body, the liver makes less cholesterol.

Proteins

About two-thirds of the dry mass of cells is protein. Proteins are macromolecules containing nitrogen, as well as carbon,

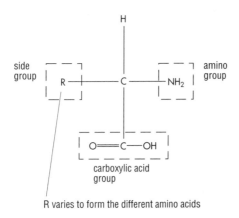

Figure 1.43   The structure of an amino acid

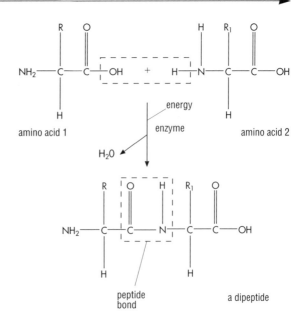

Figure 1.44   The formation of a peptide bond

hydrogen and oxygen, and sometimes sulphur. Some proteins combine with other substances to form complexes containing phosphorus, iron or other trace elements.

Proteins are a linear sequence of *amino acids* – see Figure 1.43. An amino acid has:
- an amino group —NH (basic)
- a carboxylic acid group —COOH (acid)

Both of these groups are ionised in the cell. A substance that is both acid and base is described as *amphoteric*. There are about 20 amino acids that occur in proteins.

Amino acids can react with each other in condensation reactions involving the elimination of water. Energy is required for this reaction. An amino group of one amino acid reacts with the carboxylic acid group of another to form a *peptide bond* (see Figure 1.44). When two amino acids join, a *dipeptide* is formed. If three combine, a *tripeptide* is formed. Proteins consist of chains of many amino acids joined up to form a *polypeptide*. A protein may have more than one polypeptide chain. Examples are insulin, which has 51 amino acids in two chains, and haemoglobin which has four chains each of about 140 amino acids.

The sequence of amino acids in each different protein is unique. Every protein of the same type, however, is identical. If just one amino acid is different or missing, then the protein molecule may not be able to carry out its function. The sequence of amino acids

in a polypeptide chain is called the *primary structure*.

ACTIVITY 34

1   The primary structure of a protein is determined by the chromosomes in the nucleus. Find out about how this happened, and produce a poster to show the steps involved. (Refer to the section on nucleic acids and protein synthesis.)

2   Look at Figure 1.45 which represents the sequence of amino acids in insulin. List the amino acids found in insulin by matching the symbols with the names of the amino acids in Table 1.9. There are some additional amino acids in insulin:

- Ile = isoleucine
- Gln = glutamine
- Cys = cysteine
- Asn = asparagine
- His = histidine

You will notice that the three disulphide bridges in insulin (two of which hold together the two polypeptide chains) form between the *same* amino acids in each case. Which amino acid is this?

3 Haemoglobin extracted from the red blood cells of individuals with the sickle cell trait has just one amino acid in the sequence that is different from that in normal haemoglobin. You should look again at Fig. 1.29 on p. 25 which shows the results of the electrophoresis and chromatography of haemoglobin from sickle cells.

   Find out more about sickle cell anaemia, which shows how a change of just *one* amino acid in a protein can seriously affect its function. How is it inherited?

Table 1.9 Amino acids

Amino acids
alanine
2-amino-butyric acid
arginine
glutamic acid
glycine
hydroxy-proline
isoleucine
leucine
lysine
β-phenyl-alanine
proline
serine
taurine
threonine
tyrosine
valine

Polypeptide chains also have a *secondary structure*. This is the shape which the polypeptide forms as a result of hydrogen bonding. It is most often a spiral known as the α helix. *Keratin* is a protein found in hair, skin and nails with such a secondary structure. Another pattern is a zig-zag chain, known as a β *sheet*. The protein in silk, *fibroin*, has this structure. See Figure 1.46.

Both keratin and fibroin are examples of *fibrous proteins* which have long chains running parallel to one another. They are strong, stable molecules, and are found in structures where strength is needed. Another example is *collagen*, which involves a unique triple helix. Collagen is found in connective tissue in tendons.

Many proteins have a further *tertiary structure*, held together in a compact structure by hydrogen, disulphide and ionic bonds. *Globular proteins* (see, for example, Figure 1.47) consist of polypeptide chains, mostly wound into an α helix and then folded into a spherical shape. This is the tertiary structure. Globular proteins are much less stable than the fibrous type, and have metabolic roles. All enzymes are globular proteins.

Some large complex proteins have a

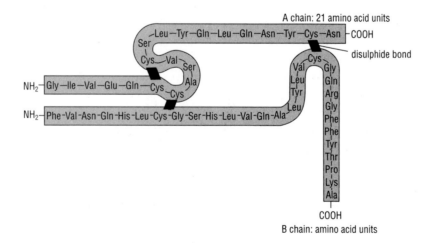

Figure 1.45 The sequence of amino acids in insulin

Source: Advanced Biology Principles and Applications, C. J. Clegg and D. G. Mackean, John Murray, 1994.

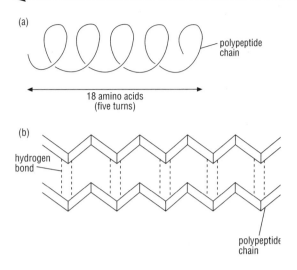

Figure 1.46 The secondary structures of proteins: (a) the α helix, (b) β sheets

quaternary structure when several globular molecules are linked together. An example is haemoglobin with four polypeptide chains, each with about 140 amino acids. You will see that a haem is bound to each globin molecule of the haemoglobin. This is an example of a *conjugated protein*. The non-protein

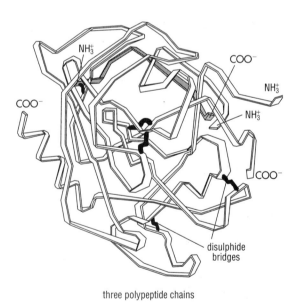

three polypeptide chains

Figure 1.47 Chymotrypsinogen – a globular protein with a tertiary structure
Source: Advanced Human Biology, J. Simpkins and J. I. Williams, Chapman and Hall, 1987; originally adapted from P. B Singer et al. in *Journal of Molecular Biology*, vol. 35, no. 143, 1968.

part is known as the *prosthetic group* – the haem in this case.

FUNCTIONS OF PROTEINS

- as enzymes: pepsin, amylase, lipase
- Contraction: actin and myosin in muscle
- Protection: antibodies, fibrinogen, prothrombin, keratin
- As hormones: insulin, somatotrophin
- Transport: haemoglobin, plasma proteins
- Support: collagen, elastin, chondrin, ossein
- Storage: myoglobin, ferritin (stores iron), casein
- Electron transfer: cytochromes

ACTIVITY 35

1 Write a short paragraph on the role of each of the proteins listed above.

2 Prepare an exhibition displaying the structure and functions of proteins.

3 Carry out the following test for the presence of proteins in liquid foods. You could test egg albumin and milk. Add a little potassium hydroxide to these to make the solution clearer, and then add a few drops of dilute copper(II) sulphate solution down the side of the test tube. Watch the surface of the liquid: if a blue ring appears, then protein is present. On shaking, the blue ring disappears and the solution becomes purple.

Test water as a control to observe a negative reaction.

ENZYMES

Enzymes are globular proteins with catalytic properties. A *catalyst* is a substance which alters the rate of a reaction without itself undergoing permanent change. Each enzyme molecule can be used many times, so they are effective in very small amounts. Enzymes cannot cause impossible reactions to occur, they can only speed up reactions which would otherwise take place extremely slowly.

Every metabolic reaction is catalysed by a particular enzyme, and there are thousands of different enzymes in every cell. These are the *intracellular enzymes*. Others that are secreted and work outside cells are called *extracellular enzymes*. Digestive enzymes fall into this latter category.

Enzymes and activation energy

Before a reaction can occur, it must be *activated*, and thus its energy level must be increased. The energy required is called the *energy of activation*. (Heat is often the source of the energy of activation, but this is not available in living organisms.) Enzymes work by *lowering the energy of activation*, so that reactions can take place at lower temperatures. See Figure 1.48. The

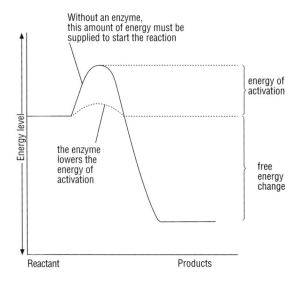

Figure 1.48 The energy of activation

example shown involves the enzyme *catalase* which breaks down hydrogen peroxide ($2H_2O_2$), the substrate, to form water and oxygen, the products. These are at a lower energy level than the substrate, and energy is released during the reaction. However, before the reaction can start, the energy of activation must be supplied. In the presence of the enzyme, the energy of activation is lowered, so more molecules react and the hydrogen peroxide breaks down more quickly. The arrow in the equation below symbolises the action of the enzyme catalase:

$$2H_2O_2 \rightarrow 2H_2O + O_2$$

The mechanism of enzyme action

The globular protein molecules of the enzyme have *active sites* within their structure. These are spaces with a particular size, shape and charge which just fit the substrate. When the substrate joins with the enzyme, it forms a temporary enzyme–substrate complex. At this stage the energy of activation is lowered, and the reaction takes place, with the release of the products, shortly after.

The specificity factor

All enzymes act on specific substrates, but there are degrees of specificity involved here. *Substrate specificity* occurs when only the *one* substrate with the particular characteristics to fit into the active site is able to form the enzyme–substrate complex and react; this means that every single reaction in metabolism can be controlled individually. *Bond specificity* is rather more general. Pepsin, for example, is able to accelerate the hydrolysis of *all* peptide bonds, irrespective of which amino acids are present. *Group specificity* is also sometimes found. An example is *phosphatase* which can remove phosphate groups from a variety of molecules.

Enzyme inhibitors

There are many substances that prevent enzymes from catalysing their reactions. These are known as *inhibitors*, and they come in two types:

1 competitive
2 non-competitive.

ACTIVITY 36

Look at Figure 1.49 which shows the comparative effects of competitive and non-competitive inhibitors on the rate of an enzyme-controlled reaction.

Describe the effect of the substrate concentration on the rate of reaction when no inhibitor is present. Then compare this relationship with the results obtained with the two different kinds of inhibitor.

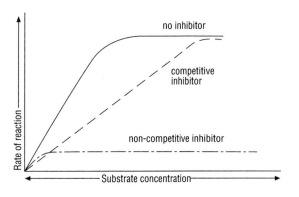

Figure 1.49 **The comparative effects of non-competitive and competitive inhibitors on the rate of an enzyme-catalysed reaction**

1 *Competitive inhibitors.* Competitive inhibitors are so called because they compete with the real substrate for the active sites on the enzyme. They are very similar in structure to the substrate, and so fit into the active site. How this happens is shown in Figure 1.70b. Here, the reaction has thus been prevented (however, an increase in substrate concentration will lead to a gradual replacement of the inhibitor molecules in the active site with substrate molecules). If, on the other hand, the concentration of substrate is increased, then the inhibitor molecules have less chance of combining with the active sites in the first place, and the reaction then proceeds at its normal rate – see Figure 1.50a.

There are several important applications of competitive inhibition in the treatment of disease. For example, drugs which slow down the undesirable reactions occurring in cancer act in this way. Another example is the use of sulphonamide drugs to combat bacterial infections. These latter drugs are very similar to a substance needed for the synthesis of vitamin B, and as a result, the bacteria cannot multiply because they are prevented from making this vitamin.

2 *Non-competitive inhibitors.* As you saw in Figure 1.49, the degree of inhibition by non-competitive inhibitors cannot be reduced by increasing the number of substrate molecules. The inhibitor molecules become attached to the enzyme at a position other than the active site, but the shape of the enzyme is so changed, nonetheless, that it cannot react.

Substances which are very poisonous to living organisms are often non-competitive inhibitors. Heavy metal ions such as mercury, silver and copper combine with the —SH groups in the enzyme and cause the disulphide bridges to break down, so disrupting the tertiary globular structure. When the globular shape breaks down like this, the process is called the DENATURATION of the enzyme. *Cyanide* is another non-competitive inhibitor, one which stops respiration.

In this type of inhibition, enzyme activity can be restored if it is purified. There is a group of inhibitors which binds so tightly to enzyme molecules that they

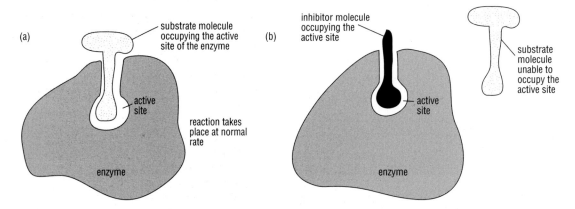

Figure 1.50 **Competitive inhibition: (a) no inhibitor present; (b) inhibitor present**

cannot be removed. This includes *organophosphorus* insecticides and nerve gases which inactivate enzymes vital to the conduction of nerve impulses.

The effect of enzyme and substrate concentration on the rate of reactions catalysed by enzymes

The active site of enzyme molecules may be used over and over again, so these molecules are effective in very low concentrations. The number of substrate molecules which can be acted on in a given time is known as the *turnover number*. This is very variable. Catalase, which acts on hydrogen peroxide, can break down many millions of substrate molecules in a minute. Some enzymes, however, only act on a few hundred substrate molecules in the same time.

In the next Activity, you will investigate the action of *sucrase* which hydrolyses sucrose. Look back at the structure of sucrose and at the Benedict's test in the carbohydrate section of this chapter.

ACTIVITY 37

Investigating the effect of enzyme and substrate concentrations on the hydrolysis of sucrose
You will need:
- water baths at 35 °C and 70 °C with metal test-tube racks
- test tubes
- a test-tube rack
- stop clocks
- syringes (1 cm^3, 5 cm^3)
- a marking pen or chinagraph pencil
- a measuring cylinder
- safety goggles
- Benedict's reagent
- distilled water
- sucrase (invertase) solution, 1%
- sucrose solution, 2%

The basic experiment
Using a syringe, place 1 cm^3 of Benedict's solution in a test tube, and place it into a test-tube rack. Then place 5 cm^3 of 2% sucrose in one test tube and 5 cm^3 of 1% sucrase in another, and put both into a water bath at 35 °C. What control should there be?

Leave both test tubes in the water bath for 10 minutes to allow their temperatures to reach the temperature of the water. Then, simultaneously, start the stop clock and pour the contents of the sucrase solution into the test tube containing sucrose solution. Swirl the contents of this test tube and rapidly put it back into the 35 °C water bath.

After 30 seconds, remove 1 cm^3 of the reaction mixture with a syringe and squirt it into the test tube of Benedict's solution in the test-tube rack. Now transfer this test tube to a water bath at 70 °C for five minutes, and during this time record both the timing of the colour changes and the approximate amount of precipitate formed.

The effect of changing enzyme and substrate concentrations: design your own experiment
Now plan and carry out an investigation, using dilutions of the sucrase and sucrose solutions provided, into the effect of altering the enzyme or substrate concentration on the rate of reaction. Write down your plan before you start. Carry out any controls necessary. Keep detailed records of what you did and the results you obtained, and be prepared to modify your technique (e.g. by allowing the reaction to take place for a minute instead of 30 seconds) to obtain more satisfactory results.

1 Write a full report on your experiment. Write a detailed description of your method, and record your results in a table; is it possible to express your results graphically? Draw some conclusions.

2 Read the explanation that follows about the effects of enzyme and substrate concentration on the rate of reactions catalysed by enzymes, and then write a discussion of your results.

The rate of reaction is directly proportional to the enzyme concentration, provided that there is an *excess* of substrate molecules. If, however, the amount of substrate present is limited, then the rate of reaction slows down. This is illustrated in Figure 1.51. For a given amount of enzyme, the rate of the reaction will increase in line with an increase in the substrate concentration up to a certain point. At low concentrations of substrate, some of the active sites on the enzyme are spare, but as the concentration increases, so more and more sites come into use. When *all* the active sites are being occupied at any one time, adding more substrate has no effect. This is shown in Figure 1.52.

The effect of different temperatures on reactions catalysed by enzymes

In the next Activity, you will be investigating the effect of different temperatures on the

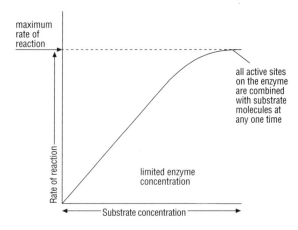

Figure 1.52 The effect of substrate concentration on the rate of a reaction catalysed by an enzyme

activity of *amylase*, an enzyme that catalyses the hydrolysis of starch. Look back at the section on carbohydrates in this chapter to remind yourself of the structure of starch and the iodine test.

ACTIVITY 38

Investigating the effect of different temperatures on amylase activity

You will need:

- test tubes
- test-tube racks
- labels or marking pens
- a stop clock
- pipettes or syringes (5 cm^3)
- a white tile
- glass rods
- water baths maintained at 25 °C, 40 °C, 60 °C and 100 °C
- thermometers
- beakers
- amylase solution (allow 100 cm^3), concentration up to 1% depending on age
- starch solution (1%) (allow 100 cm^3)
- iodine solution
- ice

The method

Label six test tubes. Measure the room temperature and the ice temperature, and

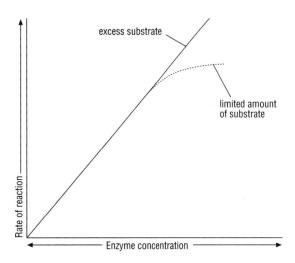

Figure 1.51 The effect of enzyme concentration on the rate of a reaction catalysed by an enzyme

check that the water baths are at 25 °C, 40 °C, 60 °C and 100 °C respectively. Add 5 cm^3 of amylase solution to each test tube.

Keep the first tube at room temperature. Place each of the remaining tubes in the ice or appropriate water bath for exactly 10 minutes. During this time, prepare a results sheet.

Once you are satisfied that the contents of each tube are at the temperature of the water bath, add 5 cm^3 of starch solution to each tube and mix with a clean glass rod.

At intervals of one minute, test each tube for the presence of starch by withdrawing one drop of the starch–enzyme mixture, placing it on a white tile and adding one drop of iodine solution. Use a separate pipette for each tube and a different one for the iodine solution. Carefully record each result as it is obtained, in terms of a consistent colour scheme. Note how long it takes in each case before a blue-back colour ceases to be obtained when iodine solution is added to the mixture.

1 For each temperature there should be a control. What should this be? Design a control and carry out a parallel experiment on it.

2 Compare your results with the controls. Draw an appropriate graph of your results.

3 If the blue-black colour takes a longer time to disappear during your experiment, does this mean that the amylase activity is greater or lower? Take this into account when designing your graph.

4 Write a full report on your investigation. What is the optimum temperature for amylase activity? Before you write your discussion, read the section following which explains the effects of temperature on reactions catalysed by enzymes.

An increase in temperature affects the rate of reaction in two ways:

1 Molecules move faster at higher temperatures: they have greater kinetic energy. The faster the molecules move, the more collisions there are between them, so that more substrate molecules react with the enzyme to make the enzyme–substrate complexes. The rate of reaction therefore increases. For most reactions, the rate roughly doubles for every 10 °C rise. The *temperature coefficient* (Q_{10}) is defined as:

$$Q_{10} = \frac{\text{rate of reaction at } (x + 10) \text{ °C}}{\text{rate of reaction at } x \text{ °C}}$$

and for most reactions:

$$Q_{10} \simeq 2$$

(i.e. Q_{10} is approximately equal to 2).

2 The hydrogen bonds which hold the globular structure of the protein in place are broken because the atoms in the enzyme molecule vibrate. The three-dimensional structure alters, and the active sites are lost (denaturation of the enzyme). The activity of the enzyme ceases.

These two factors combine so that the actual net effect of a temperature increase is first an increase in the rate of reaction and then a *decrease*. This is illustrated in Figure 1.53.

The effect of pH change on the rate of a reaction catalysed by an enzyme

The active sites of an enzyme have particular charges that attract the specific substrate, and the protein of an enzyme is mostly held together by hydrogen bonds, which depend on attractions between negative and positive parts of the molecule. So it is to be expected that changes in pH might affect enzyme reactions. Read the section again on pH earlier in this chapter.

A change in pH affects the reaction in two ways:

1 Hydrogen bonds which hold the secondary and tertiary structure in place are broken,

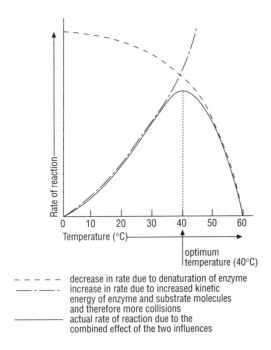

– – – – – decrease in rate due to denaturation of enzyme
—·—·— increase in rate due to increased kinetic
energy of enzyme and substrate molecules
and therefore more collisions
————— actual rate of reaction due to the
combined effect of the two influences

Figure 1.53   The effect of temperature on the rate
of a reaction catalysed by an enzyme

so that the enzyme becomes denatured and
the active sites are lost.

2 There are changes within the active site
itself, so that the substrate may no longer
fit very closely.

These changes can be reversed provided the
pH change has not been too drastic. Each
enzyme has its own optimum pH. Figure 1.54

shows the optimum pH for activity for four
common enzymes. You will see that enzymes
are only active over quite a narrow range of
pH values.

Classes of enzymes

1 *Oxidoreductases.* These catalyse the transfer of
oxygen or hydrogen atoms, or electrons,
between molecules. They are called *oxidases*
or *dehydrogenases*, and are very important in
respiration. Examples are described earlier
in this chapter on p. 14.

2 *Hydrolases.* These catalyse hydrolysis
reactions, which are discussed on p. 16.
Pepsin, amylase and sucrase are examples,
and these enzymes are important in
intracellular and extracellular digestion.

3 *Transferases.* These catalyse the transfer of a
chemical group from one substance to
another. *Transaminases* are important in
making amino acids.

4 *Isomerases.* These enable groups within a
molecule to be rearranged. They are
particularly important in carbohydrate
metabolism. Look back at the section on
monosaccharides (p. 32) to remind
yourself about isomers.

5 *Lyases.* These catalyse the removal or
addition of a chemical group by means
other than hydrolysis. *Decarboxylases* are one

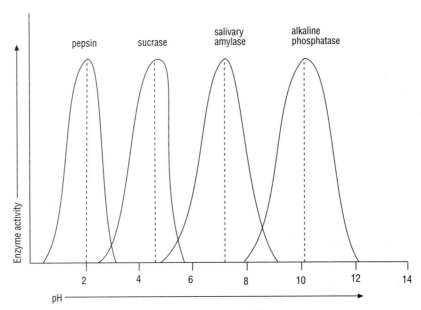

Figure 1.54   The effect of pH on the rates of reactions catalysed by enzymes

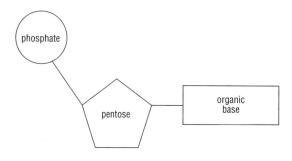

Figure 1.55 The structure of a typical nucleotide

example. These remove carbon dioxide from molecules, and are important in the formation of ethanol and carbon dioxide from glucose in fermentation processes.

6 *Ligases*. These use adenosine triphosphate (ATP) to provide energy to make new bonds between two molecules. They are important in the synthesis of proteins, polysaccharides and lipids.

Nucleic acids

Nucleic acids are polymers made of *nucleotides*. A nucleotide has three parts:

1 a phosphate group
2 a pentose monosaccharide
3 an organic base

(see Figure 1.55). There are five types of organic base, all of them ring structures containing nitrogen, carbon, hydrogen and oxygen. These types are divided into two groups:

1 *Adenine* and *guanine* are double-ring structures called *purines*.
2 *Cytosine*, *thymine* and *uracil* are single-ring structures called *pyrimidines*.

(See Figure 1.56 on p. 50.) There are two main types of nucleic acid:

1 *Ribonucleic acid* (RNA) has *ribose* as the pentose and contains the organic bases adenine, guanine, cytosine and uracil. There are three types of RNA. Some RNA is stored in the nucleus, but most is found in the cytoplasm.
2 *Deoxyribonucleic acid* (DNA) has *deoxyribose* as

the pentose and contains the organic bases adenine, guanine, cytosine and thymine. DNA is found in the chromosomes, together with proteins, which remain in the nucleus.

The organic bases of nucleic acids have the property of forming links with each other in certain patterns. This phenomenon is known as *base pairing* and is very important in the structure of DNA, which consists of two polynucleotide strands. In Figure 1.57 you will see that cytosine links with guanine (via three hydrogen bonds) and thymine links with adenine (via two hydrogen bonds). Hydrogen bonding is important in maintaining these links. Figure 1.58 shows that the ladder-like structure of DNA is wound into a double helix.

ACTIVITY 39

1 List four differences between RNA and DNA.

2 Make a model of DNA, using any materials you like to represent the deoxyribose molecules, the phosphates and the four bases.

The base-pairing mechanism is very important in the two main functions of nucleic acids:

1 chromosome multiplication
2 protein synthesis.

CHROMOSOME MULTIPLICATION IN CELL DIVISION

This occurs in two ways:

1 *Mitosis*: when a cell divides, for example during growth, and the chromosome number in the two new cells is the same as that in the original cell.
2 *Meiosis*: when a cell in the ovaries or testes divides to form four cells in the production of eggs or sperm. The chromosome

(a)

(b)

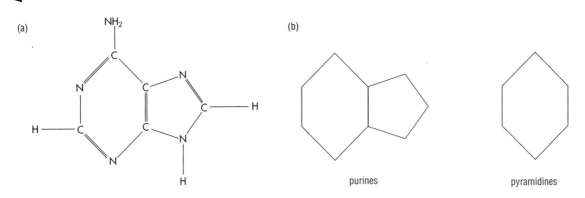

purines

pyramidines

Figure 1.56   (a) adenine (a purine); (b) representative shapes

number in the eggs and sperm is half the original number. The full number of chromosomes is restored upon fertilisation.

Deoxyribonucleic acid is important in passing hereditary characteristics from cell to cell, and from generation to generation. Genes which carry the characteristics are in fact portions of DNA. How DNA produces more of itself, a process called *replication*, is shown in Figure 1.59. The enzyme *DNA polymerase* is involved. You will see that the base-pairing properties are central to replication. The process is called *semi-conservative replication*.

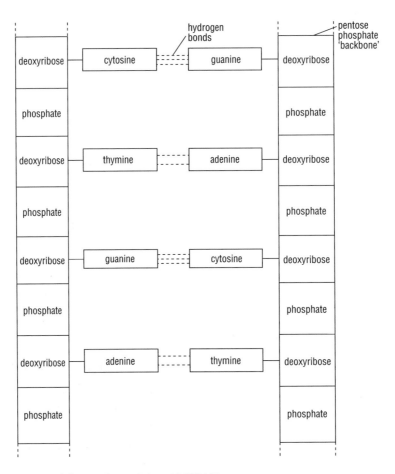

Figure 1.57   The structure of deoxyribonucleic acid (DNA)

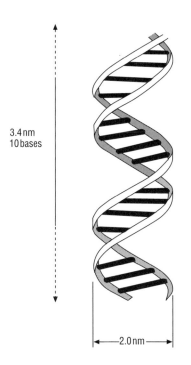

3.4 nm
10 bases

←2.0 nm→

Figure 1.58 The DNA double-helix structure

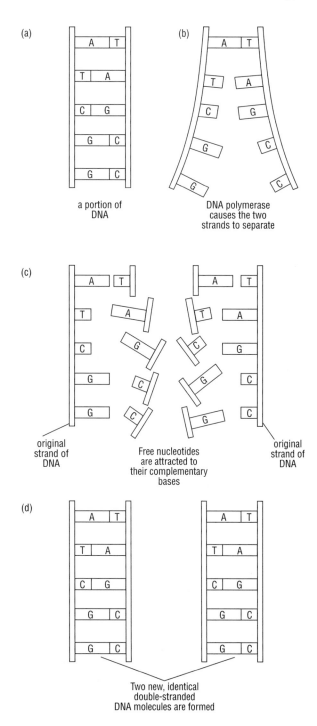

(a)

a portion of
DNA

(b)

DNA polymerase
causes the two
strands to separate

(c)

original
strand of
DNA

Free nucleotides
are attracted to
their complementary
bases

original
strand of
DNA

(d)

Two new, identical
double-stranded
DNA molecules are formed

Figure 1.59 DNA replication

ACTIVITY 40

1 Look at Figure 1.59 and summarise the information shown there. Why is DNA replication called 'semi-conservative' replication?

2 Revise, and write a brief account of, mitosis and meiosis, emphasising the stages where chromosome multiplication occurs.

PROTEIN SYNTHESIS

Both DNA and RNA are involved in protein synthesis. There are three types of RNA, all made from DNA using the base-pairing mechanism that is used when DNA replicates during cell division. All RNA is basically *single stranded*, so an important difference is that only one strand of DNA is copied in RNA formation. This copying process is called *transcription*.

The three types of RNA are:

1 *Messenger RNA*. This is a copy of a portion of one strand of DNA, usually corresponding to one gene. This carries the information necessary to line up the amino acids of one protein in the correct sequence.

2 *Transfer RNA*. This carries amino acids to the ribosomes, the site of protein synthesis. ATP provides the energy for the attachment of the amino acid to its own specific transfer-RNA (tRNA) molecule. This energy will eventually be used to make a new peptide bond.

3 *Ribosomal RNA*. This is part of the structure of the ribosome, but it has no role in lining up amino acids in the right sequence.

The genetic code and protein synthesis

We saw that for proteins to carry out their specific function, it is important that the amino acids be in the correct sequence in the primary structure. It has been found that there are three bases in a row in the messenger RNA (mRNA) code for a particular amino acid. Some amino acids have more than one such code. Where uracil = U, adenine = A, cytosine = C and guanine = G, examples of the genetic code are as follows:

- UUU = phenylalanine
- AAA = lysine
- UGU = cysteine
- GCU = alanine

The transfer RNA carrying the amino acid phenylalanine has three special bases (AAA) in its structure which recognise the code UUU on the mRNA. The base-pairing mechanism is important here as well.

ACTIVITY 41

Look at Figures 1.60 and 1.61 on pp. 53 and 54; write a brief account of protein synthesis. Explain the source of the energy required to make the new peptide bonds. Mention the roles of the following in this process:
- DNA in chromosomes
- RNA polymerase
- messenger RNA
- ribosomes
- transfer RNA
- the genetic code

SAFETY IN THE LABORATORY

The Health and Safety at Work Act 1974

The above Act relating to health and safety at work is outlined in Chapter 2. This legislation also covers experiments carried out in laboratories.

The Control of Substances Hazardous to Health Regulation and the Management of Health and Safety at Work Regulations require an employer to carry out risk assessments. A risk assessment must be made for every experiment, and then protective measures must be taken to control any risks discovered. In drawing up *general risk assessments*, various assumptions are made about good laboratory practice.

Good laboratory practice

- Practical work is conducted in a properly equipped and maintained laboratory
- Rules for student behaviour are strictly enforced
- Field work takes account of any guidelines issued by the employer
- Mains-operated equipment is regularly inspected and properly maintained, and appropriate records are kept
- Care is taken with normal laboratory operations such as heating substances and handling heavy objects
- Good laboratory practice is observed when chemicals, living organisms and materials of living origin are handled
- Eye protection is worn whenever there is any recognised risk to the eyes (including activities involving heating substances, those involving toxic, corrosive or flammable chemicals, and those in which heat may be generated in a chemical reaction)
- Any fume cupboard required operates at least to the standard of the DES Architects

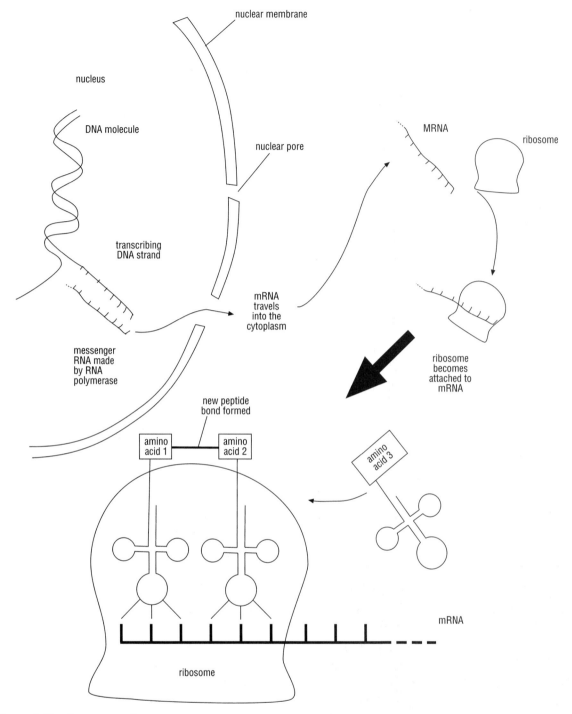

Figure 1.60 Protein synthesis

and Building Group Design Note 29, *Fume Cupboards in Schools* (HMSO, 1982)

- Students are taught safe techniques that minimise hazards for such activities as heating chemicals, smelling them, pouring from bottles or handling micro-organisms
- Hand-washing facilities are available in the laboratory

Working with chemicals

As well as the specific protective measures to be taken when hazardous chemicals are being used, there are also general procedures to be observed in chemistry laboratories at all times:

- Chemicals you use should be in clearly

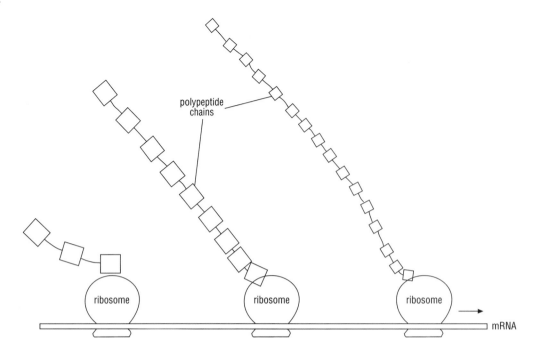

polypeptide chains

ribosome

ribosome

ribosome

mRNA

Figure 1.61 Polypeptide formation

labelled stock bottles, with the name of the chemical, details of any hazards and the date of acquisition or preparation shown on the label. In taking chemicals from a bottle, remove the stopper with one hand, keeping the stopper in your hand whilst pouring from the bottle. The stopper should then be replaced at once and remain uncontaminated. Pour liquids from the opposite side to the label, so that it does not become damaged by corrosive chemicals

- Do not let clothes and hair hang freely, where they could be a fire hazard. Wear a laboratory coat
- In areas which could be contaminated with hazardous chemicals, it is contrary to the Control of Substances Hazardous to Health Regulations to permit eating, drinking, smoking or the application of cosmetics
- Wear eye protection whenever a risk assessment requires it, or whenever there is any risk to your eyes. This includes, for example, when you are washing up at the end of the session
- Carefully study the best techniques for safely heating chemicals. Small quantities of solid can be heated in test tubes. Liquids

must be heated very carefully, because of the risk of 'bumping' and 'spitting'. Boiling tubes are safer than test tubes, but should be less than one-fifth full. Point test tubes away from your own face, but do remember the need to do the same for your neighbours. Use a water bath to heat flammable liquids – never use a naked flame

- When testing for the odour of gases, the gas should be contained in a test tube (not a larger vessel) and the test tube held about 10–15 cm from your face, pointing away from you. Slowly bring the test tube nearer. If you are asthmatic, you should not smell gases
- Clear up chemical spillages straight away. Most minor spills can be dealt with by a damp cloth or paper towels. Wash cloths and dispose of paper towels carefully. A few spills, especially larger ones, may need chemical neutralisation or similar treatment
- If you get a chemical in your eye or on your skin, flood the area with large quantities of water and keep the water running for at least 10 minutes – directing the water with rubber tubing fixed to a tap is the most convenient way of doing this

- Treat a burn from an apparatus, scalding liquids or steam by immersing the area in cool water for at least 10 minutes. Preferably use running water

ACTIVITY 42

1 Find out about the Health and Safety at Work Act 1974. Divide into four groups, and let each group investigate different aspects of the Act, as shown just below. Give a presentation to the rest of the class.
   - *Health*: Control of Substances Hazardous to Health Regulation; manual handling; display screens; noise at work
   - *Environment*: environmental legislation; control of pollution
   - *Welfare*: first aid; workplace health and safety welfare; Management of Health and Safety at Work Regulations
   - *Safety*: personal protective equipment; electricity at work

2 Define each of the following hazard terms, and give an example of each:
   - *Biological*: pathogen, irritant, carcinogen, mutagen, teratogen, harmful to the environment
   - *Chemical*: explosive, oxidive, flammable, toxic, harmful, corrosive, irritant, carcinogen, mutagen, teratogen, harmful to the environment
   - *Physical*: Equipment, radiation, electrical
   - Fire

3 *Identifying the hazards of working in laboratories*
   - Consider this question: 'What can make a laboratory a dangerous place in which to work?' In groups, write down as many things as you can think of which may be hazardous in a laboratory

   - Now agree to a set of rules to reduce the dangers, and produce a list of these rules

4 *Hazard symbols*
   Match the following warnings to the hazard symbols in Figure 1.62:
   - highly flammable
   - toxic
   - explosive
   - corrosive
   - radioactive
   - wear hand protection
   - harmful

Figure 1.62 Hazard symbols

5 Carry out a chemical risk assessment on one of your experiments. Risk assessments are made on a standard form (see Figure 1.63), and the steps for making such an assessment are as follows:

   - Write down the procedures you will be using, chemicals used or made, quantities, techniques and any non-chemical hazards
   - Use reference sources to identify any hazardous chemicals you are planning to use or make. The appropriate warning symbol should be shown on reagent bottles and in suppliers' catalogues

- Record the nature of the hazards involved and the way you might be exposed to the hazard. There are standard reference sources with this information, such as the 'Hazcards' published by CLEAPSS
- Decide what protective or control measures to take so that you can carry out your practical work in safety
- Find out how to dispose of any hazardous residues from your practical work

ASSESSMENT OPPORTUNITY

1 Write reports on practical experiments, to cover:
   - two investigations into the structure and properties of biologically important compounds and elements
   - investigations into the features of three specific enzyme-controlled reactions

2 List the safe procedures and precautions which were followed in the practical investigations.

3 Prepare a report which explains the properties and functions of biologically important compounds.

4 Prepare a list of the principal features of enzyme-controlled reactions, giving an example in each case to illustrate the feature in question.

5 Write a summary of the structure and functions of nucleic acids.

6 Write an account of the legislation which covers working in science laboratories.

7 Produce a statement signed by the assessor to verify that you have followed safe procedures during practical investigations, having undertaken a full risk assessment of each experiment.

Title of the practical activity			
Outline of the procedure			
Hazardous substance being used or made	Nature of the hazards (e.g. toxic, flammable)	Exposure limit	Quantities being used or made
Any non-chemical hazards		Steps to minimise risks from non-chemical hazards	
Emergency action			
Disposal of residues			

Figure 1.63 A risk-assessment form for working with chemicals

REFERENCES AND RESOURCES

For safety in the laboratory, consult the following:

CLEAPPS School Science Service (1995), *Hazcards*, available to members only, new edition in preparation for 1994, School Science Service, Brunel University.

Topics in Safety (1988), 2nd edn, The Association for Science Education, College Lane, Hatfield, Herts.

SSERC (1979), *Hazardous Chemicals: a Manual for Schools and Colleges*, Harlow: Oliver & Boyd.

Microbiology: an HMI Guide for Schools and Further Education, (1990), Department of Education, HMSO.

CLEAPSS (1989, and later supplements), *Laboratory Handbook* available to members only, Brunel University.

SSERC (1991), *Preparing COSHH Risk Assessments for Project Work in Schools*, 24 Bernard Terrace, Edinburgh EH8 9NX.

Vincent, R. and Borrows, T. P. (1992), 'Science department safety policies', *School Science Review*, vol. 73, no. 264.

Taylor, P. (1992), 'Reaction and over-reaction: risk assessment in teaching', *School Science Review*, vol. 74, no. 267.

Department of Education and Science (1982), *Fume Cupboards in Schools*, DES Architects and Building Group Design Note 29, Norwich: HMSO.

USEFUL ADDRESS

For information on SATIS 16–19 Unit 6 (Science & Technology in Society 1990), contact:

Association of Science Education
College Lane, Hatfield, Herts. AL10 9AA

2

ENVIRONMENT AND HEALTH

ENVIRONMENTAL HEALTH PROVISION

Food hygiene and the sale of food

THE NEED FOR LEGISLATION

Legislation on food safety has three major functions:
- the protection of the consumer
- the protection of the honest trader
- the promotion of freedom of choice and fair competition

The protection of the consumer by preventing illness and the spread of disease is a very important aspect of this legislation. Food-poisoning bacteria and viruses, as well as micro-organisms causing more serious illnesses such as typhoid, may be carried by food. Contamination by metals such as lead and mercury can also cause poisoning and serious damage.

Other measures designed to ensure food safety involve regulations relating to the composition of food, including controls on ingredients – especially food additives. Procedures for processing and preserving food are also strictly controlled. There are restrictions on the amounts and types of chemicals which may be added to food. Storage methods are also covered by the laws.

As well as protecting the public from disease and damage to health, the legislation also ensures that the food is of the expected quality. It should not be damaged or spoiled. Advertising, the labelling on packets and other descriptions of food should properly describe the food and not be misleading in any way. The quantities of the ingredients should also be recorded accurately. The public is entitled to accurate nutritional information.

These laws will also protect the honest food trader as it will obviously cost more to produce and store good-quality food. Illegal actions, for example adding large amounts of preservative, will cut costs, as will substituting inexpensive ingredients.

THE LEGISLATION

The UK's legislative arrangements are the responsibility of central government and are shared between three departments. These are the Ministry of Agriculture, Fisheries and Food, and the Departments of Health and Social Security.

While the food laws are generated centrally, their enforcement is devolved to local government. Trading-standards officers and environmental health officers have responsibility for:
- advising food producers, processors and retailers on food law
- monitoring the quality of food sold in the local area
- prosecuting those who fail to meet the required standards

The Food Safety Act 1990

The Food Safety Act 1990 contains most of the legislation relating to the safety and quality of the food that we buy. The Act is part of the criminal law, and the offences it covers are absolute. This means that people in the food production and sales business can be prosecuted for breaking the law even if they did not intend to do so.

The Food Safety Act 1990 is based on the fact that the producer and distributor of food are held to be responsible for the safety and quality of the food on sale to the public. The Act defines 'food', 'food business', 'food premises' and 'food source', and specifies what food is intended for human consumption. It also establishes the role of the local authority in the enforcement of the Act through the work of authorised food-inspection officers.

The Act further refers to the preparation and sale of *injurious food*. A person is guilty of an offence who

- adds any substance to a food
- uses any substance as an ingredient in the preparation of food
- abstracts any constituent from food
- subjects food to any other process or treatment

so as to render the food injurious to health, with the intent that the food shall be sold for human consumption in that state.

It is also an offence to sell food that does not comply with food safety requirements. This is food that has been rendered injurious to health, which is unfit for human consumption or is so contaminated that it would not be reasonable to expect it to be used for human consumption. Food suspected of not complying with food safety requirements may be inspected, seized and condemned. A food-inspection officer may serve an improvement notice to a proprietor of a food business where it is believed that an offence has been committed. Prohibition orders may be issued to prevent commercial operations where there is a risk of food being sold which may be injurious to health.

Further offences relate to the sale of:

- food which is not of the nature, substance or quality demanded by the consumer
- food which has a false or misleading description or advertisement

'Not of the nature' applies mainly to natural foods such as fish or fruit. For example, if coley is sold as cod, an offence would be committed. 'Not of the substance' refers to the composition. For example, a ham may contain a very large amount of water. 'Not of the quality' refers to possible contamination with foreign bodies or micro-organisms.

There are also sections of the Act relating to labelling and controls on ingredients, including additives.

Furthermore, powers exist to issue regulations under the Act on:

- food composition
- residues in food sources, for example live animals
- microbiological standards
- hygienic conditions and practices
- food processes or treatments
- European Community provisions
- imported foods
- the registration and licensing of food premises

Codes of practice may also be issued to help food traders to carry out procedures to ensure that food is safe and of a high quality.

INSPECTION AND THE ENFORCEMENT OF FOOD-SAFETY LEGISLATION

The Food Safety Act 1990 empowers the local authority to appoint environmental health officers with special duties of food inspection. They have powers of entry, and can enforce all aspects of the Act.

Public analysts can be appointed, and microbiological laboratories can be set up. Arrangements can be made to collect and analyse samples.

Local authorities can seize and condemn suspected food, serve improvement and prohibition orders, and prosecute offenders.

Weights-and-measures officers also play a role in ensuring that the weights-and-measures legislation is implemented.

ACTIVITY I

1 Contact your local environmental health department.
   - Arrange for a food inspector to visit your class to explain the work of the department
   - Find out how many prosecutions there have been in your area in the last five years. What has been the level of fines?
   - Collect codes of practice issued by the local environmental health department to local food traders

2 Visit local food shops, supermarkets and other outlets, and observe what special precautions are taken to avoid the decay and contamination of food. You could especially investigate:
   - a large supermarket
   - a fish shop
   - a bread and cake shop
   - an ice-cream stall
   - a hamburger stall
   - a self-service restaurant

3 Each person in the group should collect five food packages and note the descriptions that are recorded on them. Then, in groups, compare the range of detail included for the different foods. Note additives that are used to preserve or colour food. Find out more about permitted additives. What are 'E numbers'?

Protection from fire risks

THE FIRE PRECAUTIONS ACT 1971

This is an Act that was passed to protect people from fire risks in almost every environment to which the public has access, except their own homes. The fire authority, almost always the local authority, is able to grant fire certificates where premises reach specific safety standards relating to fire risks. All the following places are covered by this legislation:
- institutions providing treatment or care
- places of work
- premises used for entertainment, recreation or instruction, or for clubs and societies
- hotels, hostels and anywhere providing sleeping accommodation
- schools and premises used for training or research
- any building to which members of the public have access, including shops

Applications for fire certificates have to contain full details of the premises and the intended purpose, and the protection provided for people against fire risks must be fully described.

The most important fire safety points mentioned in the Act are as follows:
- the means of escape in case of fire
- the means of fighting fires, and how this equipment will be maintained in efficient working order
- how fire warnings will be given to people in the building
- the training that people employed in the building must receive in what to do in the case of fire

The fire-authority inspector will visit the premises to make an assessment of fire safety, and will either grant the fire certificate, or, if they are not satisfied that the safety standards have been reached, refuse it. If the application is turned down, then advice will be provided about what steps have to be taken in order to gain a certificate. If, on the other hand, the fire certificate is granted, it will specify the precise functions of the premises covered and give details of all the fire precautions expected to be found there.

INSPECTION AND THE ENFORCEMENT OF FIRE SAFETY LEGISLATION

Inspections of places of work for fire safety purposes are often arranged in conjunction with the Health and Safety Commission. Such inspections can also be carried out by officers of the fire brigade if so authorised by the fire authority.

Inspectors have powers to enter premises and require the production of a fire certificate. They can carry out fire safety checks to make sure that all the requirements of the certificate are in place. It is an offence to obstruct a fire inspector who is trying to carry out an inspection. The occupier of premises which should have a fire certificate commits an offence if such a certificate has not been obtained. It is also an offence to contravene any of the conditions and requirements laid down in the fire certificate. Fines or imprisonment may be imposed.

In addition to prosecuting offenders, the Act also enables codes of practice to be produced to help occupiers make their premises safe against fire hazards. Furthermore, improvement notices may be issued if fire precautions need upgrading or are slightly deficient. Sometimes, when serious fire risks are discovered in a premises, a prohibition notice is issued specifying the particular hazard. This will prevent use of the premises until the hazard is rectified.

Another way in which fire safety in buildings is enforced is through the power that local authorities have when they grant planning permission for new buildings. There are rules that specify that new buildings, and alterations or additions to existing buildings, must be safe against fire hazards.

ACTIVITY 2

Find out about the fire safety precautions in your school or college.
- How will you escape if there is a fire?
- Where is the fire-fighting equipment located?
- How is it maintained?
- Is the fire warning system in place?
- Who is trained about what to do in the case of fire?

If you go to a hospital or residential home on a visit or for work experience, find out about the fire safety precautions there. Contact your local authority and fire brigade for information as well.

Health and safety at work

THE NEED FOR LEGISLATION

In 1970 a Government Select Committee was set up to investigate health and safety at work. It was found that the UK had the best legal and regulatory system in the world, but that it was not effective in preventing accidents at work. The law was very difficult to interpret and was often out of date. There were too many enforcement authorities, and inspection was not systematic. Apathy was deemed to be the main cause of accidents at work.

A new Act was introduced after the Select Committee produced a report on the situation. This was the Health and Safety at Work Act 1974. It is still in force, together with the Factories Act 1961 and the Offices, Shops and Railway Premises Act 1963, which have very detailed requirements for health and safety. European Community directives have further helped to shape the UK laws on health and safety over the last 10 years, and from 1992 there have been 10 such directives, which must be implemented in all member states.

For the first time, the *Annual Report of the Health and Safety Commission 1990–91* gave some statistics for the UK that showed the need for health and safety legislation.
- There are 700,000 workplace accidents a year that result in absences from work of over three days
- There are 1,500,000 workplace injuries a year
- About 70,000 accidents a year involve absence from work for over a month
- 2,000,000 people have illnesses which they believe are caused, or made worse, by work
- Work-related injuries and ill-health cause

the loss of 29,000,000 working days a year. This is 10 times the total lost through strikes
- Back injuries and other stresses and strains to the limbs affect over a million people
- Nearly half a million suffer from stress, heart disease or depression which may be work related
- 150,000 have some hearing loss related to exposure to loud noise at work
- Over 350,000 have throat, skin or lung diseases made worse, or actually caused, by dusts and fumes at work

THE HEALTH AND SAFETY AT WORK ACT 1974

The Health and Safety at Work Act 1974 is based on the following principles:
- All employers and employees should be aware of health and safety matters. Personal responsibility is very important
- There should be one comprehensive framework which includes basic legislation, regulations covering specific hazards at work, and codes of practice
- There should be one unified enforcement authority which carries out inspections, initiates legal proceedings and gives help and advice

Eight million existing employees not previously protected by legislation came under the Act, so that now all employees are covered. Duties for employers and employees are outlined:

HEALTH AND SAFETY LAW

What you should know
Your health, safety and welfare at work are protected by law. Your employer has a duty to protect you and to keep you informed about health and safety. You have a responsibility to look after yourself and others. If there is a problem, discuss it with your employer or your safety representative, if there is one.

Your employer has a duty under the law, to ensure so far as is reasonably practicable, your health, safety and welfare at work.

In general, your employer's duties include:
- making your workplace safe and without risks to health
- keeping dust, fume and noise under control
- ensuring plant and machinery are safe and that safe systems of work are set and followed
- ensuring articles and substances are moved, stored and used safely
- providing adequate welfare facilities
- giving you the information, instruction, training and supervision necessary for your health and safety

Your employer must also:
- draw up a health and safety policy statement if there are five or more employees, including the health and safety organisation and arrangements in force, and bring it to your attention
- provide free, any protective clothing or equipment specifically required by health and safety law
- report certain injuries, diseases and dangerous occurrences to the enforcing authority
- provide adequate first-aid facilities
- consult a safety representative, if one is appointed by a recognised trade union, about matters affecting your health and safety
- set up a safety committee if asked in writing by two or more safety representatives

Employers also have duties to take precautions against fire, provide adequate means of escape and means for fighting fire.

As an employee, you have legal duties too. They include:
- taking reasonable care for your own health and safety and that of others who may be affected by what you do or do not do
- cooperating with your employer on health and safety
- not interfering with or misusing anything provided for your health, safety or welfare

(Health and Safety Executive 1989)

There are recommended safety policies, as well as a requirement for safety representatives to be appointed from the workforce. There are also approved codes of practice for every workplace and strong enforcement procedures.

THE HEALTH AND SAFETY COMMISSION

This was set up under the Act to administer the legislative provisions. It also reviews health and safety legislation and submits proposals for new and revised regulations.

The Commission appoints advisory committees which consider the following substances/areas of employment:
- major hazards
- toxic substances
- dangerous substances
- the medical sector
- nuclear safety
- dangerous pathogens
- the industrial sector – paper, oil, agriculture, health services, printing, foundries, construction, railways

A major task is to formulate safety standards for every industry and to provide regulations and guidance.

INSPECTION AND THE ENFORCEMENT OF HEALTH AND SAFETY LEGISLATION

The Health and Safety Executive

This is the major instrument of the Health and Safety Commission. It is responsible for the Health and Safety Inspectorate, through which it enforces the health and safety law. It ensures that the regulations and guidance provisions are implemented. There are 21 regional offices of the Health and Safety Executive.

There are different types of health and safety inspector:
- factories
- nuclear installations
- industry
- explosives
- alkali and clean air
- hospitals

- mines and quarries
- agriculture
- schools

The inspectors have four main roles:
- inspection and enforcement of the law
- help and advice to employers
- serving improvement and prohibition notices
- criminal proceedings (as a last resort)

Criminal proceedings result in fines and compensation for victims of accidents if the employer is shown to be negligent. Occasionally, the sentence is imprisonment if the following factors apply:
- warnings previously given and ignored
- blatant flouting of the law
- culpable neglect
- culpable ignorance
- repeated breaches
- a real risk of serious injury
- actual injury
- economic advantage placed before safety
- not the first conviction
- a failure to set up training and supervision
- serious concern in the workforce
- serious concern in the general public

ACTIVITY 3

1 Obtain from the Health and Safety Executive a copy of their leaflet *Health and Safety Law: What You Should Know* which outlines the respective duties of employer and employee in detail. Read the leaflet, and prepare a display on health and safety at work to be erected in the foyer of an industrial premises. Write to the Health and Safety Executive for any additional material you may need.

2 Consider the health and safety requirements of your own school or college and then carry out a safety audit. The following checklist can be used for this purpose. You may like to amend it

so that it applies to your own environment. You should select those items that apply to the area where you are carrying out the audit.

Rooms for students, clients or patients; entrance halls, staircases and passages; toilets; kitchens:
- Is the lighting adequate?
- Are all the lights working?
- Are fire-escape doors and routes identified?
- Are exits and escapes free from obstruction?
- Is there fire-fighting equipment?
- Is it in working order?
- Are floors clean and dry?
- Are electric sockets, plugs and leads undamaged and in working order?
- Are lifts/stairs free from obstruction?
- Are they free from rubbish?
- Are materials stored safely and tidily?
- Are fires protected and in working order?
- Is there enough space for people and equipment to move around safely?
- Are all appliances kept clean and undamaged?
- Are all doors, locks and catches in working order?
- Is there a supply of soap, towels and toilet rolls?
- Are bins emptied regularly?
- Is ventilation adequate?
- Is the water supply adequate?
- Are there guards on dangerous machines?
- Are notices displayed (e.g. 'No smoking')?
- Are knives stored correctly?
- Do the staff wear protective clothing where necessary?
- Is food stored correctly?
- Are all surfaces undamaged and clean?
- Is there any evidence of vermin or insects?
- Are chemicals/cleaning agents stored in a lockable cupboard?

- Is the temperature reasonable?

You should work with a partner. Different pairs of students could be allocated to the various areas of your school or college.

When you have completed your audit, you should prepare a report to present to the rest of the class. You could illustrate the report with drawings, photos or even taped interviews with staff who work in the area.

3 Find out what the Health and Safety at Work Act 1974 specifies about minimum standards in relation to the following conditions at work:
- heating
- fresh air and ventilation
- lighting
- electricity
- cleaning
- toilets and washbasins
- cloakrooms
- eating and drinking
- seating
- space for workers
- means of access – stairs and passageways
- workers with disabilities
- pregnant workers
- young people
- hours of work

Work in a group and prepare an exhibition, which summarises the standards, for the workforce.

HEALTH AND SAFETY REGULATIONS

The Health and Safety at Work Act 1974 and the other relevant acts outline requirements for health and safety in the workplace. In addition, there are regulations made under these acts which give even more detail about specific aspects of health and safety. Regulations have the same force in law as the acts themselves, and employers must therefore comply with them to be within the law.

Control of Substances Hazardous to Health 1988 (COSHH) Regulations

About 100,000 chemicals are in everyday use, and not all of them have been properly tested for the possibility that they might cause cancer or allergies, or have other toxic effects on the human body. Most workers are regularly exposed to toxic substances.

Substances are classed as hazardous if they cause short- or long-term harm. They include dusts, fumes and gases, liquids, pastes, powders, oils, resins, aerosols and sprays. Inks and toners can be toxic. Liquid chemicals like cleaning, antiseptic and sterilising fluids and solvents are often potential hazards which may affect care workers. Although micro-organisms are not chemicals in the sense of the rest of the substances covered by the COSHH regulations, they are nonetheless included, and this is of great importance in a care setting for it offers protection to workers.

The COSHH regulations apply to every workplace.

The prevention and control of exposure to hazardous substances

Employers must prevent the exposure of employees to hazardous substances. Sometimes, complete prevention is not reasonably practicable, in which case it is legal to use the hazardous substance providing there are proper control measures.

Preventing exposure involves eliminating the use of the substance or substituting a less hazardous substance. *Controlling* exposure, on the other hand, includes

1 totally enclosing the process;
2 using adequate ventilation;
3 using safe systems of work and handling procedures.

This third option is the most frequently used in hospitals and other care settings, as it is not usually possible to eliminate the hazard totally. As well as making sure all employees are aware of safe working practices and handling procedures, the use of personal protective equipment and clothing is also important. Information must be given to workers about the dangers of their work, and training must take place to ensure that ways of avoiding the dangers are understood.

Enforcing the COSHH Regulations

The Health and Safety Commission, which is responsible for the Health and Safety Inspectorate, enforces the COSHH Regulations. When a health-and-safety inspector visits a workplace, they have to find out whether the employer has carried out all that is required. Their checklist is as follows:

- Has a complete audit of substances been carried out?
- Have those substances identified as being hazardous to health been assessed?
- Has the employer provided copies of all relevant information to employees?
- Has a central group been set up to review all the information and agree the assessment?
- Does the evidence used for the assessment include information from all relevant bodies?
- Have all necessary preventative and control measures been implemented?
- Are the procedures being observed, and is all the necessary equipment in good working order?
- Has personal protective clothing and equipment been issued?
- Is airborne monitoring being carried out where necessary, and are the results being made available? Are occupational exposure limits being exceeded?
- Is health surveillance being carried out, and are health records being made available?
- Has full information, instruction and training about the risks of hazardous substances and precautions to be taken been given to employees?

ACTIVITY 4

1 Read about the COSHH Regulations.

2 Divide your class into groups. Let each group take a different environment where COSSH Regulations apply. This could be the school or college science laboratories, or a particular area or department in a hospital for example. Find out how risks are assessed, and by whom, and what substances hazardous to health are present. What injurious effects do they have on the human body? What control measures are adopted? Do all the employees who work in the area know about the hazards involved, and has training been given about the risks and precautions to be taken? What sort of records exist? You should plan your investigation before you start, and decide whether it would be useful to interview employees and supervisors.

3 Write a clear set of instructions for using one potentially hazardous substance in a care setting.

Health and Safety (First Aid) Regulations 1981

All workplaces must have first-aid equipment and arrangements for making sure that injured workers are treated quickly. Employers must:

- provide first-aid equipment, facilities, arrangements and personnel
- inform all employees of the arrangements for getting first aid

Self-employed people must provide their own first-aid cover.

The regulations further stipulate that first-aid arrangements must be 'adequate and appropriate'. The employer decides what should be provided, taking into account the following factors:

- the number of employees
- the nature of the work
- the size of the workplace
- the distance of the workplace from outside medical services

These factors determine what equipment and facilities must be present, such as first-aid rooms, first-aid boxes and eye-wash bottles.

First-aid boxes must be provided in a box marked with a white cross on a green background. Travelling kits should be provided where necessary. First-aid personnel must be appointed who hold a current first-aid certificate from a training course approved by the Health and Safety Executive. Two approved organisations are St John's Ambulance and the Red Cross. Trained first-aiders administer emergency first aid and know how to take charge in an emergency, for example by calling a doctor or ambulance. They should also take responsibility for first-aid equipment and facilities. Even the smallest workplace must have one first-aider on duty at all times when employees are at work. Larger employers should ensure that there is one first-aider for every 50 employees. Records should be kept in an accident book of all first-aid cases treated.

ACTIVITY 5

1 Investigate first-aid provision in your school or college. Where are the first-aid boxes, and what are their contents? Who are the first-aid personnel? What training is provided? Is there an accident-recording book? Prepare a report.

2 What is the first-aid provision in a care setting? You may be able to investigate this while you are on work placement. Write a brief report of your findings.

The Reporting of Injuries, Diseases and Dangerous Occurrences Regulations 1985 (RIDDOR)

These regulations are concerned with recording and reporting accidents and ill-health at work.

If there are more than 10 employees, then there must be an *accident book* in which are recorded
- accidents
- sickness which may have been caused by work
- dangerous occurrences and 'near misses'

Employees must tell the employer verbally or in writing as soon as possible of any such problems, and then the employer is legally bound to investigate.

Employers must report to the Health and Safety Executive or the environmental health department of the local authority whenever the following events occur:
- fatal accidents
- a major injury or condition requiring medical treatment
- dangerous occurrences
- accidents causing incapacity for more than three days
- some work-related diseases
- gas incidents

More serious accidents and dangerous occurrences must be reported immediately, and a written report provided within seven days.

There are special forms which must be completed when diseases occur, and there are 28 categories of reportable diseases including poisoning and skin and lung diseases.

Trade-union safety representatives must have access to all information relating to all these problems in the workplace. The Employment Medical Advisory Service, which is part of the HSE, gives advice and information on the reporting of diseases.

Manual Operations Handling Regulations 1992

More than a quarter of accidents occurring in the workplace each year and reported to the enforcing authorities are associated with manual handling. The vast majority of these result in people being absent from work for over three days. The injuries are commonly sprains and strains, often of the back.

For medical and health services, 55% of all over-three-day injuries are caused by manual-handling accidents. The sprains and strains arise from incorrect ways of lifting and moving loads. Many manual-handling injuries are cumulative, resulting from poor posture and excessive repetition of particular movements. Sometimes the injury is attributable to a single handling incident, but not often. A full recovery is not always made, and physical impairment or even permanent disability can result.

The Manual Operations Handling Regulations 1992 are made under the Health and Safety at Work Act 1974. These implement a European Commission (EC) directive on manual handling. There is now an ergonomic approach to this aspect of work. Ergonomics is sometimes described as 'fitting the job to the person, rather than the person to the job'.

The Regulations require employers to carry out the following measures:
- avoid hazardous manual-handling operations where possible by redesigning the task, or by automating or mechanising the process
- make an assessment of any hazardous manual-handling operation that cannot be avoided

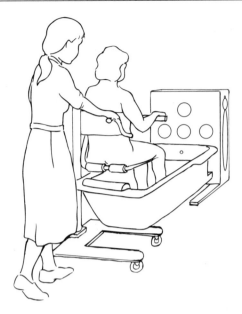

Figure 2.1 Bathing a patient using a mechanical device

- reduce the risk of injury from those operations by improving the task, the load and the working environment

Accurate records of accidents and ill-health will help identify potentially risky manual-handling operations. When a full assessment of the task has taken place, attention must then be given to reducing the risk of injury. Mechanical assistance may be possible. Figure 2.1 shows a device helping patients in and out of the bath.

Full training should be given to employees to ensure that they know how to safely carry out all the manual-handling operations required of them.

ACTIVITY 7

Find out about how heavy loads are moved around in your school or college. What mechanical assistance is provided?

SAFETY POLICIES IN THE WORKPLACE

Employers have many legal responsibilities to ensure the safety of their employees at work.

Among these duties is the provision of a *safety policy*. This must be provided in writing and communicated to all employees. The document must be revised and updated whenever necessary.

The Health and Safety at Work Act 1974 gives clear guidance about what a safety policy must contain:

1 *The general policy*
   This must state the employer's approach to health, safety and welfare and make it clear that health and safety is an important objective of the organisation.

2 *The organisation*
   There must be a clear chain of duties from employer to all employees. Every employee must know who to consult on safety matters. The employer must specify the duties of employees in carrying out the policy, but cannot transfer final responsibility for safety to employees. The duties must be clear and realistic, and the employees must be given the time and facilities for carrying out the duties.

3 *Arrangements*
   These must describe in detail the steps taken to eliminate or minimise every hazard in each job. The policy should cover the following:
   - the general environment: keeping gangways and doors clear, cleaning, noise levels, lighting, welfare facilities etc.
   - each machine, substance or process
   - special work situations, e.g. the prevention of infections, night shifts, dealing with patients, contact with the public
   - dealing with injury, fire and other emergencies
   - informing employees, training and refresher training, supervision
   - consultation with employees, assessing success, revising and updating procedures and policies

ACTIVITY 8

Work in pairs to investigate and compare safety policies in different environments. If you are doing work experience, you could find out about the safety policy at your placement. This may be a nursery, nursing home, hospital or day centre. You could also investigate catering areas at your school or college.

Evaluate your chosen policy by seeing how it matches up to the points in the following checklist.

- Do all employees have access to a copy of the policy, and is the policy up to date?
- Does the policy clearly tell employees about the safety procedures for all the work that they do?
- Does the policy name the person who is in charge of safety?
- Does the policy refer to other documents? If so, are these documents available?
- Does the policy cover all the relevant issues and hazards such as first aid, fire, noise, chemicals, the prevention of infection? Are the Control of Substances Hazardous to Health Regulations 1988 mentioned?
- If there are employees whose first language is not English, has the policy been explained in their first language? Are the most important parts translated in writing?

Write a report which includes both the safety policy itself and your evaluation of it, and present it to the whole group.

ACTIVITY 9

Since 1978, employees who belong to trade unions which are recognised by the employer have been legally entitled to appoint safety representatives and to ask their employer to set up a safety committee. Since 1993 all employees have the right under EC law to appoint and elect safety representatives. Investigate the rights of the safety representatives in their place of work, and write a brief report that outlines these rights.

Procedures designed to control infection in a care setting

HYGIENIC PRACTICES AND THE SAFE DISPOSAL OF INFECTED MATERIALS

Infection control is very important in the effective provision and management of health care services. The aim is to protect the population from avoidable infections, whether in a community or in a hospital-based group.

Over the last two decades a number of epidemiological changes have taken place that have influenced how infections caused by micro-organisms are managed and prevented. These changes include the following:

- Technological advancement has resulted in the development of complicated instruments that can be difficult to decontaminate
- New pathological micro-organisms have emerged, such as the hepatitis C virus (HCV), the human immunodeficiency virus (HIV) and *Clostridium difficile*
- Familiar organisms are showing increasing resistance to commonly used antiseptics and antibiotics, for example, *Methicillin-resistant staphylococcus aureus* (MRSA)
- People are travelling further afield, and health care workers may come back with unusual infections. There is also an increase in the use of agency nurses, so personnel are more transient
- There are more people receiving care who are particularly susceptible to infection

WHAT IS AN INFECTION?

Micro-organisms are everywhere in our environment, on our skin and in our mucous membranes and alimentary tracts. Not many of these organisms are pathogenic (cause diseases), and infection will only occur if there is an imbalance between the environment, the human body and the micro-organism. The term 'infection' is used when organisms reach a vulnerable site in sufficient numbers to create an adverse reaction. Infections can be caused by bacteria, viruses and fungi.

Endogenous infections

These self-infections occur when micro-organisms, which exist harmlessly in one part of the body, become pathogenic when transferred to another site. An example is *Staphylococcus epidermidis* which lives harmlessly on the skin but can cause serious infection in plastic joints after operations.

Exogenous infections

These are cross-infections, which occur when bacteria are transferred to the human body from another source. One particular problem in hospitals is *Pseudomonas aeruginosa*, which is pathogenic when it invades immunocompromised patients. Another example is *salmonella*, which will only cause a food-poisoning infection when 10^5 organisms are present. In those older patients who may be regularly receiving antacids, the infective dose is much smaller since the gastric pH is high and bacteria are not killed in the stomach.

Hospital environments are laden with bacteria. A hospital-based infection is known as *nosocomial*.

The transmission of infections and preventative measures

There are three elements in the chain of infection (see Figure 2.2), and infection-control principles are based on breaking this chain. The source of the infection will originate from a person carrying the infection. Usually, the symptoms of that

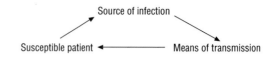

Figure 2.2 **The chain of infection**

infection will be clear, but sometimes there is no illness and people can be carriers of potentially pathogenic organisms. Examples include typhoid, HIV, the hepatitis-B virus and MRSA. Carriers can transmit the disease to others even though they themselves have no symptoms.

There are three ways in which infection can be spread:
- direct or indirect contact with the source
- carried in the air (airborne)
- vector-borne

Direct contact spread

Cross-infection occurs when an individual has direct physical contact with the source of an infected organism. This could be by contact either with infected blood and body fluids, or with the hands of health care professionals.

Dirty hands are the major method of cross-infection, particularly for organisms such as *Staphylococcus aureus*, since over 40% of the population has this bacterium in the nasal passages, axilla and groin. These micro-organisms are transmitted during routine nursing care when they are transferred to the surface of the skin of the hands of the nurse. *Staphylococcus aureus* is a major cause of the infection of wounds after surgery. The infection can take hold up to 30 days after the operation. There is the added problem that some strains of this bacterium are now resistant to the antibiotic used to combat it, *methicillin*.

Preventative measures

If blood or body fluids are splashed into the mouth, eyes or broken skin, the same procedures should be carried out as those for injuries with a used needle or other sharp implement. These are described in the next section on preventative measures for indirect infection.

Micro-organisms can be removed from hands by thorough washing and drying. Since this is so important, much research has been done to find out the best methods. Soap is the least effective, and alcohol the most effective way to kill bacteria on hands. The disinfectant *chlorhexidine* continues to destroy bacteria some time after application. In reality, however, soap is used most frequently to wash hands in hospitals and other care settings because it is the cheapest agent, and it can be quite effective if hands are washed very thoroughly. Bacteria are transferred more easily between wet surfaces than dry ones, so drying hands is also very important. Surprisingly, it has been shown that drying with paper towels is more efficient than linen, and that hot-air driers are the least effective: in fact, the nozzles and circuits of these driers become heavily contaminated and recirculate bacteria-laden air currents. It is thought that paper towels provide more friction to remove bacteria, both from the surface and deeper down, by removing layers of dead skin cells.

As far as post-operative wound infections are concerned, antiseptic cleansing agents are used before surgery, and good hygiene on the patient's part is important. Vulnerable patients, such as those who are elderly or have arterial disease or diabetes, must be identified, and a close watch must be kept on them.

Indirect spread

This is sometimes referred to as 'common vehicle spread'. There is indirect contact with the source in that an intermediate object has carried the infection. This object could be food, blood or blood products, antiseptic fluids, equipment, contaminated waste, or needles, scissors or scalpels contaminated with infected blood or body fluids. These sharp implements are commonly known as just 'sharps'.

There are numerous diseases transmitted in this indirect manner. Food may carry food-poisoning organisms, such as salmonella and clostridium, as well as more serious diseases like typhoid.

Accidental inoculations by contaminated sharps can transmit tuberculosis, malaria, syphilis, gonorrhoea, herpes, viral haemorrhagic fever, leptospirosis, streptococcus, diphtheria, brucellosis, hepatitis B and the HIV infection. There are at least 15 cases worldwide of people who have caught the HIV virus from sharps injuries. Most sharps injuries result from the incorrect disposal of sharps – in particular, of unsheathed needles.

Preventative measures

Widespread education and training is crucial to control this type of infection. Employees have a responsibility to carry out safe procedures, and employers must monitor standards.

Personal hygiene for both staff and patients is of utmost importance. Food hygiene procedures must be fully implemented. These include

- the hygienic preparation of food using clean equipment, and making sure that meat and vegetables are prepared separately, to avoid the contamination of meat by soil micro-organisms
- ensuring that there is no cross-contamination between raw and cooked food
- refrigerated storage
- thorough cooking
- adequate reheating and no slow cooling processes

All medical equipment should be decontaminated and sterilised before use. Medical staff at risk from blood splashes should wear gloves, waterproof aprons, face masks and eyewear.

Training programmes should be compulsory, so that the correct procedures are used when, for example, taking blood.

Employers must draw up policies on procedures for dealing with injuries and display them prominently at places of work. Staff must be informed what to do if they are injured by a sharp or are exposed to blood or body fluids.

Contaminated waste should be dealt with safely and incinerated whenever possible.

The safe disposal of sharps is of great importance. The British Medical Association has produced the following code of practice:

- You used it, you bin it
- Do not resheath needles
- Discard the needle and the syringe as one unit
- Dispose of sharps into a safe container immediately after use (do not dispose into a polythene bag)
- Do not leave sharps lying around
- Do not overfill sharps containers
- Get immunised against hepatitis B

Airborne spread

Micro-organisms which are spread in the air come from two sources

- respiratory droplets from humans in coughs and sneezes, e.g. tuberculosis
- bacteria spores in dust, heating or air-conditioning systems, humidifiers and other equipment, e.g. legionella

Vector-borne spread

This refers to the mechanical transfer either in or on the body of a vector. Examples include shigella and salmonella, which can be transmitted by flies. Malarial parasites are carried within the mosquito.

VACCINATION PROGRAMMES

It is usual that staff working in a care setting will have been immunised against diphtheria, whooping cough, tetanus, rubella, polio, measles, mumps and tuberculosis. These vaccinations are provided as part of the immunisation programme for children in the UK (see pp. 166–167). In addition, there has been a mass vaccination programme to immunise certain care workers against the highly infective hepatitis B. Those staff in accident and emergency departments, hospital laboratories, surgical areas and maternity wards are at particular risk.

ACTIVITY 10

1   For this Activity, you will need to refer to Tables 2.1 and 2.2. For Table 2.1, calculate (i) the percentage of total accidents (column 4) and (ii) the annual incidents per 1,000 employees (column 5), and then place the job classifications in rank order of danger of accidental inoculation (column 1). For Table 2.2, calculate the number of accidents for each type of activity as a percentage of the total number of accidents.

Illustrate the two sets of data graphically. Summarise the results, and note which staff are most at risk and which activities are the most dangerous ones.

2   Look at the BMA Code of Practice for the safe disposal of sharps, and give a reason for each of the precautions noted.

3   Produce a report which outlines measures to prevent airborne and vector-borne infections in a care setting.

4   When you are visiting, or carrying out your work placement in, a hospital or other care setting, study the hygienic practices and write a report on your findings. Find out which infections each hygienic practice is designed to control.

The reporting of illnesses

Legislation exists to ensure that diseases are reported to the relevant authority. Employers have a duty to report accidents, injuries and work-related diseases to the Health and Safety Executive or the local authority's environmental health department. The Reporting of Injuries, Diseases and Dangerous Occurrences Regulations 1985 (RIDDOR) are described earlier in this chapter.

In addition to these procedures, legislation exists which is designed to record and control

Table 2.1 The incidence of accidental inoculations by job classification

Rank order	Classification	No. of employees	Reported no. of accidents	% of total	Annual incidents per 1,000 employees
1		2	3	4	5
	Trained nurses	886	57		
	Learners	298	25		
	Nursing auxiliaries	284	7		
	Doctors	56	5		
	Lab staff	67	6		
	ODAs	20	2		
	Porters & HSDU	73	6		
	Domestics	256	13		

ODA: Operating Department Assistant
HSDU: Hospital Sterilising Disinfecting Unit

Reproduced by kind permission of *Nursing Times* where this table first appeared in the article 'Point Taken?' on December 2nd 1987.

diseases which are not necessarily related to the place of work. Diagnosed cases of HIV and Aids are reported in anonymous returns to the Centre of Communicable Diseases which is attached to the Department of Health. This centre is responsible for keeping statistics on HIV, Aids and many other diseases.

Table 2.2 Accidents by type

Activity associated with accidents	Total no. reported accidents	As % of total
Collection/disposal of refuse	20	
Disposal of needles	17	
Clearing trolley & equipment	13	
Assisting doctor	13	
Bite by patient	11	
Obtaining blood	10	
Re-sheathing needles	9	
During procedures	8	
After giving injection	6	
Contamination of skin	6	
Contamination of mucous membrane	5	
Sharps bin too full	3	

Reproduced by kind permission of *Nursing Times* where this table first appeared in the article 'Point Taken?' on December 2nd 1987.

Under public health legislation, it is the duty of the general practitioner to inform the Department of Health of the occurrence of certain diseases which are designated 'Notifiable Diseases'. These include the following:
- Anthrax
- Cholera
- Cryptosoridiosis
- Diphtheria
- Dysentery
- Encephalitis
- Food poisoning
- Hepatitis A, B, C
- Impetigo
- Infective jaundice
- Lassa fever
- Leprosy
- Leptospirosis
- Malaria
- Measles
- Meningitis
- Paratyphoid fever
- Plague
- Poliomyelitis
- Rabies
- Relapsing fever
- Scarlet fever
- Smallpox
- Tetanus
- Tuberculosis
- Typhoid fever
- Viral haemorrhagic fever
- Whooping cough
- Yellow fever

The aims of these notification procedures are as follows:
- to keep records of numbers and types of infections in the community at any given time
- to allow preventative measures to be introduced immediately
- to allow local doctors to be informed and reminded of symptoms
- to allow the provision of adequate treatment facilities like hospital beds
- to allow research to be carried out

SOCIAL AND ECONOMIC INFLUENCES ON THE ENVIRONMENT

Social factors

- Environmental pressure groups have become important in the last decade. Examples include Friends of the Earth and Greenpeace
- The World Health Organization and governments organise education campaigns to increase awareness of environmental health issues
- Media involvement in the environmental debate has increased, and ecological issues now receive more public attention
- Individual responsibility for the environment is encouraged. Recycling schemes are now commonly organised by local authorities
- 'Environmental poverty' can occur where a high density of population, combined with low incomes, results in an unhealthy environment. (There is more about the effects of urbanisation later in this chapter.)

Economic factors

The economy and environmental concerns are closely linked. Increased industrialisation requires more use of non-renewable resources to supply energy and raw materials. More land is taken to provide for new buildings, roads and airports to sustain industry, and as a result there will be more pollution and waste. There is thus a conflict between profit-making and maintaining the environment.

The report of the World Commission on Environment and Development to the UN in 1987 and the Earth Summit in Rio de Janeiro in 1992 brought these issues to the attention of the public and world governments.

WHO PAYS FOR THE REDUCTION OF POLLUTION?

Although recent UK and European laws and international agreements are demanding more rigorous standards for pollution control, it is clear that levels of pollutants and toxic waste in the environment are still high and a danger to human health. It is very difficult to ensure that the new standards outlined in the laws are being enforced. The debate is now centred around who pays for cleaning up.

ACTIVITY 11

1 Find out about the activities of the various environmental pressure groups and international bodies. You could work in groups to cover a wide range. Collect information and prepare a presentation for the class. Mention changes in public awareness or legislation which might have been influenced by the activities.

2 Investigate examples of how media involvement has influenced environmental awareness. Each member of the class should find one example to present.

GOVERNMENT MAY IMPOSE TAXES TO REDUCE POLLUTION

The government may impose environmental taxes on motoring, electricity, fuel, water, household rubbish and industrial waste, the Secretary of State for the Environment, said yesterday.

Ministers now preferred to use taxation, financial incentives and other economic instruments instead of regulations to conserve natural resources and curb pollution, he told a press conference ...

To date, just one such economic instrument is well established – cheaper lead-free petrol, and most cars on the road still take leaded fuel.

(The Independent, 2 October 1992)

The Confederation of British Industry was yesterday accused of seeking to avoid industry paying the bill for contaminated land when it launched its proposals for environmental liability.

Introducing the CBI's plans, published as Firm Foundations, director-general Howard Davies said environmental liability was an extremely important issue which had to be handled carefully if action was not to be counter-productive.

'It is a matter of public concern and a matter of business concern,' he said. 'But we have to be concerned about the cost impact on business. There is a need to target resources on the highest priorities. The case for cleaning up is not contested, but the costs and benefits must be assessed.'

The CBI approach was met with scorn by pressure group Friends of the Earth, which said the industry organisation was trying to make taxpayers pay for industrial pollution and wanted lower environmental standards in Britain that in the rest of Europe.

'The public has a right to expect the government to ensure the cost of cleaning up is borne by the polluter, not the polluted,' said one campaigner. 'The CBI is calling for British industry to be given a competitive advantage in Europe at the expense of the public and the UK environment' . . . .

While accepting that businesses should pay for future contamination, the CBI argues that the UK government and the European Community should pay for past pollution through regeneration grants . . .

The cost of totally restoring all affected land is estimated at anything from £20 billion to £60 billion, but CBI environmental director John Cridland said this sum did not need to be spent. He suggested the cost of urgent rectification would be much smaller.

(The Guardian, 3 November 1993)

ACTIVITY 12

1 Read the above extracts from The Independent and The Guardian on paying for pollution.

2 Discuss the following dilemmas:
- Why are bodies like the CBI resisting bearing total responsibility for pollution control? What would be the social and economic consequences if the total costs were to be borne by the polluters?
- Who should pay for cleaning up the consequences of past pollution? Should it be the government giving grants from taxpayers' money, or should it be the industries that caused the problem?

ASSESSMENT OPPORTUNITY

Write a report which explains
- the importance of legislation in maintaining environmental health standards
- the roles of inspection and enforcement agencies in environmental health in a care setting
- health and safety policy in a care setting
- procedures for controlling infection in a care setting
- social and economic influences on the environment

THE HARMFUL EFFECTS OF HUMAN ACTIVITY ON THE ENVIRONMENT AND HEALTH

Pollution

The effect of human activities on the environment is proportional to the size of the human population, which is increasing at the rate of about 100,000,000 each year. The waste products that result from these activities are often added to the environment at a rate faster than it can accommodate. Sometimes these products are substances that are already naturally present in the environment, but we call them *pollutants* if they reach critical levels and if they are potentially harmful to life. Waste products which are potential pollutants can be in solid, liquid or gaseous form. But waste does not always consist of *materials*: forms of energy like sound, heat and radioactive particles can be pollutants as well.

It is convenient to divide the environment into air, water and land to investigate pollution, but all parts of the environment are linked, and a substance produced as a waste product from a process on land may pollute both air and water.

AIR POLLUTION

The *atmosphere* is a layer around the earth of approximately 2,000 km. Most of this layer comprises the *stratosphere*. The *troposphere* extends 8 km above the earth, and the proportions of gases in it are as follows:

Nitrogen	78.08%
Oxygen	20.96%
Argon	0.93%
Carbon dioxide	0.03%

There are also variable amounts of carbon monoxide, ammonia, methane, helium, krypton, sulphur dioxide, hydrogen sulphide and nitric and nitrous oxides. These are present as part of natural recycling processes.

Burning fossil fuel in the home, in industry and in internal-combustion engines has altered the proportions of atmospheric natural gases, and new technology has added new gases to the atmosphere which are destroying the ozone layer (in the stratosphere) which absorbs ultraviolet and infrared radiation and thus prevents damage to living organisms from this radiation: ultraviolet rays can cause mutations, and infrared rays can cause an increase in body temperature.

Smoke and other particles

Smoke comprises very small particles of carbon. Larger particles include soot and ash. These are produced by burning coal and oil, and are released into the air. Smoke can affect the alveoli of the lungs by damaging their epithelial linings. It causes respiratory problems and aggravates bronchitis. It can reduce light intensity at ground level and lower the rate of photosynthesis in plants, which may be even further decreased if there are deposits of soot coating leaves and blocking stomata thereby preventing gaseous exchange.

Sulphur dioxide

Sulphur dioxide is released into the air both when fossil fuels are burnt and during the smelting of ores. It is normally present in concentrations of $0.3–1.0 \ \mu gm^{-3}$, and is produced both by volcanoes and from other natural processes. In industrial areas it can reach a concentration of $3,000 \ \mu gm^{-3}$. Sulphur dioxide is oxidised to sulphate ions in the air. When it returns to the earth in rain, it can enrich deficient soils, and plants can take up the sulphates through their roots. However, sulphur dioxide in air is mostly damaging to plants as it combines with water to form *sulphurous* and *sulphuric acid*. This is then precipitated as 'acid rain', so called because it is rain with a low pH. This damages trees and kills life in lakes. The most damage has occurred in Scandinavia since the prevailing winds carry the sulphur dioxide from the UK and the rest of Europe to that area. (Figure 2.3 shows conifers with acid-rain damage.)

The human respiratory system also is affected by sulphur dioxide: extra mucous is produced by the goblet cells in the linings of the bronchi and bronchioles. Also, the cilia stop beating and are now no longer able to remove the mucous with the particles and bacteria it contains (normally, this is constantly removed from the lungs). This mucous then prevents gaseous exchange occurring in the alveoli where the epithelial linings can also be damaged.

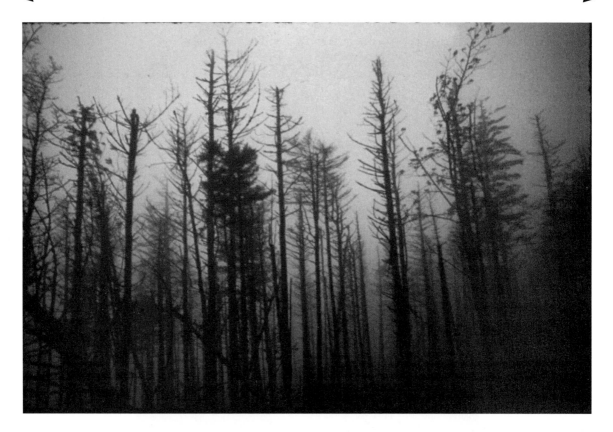

Figure 2.3 The effects of acid rain on conifers

Bronchial conditions can result from an exposure to sulphur dioxide. Figure 2.4 shows the effects of sulphur dioxide on the lung.

Smog

Smogs occur in special environmental conditions which cause fog to remain static and hang over an area. In a large urban area where fossil fuels are being burnt, smoke and sulphur dioxide are produced. These pollutants then become trapped in the fog, causing damp and dirty smog. These were common in London in the 1950s. In 1952 there was an especially bad one, during which there were many deaths. This was the trigger for the modern air-pollution-control legislation. Figure 2.5 shows the effects of smog in London.

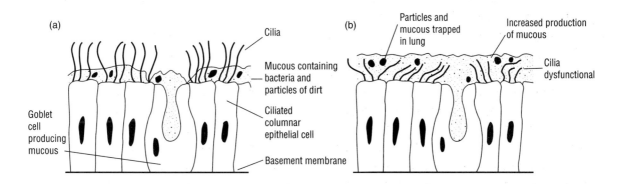

Figure 2.4 The effects of sulphur dioxide on the lung: (a) normal lung – lining of the bronchiole; (b) the effects of sulphur dioxide on the lining of the bronchiole

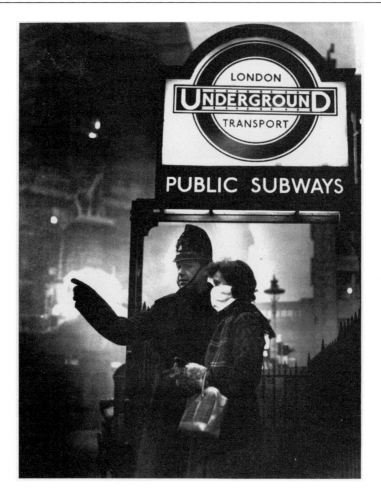

Figure 2.5   The London smog of December 1952

ACTIVITY 13

Look at the data in Table 2.3. Illustrate this in graphical form, and then answer the following questions:
- What conclusions can be drawn from the data?
- How significant are the results and conclusions? (Suggest a control which should be carried out)
- Discuss the effects of sulphur dioxide and smoke on human health

Carbon dioxide

The burning of fossil fuels such as coal, oil and natural gas releases carbon dioxide. Data collected from different sites around the world shows that the level of this gas has been

Table 2.3   The health effects of sulphur dioxide and smoke in December 1952 during the London smog

Date in December	Deaths per day	Smoke $\mu g/m^{-3}$ air	Sulphur dioxide $\mu g/m^{-3}$
1	250	200	350
2	260	300	400
3	300	400	620
4	260	350	520
5	325	1,100	1,000
6	600	1,600	1,520
7	875	1,700	1,850
8	900	1,580	2,000
9	850	1,000	1,500
10	600	300	350
11	550	200	360
12	500	200	350
13	520	300	350
14	450	300	375
15	400	250	350

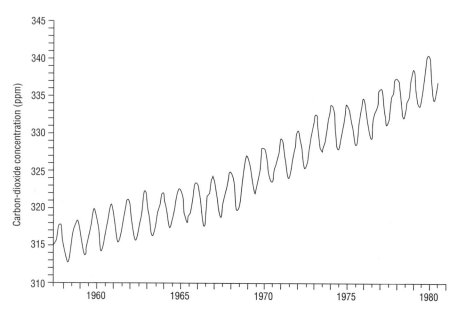

Figure 2.6 Increasing levels of carbon-dioxide concentration in the atmosphere as measured at Mauna Loa, Hawaii
Source: Holdgate et al., 1982.

steadily increasing. (Figure 2.6 shows data collected from Hawaii, in the Pacific.) Increases in carbon dioxide may stimulate photosynthesis in plants, but at the same time, other environmental factors are working *against* an increase in plant growth. In fact, because of the depletion of tropical rainforests and other vegetation, there is likely, overall, to be less photosynthesis in the world. Some of the extra carbon dioxide is also absorbed into the sea.

Carbon dioxide is known as a 'greenhouse gas' as it enables the atmosphere to absorb the earth's heat and re-radiate it back to earth. If it were not for this 'greenhouse effect', the earth would be too cold to sustain life. However, if the level of carbon dioxide increases too much, then too much global warming could result.

Other greenhouse gases, and ozone depletion

Carbon dioxide has already been mentioned as a greenhouse gas. Others include:
- chlorofluorocarbons (CFCs) from aerosol sprays, refrigerators and bubbles in plastic foams
- methane from bacterial activities and the use of natural gas

- nitrous oxide from fertilisers
- ozone from car-exhaust fumes

CFCs are also responsible for destroying ozone in the stratosphere. There are now holes in the ozone layer over the Arctic and Antarctic, as a result of which damaging ultraviolet and infrared light can come through. Even the UK has been trapped under a 'mini-hole' in the ozone layer.

Britain has been trapped under a 'mini-hole' in the ozone layer for much of this month – and the Government has failed to tell the public.

Measurements taken last Monday showed that about a quarter of the atmospheric shield – which protects all life from the sun's harmful ultraviolet rays – had disappeared over Scotland. But the next day an Environment Minister assured Parliament nothing out of the ordinary was happening.

Record lows in the ozone layer have been found over Norway, Sweden, Finland, Canada and Japan during the last six weeks – and in each of these countries the public was promptly informed . . .

This is the second successive winter in which ozone levels over the northern hemisphere have been alarmingly low, raising fears that a full hole may open up next month. This would be much more dangerous than the Antarctic ozone hole, as it would expose some of the most densely populated areas on Earth.

(The Observer, 28 February 1993)

Carbon monoxide

Carbon monoxide occurs in car-exhaust fumes and cigarette smoke. It has an affinity for haemoglobin which is 250 times greater than that of oxygen. It forms a stable compound with haemoglobin and prevents oxygen combining with it.

Nitrogen oxides

Nitrogen oxides, like nitrogen dioxide and nitric oxide, are produced by the burning of fuel in car engines, and are emitted in car exhausts. They can combine with other chemicals in sunlight and form peroxyacyl nitrates (PANS) which result in photochemical smogs.

These nitrogen-containing gases are all very poisonous, and cause breathing difficulties.

Lead

This is the most serious heavy-metal pollutant in the atmosphere. The lead in car-exhaust fumes accounts for 80% of this. It is added to petrol as tetraethyl lead (TEL), which serves as an anti-knock compound, and it comes out as lead chlorobromide. There is an increasing worry about lead affecting the brains of children. Lead is also taken into the body in food, and it is possible that the lead which contaminated the food came from car exhausts originally.

LEAD LEVEL IN CHILDREN 'NEARING DANGER POINT'

Thousands of Bradford schoolchildren have dangerously high levels of lead in their blood, according to a report commissioned by the area

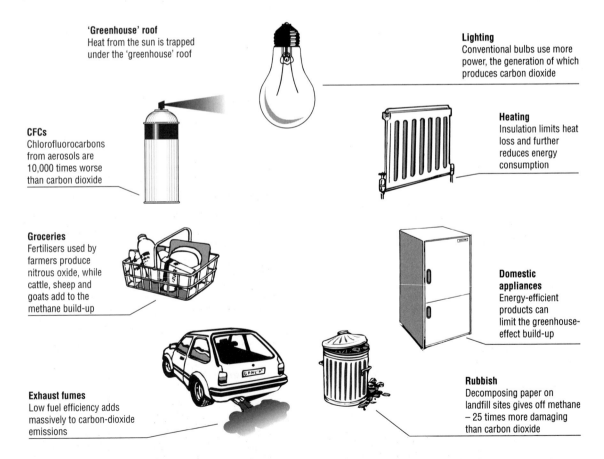

'Greenhouse' roof
Heat from the sun is trapped under the 'greenhouse' roof

Lighting
Conventional bulbs use more power, the generation of which produces carbon dioxide

CFCs
Chlorofluorocarbons from aerosols are 10,000 times worse than carbon dioxide

Heating
Insulation limits heat loss and further reduces energy consumption

Groceries
Fertilisers used by farmers produce nitrous oxide, while cattle, sheep and goats add to the methane build-up

Domestic appliances
Energy-efficient products can limit the greenhouse-effect build-up

Exhaust fumes
Low fuel efficiency adds massively to carbon-dioxide emissions

Rubbish
Decomposing paper on landfill sites gives off methane – 25 times more damaging than carbon dioxide

Figure 2.7 An everyday guide to greenhouse gases
Source: The Observer, 24 September 1989.

health authority, details of which have been passed to *The Observer*.

More than a hundred youngsters are suffering from lead poisoning, with nearly 10 per cent of the primary school population considered 'at risk'.

There is considerable evidence that lead can damage the brains of young children and lead to intellectual retardation. In another study, Dr Neil Ward of Surrey University last week claimed to have established a link between high levels of lead in children and poor reading.

In September, school inspectors will monitor the reading ability of young children following a leaked report earlier this month from nine education authorities which showed a dramatic decline in standards . . .

The Bradford study shows children from poor families to be at greatest risk. Richard Stainton, a senior official of the National Union of Teachers, said yesterday the survey illustrated the link between the environment, poverty and educational performance . . .

Lead poisoning is widespread in Victorian, industrial cities because of old housing stock with lead plumbing often decorated with lead paint. Dr Ward's findings, however, are based on research with children in non-industrial Berkshire. He sampled hair and saliva taken from 31 primary school pupils from a new housing development built without lead pipes, next to a dual carriageway.

'About half the group had a high level of lead and low reading ability,' said Dr Ward, 'The children with the highest lead content had the lowest reading ability.' . .

(The Observer, 1992)

ACTIVITY 14

TEST THE AIR

1 The card test
You can check levels of air pollution in your area with a 'white-card test'. Obtain four pieces of white card (each 15 cm square) with at least one shiny side. Number the cards 1 to 4 and smear the shiny side of each with a thin layer of Vaseline.

- Leave Card 1 indoors
- Leave Card 2 near a busy road
- Leave Card 3 in a garden or your school grounds
- Leave Card 4 underneath a tree

Stand each card upright with the Vaseline side facing outwards. Secure the cards with string or sticky tape and make a note of the time, date and place you left them. After three or four days, fetch the cards and compare each with Card 1 to decide which is the dirtiest. Most air pollution is caused by cars and factories. This may help to explain your results.

Using the white-card test, it is easy to make a pollution map of your area. Simply draw a local map, or take a copy of a printed one, and mark the places where you left cards.

2 Leaf-washing
A quicker way to test for pollution in public areas is gently to wipe some dirt from a surface – of a park bench, for example – with a clean, damp piece of cotton wool. Wipe the surface only once and place the cotton wool in a clear polythene bag. Remember to use a new piece of cotton wool for each test and to keep a record of your tests in order to compare the dirtiness of the samples. You could use colours on your pollution map to show different levels of pollution.

Leaves in badly polluted areas often appear covered in soot and grime. This can be a problem because plants need sunlight in order to make food. The sunlight falling on the leaves may be blocked out if they are covered with too much dirt.

When the weather is dry, you can investigate this problem further with a 'leaf-washing test'. Collect a filter paper and funnel, jamjar, pencil, clean paintbrush and notepad, and half-fill the jamjar with water. Identify some leaves to wash: the best ones to choose are those on plants, trees, bushes or hedges which do not lose their leaves in winter.

1 Choose a leaf which is neither too high nor too near the ground. Dip it in the water and gently wash both sides using the paintbrush. Try not to remove the leaf from the plant.
2 Now repeat the process with 14 more leaves.
3 Pour the dirty water through the filter paper. When the water has drained away, remove the filter paper and allow it to dry.

The dirt which you have washed from the leaves will be left on the paper. You could repeat the leaf-washing test to compare plants growing in different places, such as near a busy road or in your school grounds. Be careful when you are collecting leaves on or near roads. Add your results to your pollution map. It is only a fair test if you use plants with leaves of similar sizes. Try and work out why.

(Adapted from The Guardian, *14 May 1991)*

WATER POLLUTION

Pure water rarely exists naturally: rainwater absorbs chemicals as it passes through the air; water that runs into rivers carries with it materials that have been leached from the soil; and as rivers flow towards the sea, organic matter and silt are picked up. The sea itself contains salt, other minerals and organic materials. Many additives are therefore natural products. Often, though, materials in quite high concentrations are released directly or indirectly into water as the result of human activity, and these additives are considered as pollutants. (The problems of acid rain have been considered earlier in this chapter.) Domestic, industrial and agricultural effluents are released into rivers and seas. These nclude sewage, toxic chemicals and farm wastes.

ACTIVITY 15

1 Design a poster to show the natural water cycle, including rain, rivers and the seas. Show the role both of vegetation and of the human removal and return of water. When you have read this section on water pollution, you can add the sources of human pollution to your poster.

2 List at least eight uses of water by humans. Remember that each individual in the UK uses about 150 litres of water a day for domestic use alone.

Why we need clean water

Humans need water for a wide variety of uses. It must be clean, and not be contaminated with pollutants, in order to prevent infectious disease and poisoning. Water-borne disease-causing organisms include various parasitic worms and also protozoa like *entamoeba histolytica*, which causes amoebic dysentery. Pathogenic bacteria causing intestinal infections and more serious diseases like cholera and typhoid are also carried in water, as are many viruses. The poliomyelitis virus is an example.

Toxic chemicals in industrial waste are common pollutants of water. These are poisonous to humans as well as to aquatic flora and fauna. They may enter humans directly, in water, or they may be in our food. Chemicals like heavy metals accumulate in food chains and become concentrated in organisms that we eat, like fish.

Animals and plants that live in water are in balance, and rely on each other to remain alive. Plants capture the energy from the sun via photosynthesis to make nutrients, some of which will feed animals. There is a balance of oxygen and carbon dioxide brought about through the processes of respiration and photosynthesis. Both organic and inorganic pollutants upset this balance, and ecosystems will be damaged. In some cases of pollution, the relative levels of plants, animals and decomposers change, and the death of most of the plants and animals involved will eventually occur. This is not only a serious environmental consequence: in addition, the water will be rendered unacceptable for use by humans.

Purification is carried out before water is used, but although the treatment can remove organic waste and some bacterial contamination, it cannot cope with heavy chemical pollution.

Industrial pollutants

Water pollution by industrial waste can reach water either directly or indirectly, leached from landfill waste deposits. Some examples:

1 Mercury can be changed to dimethyl mercury, a neurotoxin. This accumulates in marine food chains, and becomes concentrated in fish, and when this is then eaten by humans, it concentrates in the kidneys, liver and brain. It can cause paralysis, numbness, convulsions and blindness, and even death. In Japan in the 1950s, there was a mercury poisoning incident in which over 160 people died. Today, the level of mercury in fish in Liverpool Bay is a cause for concern. Mercury is discharged into the Mersey river by industries there.
2 Lead is taken into humans via air, food and water. It concentrates in the liver, kidneys and bones. There is evidence that it can cause mental retardation.
3 Aluminium poisoning causes many symptoms, and it is thought that Alzheimer's disease may be linked to aluminium in water, taken in over a long period.

Fertilisers

Fertilisers contain nitrates and phosphates. These are frequently leached out of the soil and then carried to lakes in water run off from the land. Once in the lake, they cause an increase in algal growth, particularly in blue-green algae, and they become so dense on the surface waters that light is unable to penetrate to the layers beneath. As a result, algae lower down in the water cannot photosynthesise, and eventually die. The saprophytic bacteria which decompose these dead algae multiply and use large amounts of oxygen in their activities, thus causing an increase in the biological oxygen demand (BOD). The oxygen level in the water is then severely depleted, and fish and other animals die. Anaerobic bacteria, which can thrive in the absence of oxygen, feed on the decaying material and produce ammonia, methane and hydrogen sulphide. This process is called eutrophication. The water is made unfit for most forms of life, and is certainly not safe for human consumption. It is usually still bodies of water that undergo eutrophication, but this can also happen in short stretches of river and even in seas. Some localised areas of the Baltic and Mediterranean seas are examples of the latter.

Sewage

Sewage-treatment works exist throughout the country to deal with sewage before it is released into water courses. In 1985–86 it was shown that one in five sewage works failed to keep effluent quality up to the standards set by the government. Leakage, overflow and general inefficiency causes sewage to enter rivers. In some parts of the country untreated sewage is still released directly into the sea. Sewage does eventually break down, but if too much enters water at one time, bacteria present in the sewage reduces oxygen to a low level, causing aquatic wildlife to suffer. Eutrophication can occur in stretches of a river below the outfall where the sewage comes in.

Even where sewage is treated successfully, large quantities of sludge are still left behind. This can be dumped on land, and is sometimes used as fertiliser, though this is not always possible because it can contain high levels of toxic heavy metals, like lead, resulting from industrial waste which is processed along with domestic waste by the sewage works. Some sludge is taken to the sea and dumped under government licence. Sludge can be digested to release methane which can be used to make electricity, but this process is not very common.

Wastes from factory farming

Over half the prosecutions for the serious pollution of rivers are now against farmers. Two products of modern farming are particularly to blame. Slurry is the heavy liquid excrement from poultry, cattle or pigs kept indoors. This is kept in storage tanks for safe disposal, but may contaminate rivers. Silage is grass cut while it is still green and left to ferment in silos, later being made into cattle feed. This creates a highly acid product which can be very toxic if it pollutes rivers.

Marine pollution

Sea water moves continuously, and pollutants can be carried away and dispersed provided they are not too concentrated. Polluting effects are more likely in shallow enclosed seas where eutrophication can occur as a result of sewage or fertiliser pollution.

Organochloride insecticides are thought to be responsible for the decline in marine predatory birds such as the herring gull, osprey and brown pelican. DDT (dichlorodiphenyltrichloroethane) is such an insecticide, and it can be concentrated by as much as 70,000 times in oysters – as little as 0.001 ppm can reduce their growth. DDT concentrates in the tissues in predatory birds at the top of the food chain, and reduces their reproductive capacity.

Oil pollution is also a hazard: up to 10 million tonnes of crude oil are released annually into the sea. Sometimes there are large spillages. Examples include the *Torrey Canyon* which went aground off Land's End in 1967, the *Amoco Cadiz* which foundered off the coast of France in 1978, the big disaster of the *Braer* which released 85,000 tonnes of oil off the Shetlands, and the *Sea Empress* disaster, in which over 70,000 tonnes of crude oil seeped into the Pembrokeshire sea. The worst casualties are the fish-eating birds: the birds

settle on the slick of oil and their feathers become clogged. Seaweeds, molluscs and crustaceans are also killed by oil.

It is thought that the water in the North Sea can be replaced every two years, so theoretically pollution should not build up. However, the current level of pollution is a matter of great concern. The article featured in Activity 17 shows how polluted the North Sea is today.

Heat

The thermal pollution of rivers and lakes occurs when hot water is released from the cooling processes of electricity generation in power stations. Water is discharged at a temperature 10–15 °C higher than when it was removed from the river or lake. Since most aquatic organisms live within a fairly narrow range of temperatures, this can have the effect of favouring warm-water species at the expense of cold-water ones. Coarse fish such as roach and perch may replace salmon and trout. Plant growth is also affected by warm water.

Detergents

Back in the 1950s, detergents with synthetic ingredients (derived from petroleum) caused banks of foam to float down rivers and streams. The problem largely went away when the detergent manufacturers changed to biodegradable products. However, detergents still contain phosphates as a water-softening agent, and such detergents enter rivers in domestic sewage and industrial waste. Eutrophication, already described earlier in this chapter for fertilisers, is a result.

ACTIVITY 16

1 *The effects of sewage on a river*
Figure 2.8a shows the effects of sewage on ammonia, nitrate and oxygen levels in a river. You can see the levels that exist in a clean river and then how they change downstream from the sewage outfall. Figure 2.8b shows the effects of

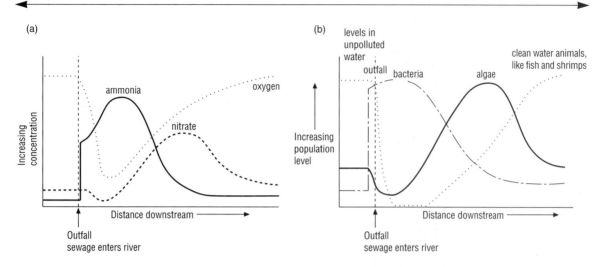

Figure 2.8 The effects of sewage effluent on a river below the outfall: (a) changes in chemicals; (b) changes in numbers of plants and animals
Source: The Biology of Polluted Water, Hynes, Liverpool University Press, 1978.

sewage on the levels of bacteria, algae and animals. The clean river levels are shown, plus the changes that are caused by the sewage.

(a) Describe what happens to the levels of ammonia, nitrate and oxygen downstream from the sewage outfall.

(b) Describe what happens to the levels of bacteria, algae and animals downstream from the sewage outfall.

(c) Explain these changes. You will need to reread the section on eutrophication and look up some details about the nitrogen cycle. In particular, consider the following points:

• Why is there an increase in the level of ammonia downstream from the outfall, and an increase in nitrate even further down?

• Why is there a sudden increase in the level of bacteria at the point of the outfall?

• Why does the oxygen level fall shortly after the outfall point?

• Why does the algae level increase further downstream?

• Why does the animal life first decrease and then regain its former level further downstream?

Link the changes in living organisms with the changes in the levels of oxygen, ammonia and nitrate.

2 *Is your river polluted? Experiments to test the purity of river water*
One way to measure the purity of a water sample is to find out how much dissolved oxygen is present: the more polluted, the less oxygen. Organic matter can enter water in sewage or farm waste pollution. We have seen that bacteria use up the oxygen in water as they decompose organic matter. Because organic matter provides food for bacteria, its presence will stimulate their growth. Therefore, the levels of oxygen present are related to the amounts of polluting organic matter present. Low levels of oxygen indicate high levels of polluting organic matter and bacteria.

Collect samples of water to be tested in 500 cm^3 bottles. For example, you could collect samples from a river at points above and below a sewage outfall or near a farm. Collect two bottles full of water at each collection site.

(a) *The measurement of biological oxygen demand (BOD)*

The BOD is defined as the amount of dissolved oxygen, in grammes per cubic metre, taken out of solution by a sample over five days at 20 °C. It can be measured using a dissolved oxygen electrode or oxygen meter. Take measurements as soon as you bring your samples back into the laboratory. Then, store the samples in the dark at 20 °C for five days. Repeat the measurements. Calculate the differences in oxygen levels in your two measurements, and work out the BOD of the samples. Is there any difference in the samples you have collected? Can you explain any differences? (Sewage effluent should not exhibit a BOD of more than 20 g/m^{-3} over five days. The BOD of the river water below the sewage effluent outfall should not be more than 4 g/m^{-3}.)

(b) *The methylene blue test to indicate oxygen levels*

This is a simpler test, and can be carried out if you have not got access to an oxygen meter. Methylene blue is added to a water sample. The solution remains blue if there is a high level of oxygen but will go colourless with low levels of oxygen.

Pipette 50 cm^3 quantities from each of your samples into suitable-sized flasks or bottles which can be corked. Add 5 cm^3 methylene blue and incubate the bottles at 20 °C for five days. Observe the colour changes over these five days. In clean water with a high dissolved-oxygen content, little polluting organic matter and few bacteria, the methylene blue will retain its blue colour over the five days. This water can be said to have passed the stability test. Where water has a high organic content, on the other hand, bacteria will thrive and use up the oxygen, and the blue colour will disappear more rapidly.

3 How clean is your stream?

You will need:
- Hand net
- White tray
- Hand lens
- Wide-mouthed pipette
- Petri dishes and specimen tubes
- Record sheet
- Key to freshwater animals

Method:
Divide into pairs and take different parts of the stream to study. Look carefully to see if there is any effluent running into it. Record exactly where your samples will be taken. Using the hand net, take 10 samples from the water. Sweep close to the bottom of the stream. You will probably collect mud and debris as well as samples of small freshwater animals. Tip all the samples into the tray. You can take the animals out and put them into petri dishes with the pipettes for identification.

Results:
Look carefully at your samples and count the numbers of each species. Compare the results with the following tables of species able to live in very poor, poor, moderate or only very clean water.

Animals found only in very clean water:
- Mayfly larvae
- Freshwater shrimps
- Flatworms
- Frogs
- Stonefly larvae
- Caddis larvae
- Newts
- Toads

Animals tolerating water of moderate quality:

- Spire-shell snail
- Orb shell
- Damselfly larvae
- Beetles
- Fish
- Ramshorn snail
- Pea shell
- Greater waterboatman
- Beetle larvae

Animals tolerating poor-quality water (recovering from pollution):
- Other pond snails
- Alderfly larvae
- Water flea
- Pond skater
- Waterlouse
- Lesser waterboatman
- Leech
- Pond measurer

Animals found in water of very poor quality (polluted):
- Sludge worm
- Cranefly larvae
- Midge larvae

Collect all the class results together and decide what conclusions you can come to. Prepare an exhibition of your findings.

4 *Pollution in the North Sea*
Read the article below from *The Observer*:

RISE IN POLLUTION CALLS FOR DRASTIC MEASURES

Efforts to protect the North Sea from devastating pollution have failed. A shocking report on the quality of its water is to be discussed in Denmark next month by European Ministers, but the outline of the report has already been accepted.

The Quality Status Report ... says chemicals such as hexachlorocyclohexane (HCH), polychlorinated biphenyls (PCBs) and tributyl tin (TBT) have reached alarming levels. Discharges of pesticides, oil and poisonous metals – such as cadmium – have risen unchecked and pose disturbing problems.

'More stringent goals and measures are urgently needed,' says the report: only radical action will halt a decline that is turning the sea into the waste dump of northern Europe.

The measures to be discussed by Ministers will include drastically reducing the use of the fertilisers now leaching into rivers; halting industrial pollution; and stopping the overfishing of cod, haddock, sand eels and sprats.

Such moves would, however, also have a dramatic impact on farming, fishing and manufacturing throughout the northern countries of the European Union. Fertilisers are used to sustain high agricultural yields and anti-pollution controls would make factories more expensive to run, while fishing often provides the only income for many communities around the North Sea.

Discussion of the report could be protracted. Nevertheless, the eight nations are committed to reducing by 1995 emissions that are killing the sea. This gives Ministers little time to act.

The report admits: 'It is expected that the goal of a 50 per cent reduction in inputs of nitrogen (from fertilisers) to potential problem areas will not be realised by 1995.' Additional measures and better controls are therefore urgent, it concludes ...

The report concludes that, although scientists have uncovered a depressing list of ailments that are killing the North Sea, more research is required to pinpoint other threats.

(The Observer, 13 March 1994)

(a) Name six pollutants which are causing concern.
(b) What three measures are proposed 'to halt a decline that is turning the sea into the waste dump of Northern Europe'?
(c) Why would these measures have a dramatic impact on farming,

fisheries and manufacturing in the northern countries of the European Union?

(d) What date has been set as a target to improve the situation?

What are sound and noise?

Sound and noise are really the same phenomenon. Noise can be defined as an unwanted sound. We detect sound using our ears. We are sensitive to changes in sounds in our environment, and we are able to react in an appropriate way. We can communicate with each other through sound and also recognise and react to dangerous sounds. These are only two examples of the importance of sound in our lives.

SOUND LEVELS

Sound is caused by a change in air pressure which is detected by the ear and registered in the brain. Normal atmospheric pressure is at about 100,000 newtons per metre^2. The ear is a very sensitive detector, and registers a pressure change of only 0.00001 N/m^2 as a very quiet sound. Pressure changes as great as 1,000 N/m^2, on the other hand, are recognised as a loud sound, and very loud sounds can damage ears. A special way of indicating sound levels has had to be devised because the ear can detect such a very great range of pressure changes. Sound levels are given in *decibels* (dB) – see Table 2.4 for some examples (and Figure 3.23 on p. 151 of Chapter 3).

Since the decibel scale is based on logarithms, a sound of 60 dB is not twice as loud as a sound of 30 dB: it is very much louder. Very roughly, a sound increase of 10 dB is heard by the ear as a sound about twice as loud. If there is one sound of 30 dB and another of 60 dB, then the 60 dB sound is very approximately $2 \times 2 \times 2 = 8$ times louder than the 30 dB sound.

Table 2.4 The sound intensity level (dB) for selected sources

dB	Source	
140	Jet engine (at 25 m)	Injurious range
130	Rivet gun	
120	Propeller aircraft (at 50 m)	
110	Road drill	Danger range
100	Metal-working shop/foundry	
80–90	Heavy lorry	
80	Busy street	Safe range
60–70	Private car	
60	Ordinary conversation (at 1 m)	
50	Low conversation (at 1 m)	
40	Soft music	
30	Whisper (at 1 m)	
20	Quiet town dwelling	
10	Rustling leaf	

ACTIVITY 17

1 Discuss other reasons (than the two examples given above) why it is important for humans to be able to respond to sounds.

2 Read the above section on sound levels and answer the following questions:
- What is sound?
- What range of pressures can the ear detect?
- Why has a special way of indicating sound levels been invented?
- What are the limits of the safe, dangerous and injurious sound ranges?
- How much louder is 40 dB compared to 30 dB?

NOISE POLLUTION

Sound is required for human life. However, unwanted sounds or noise can be a health hazard. It is for this reason that noise can be considered as a form of pollution.

Look again at Table 2.4. This shows which sounds will not cause damage to hearing

(0–80 dB) and which sounds are in the danger range (90–110 dB). These louder sounds can cause permanent damage and deafness if exposure is over a long period. The effect on hearing is greater the longer the exposure to the loud noise. 140 dB is at the threshold of pain. Really loud sounds can cause physical damage: 190 dB will cause rupture of the eardrums and damage the ossicles. On the other hand, low-intensity sounds which are not likely to cause damage to hearing may nonetheless be psychologically damaging and cause stress. Then there can be tiredness, loss of concentration and even sickness. At work, a lack of concentration could cause accidents.

Some of the main noise 'polluters' are aircraft, motor vehicles, greatly amplified music and many types of machinery, including factory and domestic appliances. There is evidence that noise in the workplace can cause damage to hearing.

ACTIVITY 18

This is a major practical assignment which will enable you to measure noise levels in your own environment. You will be able to decide whether noise levels that you encounter are just a nuisance or could actually cause damage to your hearing. You will be able to investigate both the legislation that controls noise and measures that must be taken to protect workers from hearing damage. It is better that you work in a group to collect as many measurements as possible and then write up the report individually.

1 *Rationale*
In this assignment you will investigate noise levels in the outside environment and within your college or school. There are three aims:
  (a) To measure the noise level of traffic in the environment of the building.

Is the level of noise damaging to hearing or merely an environmental 'nuisance'?
  (b) To measure noise levels in the library/study areas at your college or school. Are these designated study areas suitable for successful study without stress? What level of noise is likely to cause stress?
  (c) To measure the noise level in a very noisy environment, for example outside a bus station, near the airport, drilling at a building or road works site.

2 *Resources*
A sound-level meter is required.

3 *Measuring sound levels*
Follow the instructions provided on how to operate the sound-level meter.
  Precautions:
  • Hold the noise meter at arm's length
  • When measuring sound from objects, you should be at least 100 cm from the source
  • When measuring traffic sound, you should hold the meter 100–150 cm above the ground
  • You should be in the centre when measuring sound in a room
  • For periodic sound, measure the highest value on several occasions and obtain an average value
  • For sound which shows a varied level, take several measurements and obtain an average value

4 *Investigations*
When measuring noise levels, follow the instructions about operating the noise meter. You will have to decide exactly how to take measurements since the precise method required depends on the nature of the noise. For example, if the noise is fluctuating (i.e. periodic), you could measure the highest value every two minutes so that you obtain an

average of three results. This would not be a suitable method, however, when measuring the noise of an aeroplane taking off, for here you need to measure the duration of the noise as well as the noise level. When recording noise measurements, you may like to make extra observations. For example, when measuring traffic, you could record changes in noise levels when heavy lorries go past. In libraries, you could note changes in noise levels when people whisper or speak.

(a) Design and carry out an investigation to show whether traffic noise within the vicinity of your college or school is likely to cause damage to hearing or is merely a nuisance. You could compare a main road with a quiet residential road. Try recording noise levels at different times of the day.

(b) Design and carry out an investigation to show whether the study areas in your college or school are suitable for studying purposes. Again, taking readings at different times of the day may give some interesting results.

(c) Design and carry out an investigation to show the level of noise at a really noisy site, like a roadworks, an airport or a disco.

5 *The report*

In the report there should be an introduction which outlines the aims of the investigations. The method should follow, with very precise details of what you did. The results should be in tabular form, and you should illustrate them graphically as well. Any written observations should also be included. Finally, the conclusions should be drawn from your own results.

In the discussion afterwards, there is plenty of scope for further research, and

you could include a consideration of the following points:

• Are the noise levels you have found in your investigations damaging to hearing or just a nuisance?
• What effects can 'nuisance' noise have on people? How does stress affect people at work and at home?
• How can loud noise damage hearing?
• What is the legislation that controls noise in the environment?
• How are the noise laws enforced?
• Are there any health-and-safety leaflets or guides to complaints procedures issued by your local council? Consult your local environmental health department.

Intensification of agriculture

Humans began to change the environment when they adopted agriculture as a way of life. Forest, woodland and scrub were cleared to provide the land required to grow enough food for the growing population. Deforestation still goes on today in developing nations. For example, vast tracts of tropical forest in the Amazon basin have been cleared in recent years, and poor Brazilian families have been given financial inducements to settle as farmers in the cleared areas. This plan has not succeeded, however, because the soil is infertile and the population cannot afford fertilisers. Tropical storms have washed away most of the bare soil which had previously been held in place by the roots of trees.

Soil erosion is common worldwide. The Yellow River in China is so called because its colour comes from soil washed away from the surrounding land. In dry areas the wind has eroded soil from farmland, creating dust storms – this occurred in the USA in the 1930s. Wind and rain have also caused erosion in North Africa, where goats and cattle have overgrazed the vegetation for centuries.

Wetlands have been drained to increase the areas available for agriculture, and as a result, bogs and fens have disappeared. In the UK, East Anglia gives a good example of this.

Intensive methods of farming require large machines like combine harvesters to work efficiently, and so hedgerows have been removed to allow extra space. The large fields thus created are used to raise monocultures, that is crops of a single species such as wheat. This depletes the soil of the same nutrients year after year. The rotation of crops used to allow some return of nitrogen to the soil.

Ecologists are concerned that the intensive practices of modern agriculture have caused habitats to disappear, and that some unique species may now become extinct.

ACTIVITY 19

Divide into groups in your class and each choose an area where modern intensive agricultural practices have been introduced. Prepare a presentation to the rest of the class which explains both the intensive farming methods involved and the ecological problems that have been encountered.

FERTILISERS

Fertilisers in the form of ammonia, potash and rock phosphate are commonly used to promote crop growth. Potash and phosphate are firmly held in the soil, but ammonia is converted into nitrate. Approximately 30% of nitrates found in rivers comes from fertilisers leached out by rainwater. The effect of fertilisers on rivers and lakes is discussed earlier in this chapter.

PESTICIDES

A wide range of toxic chemicals are used to control or eradicate pests and weeds. Some examples include:

- Mercuric chloride: a fungicide used for dusting seeds. Mercury is toxic
- Copper compounds: fungicides that are in general use. Copper is toxic
- Sodium chlorate: a herbicide used to clear paths of weeds. Not very toxic
- Organo-phosphorous compounds, e.g. Parathion: insecticides that are very toxic but not persistent. Can kill useful insects like bees
- Organo-chlorine compounds, e.g. DDT, dieldrin: these are insecticides. DDT is persistent and accumulates in food chains. It also affects reproductive capacity
- 2.4 D (dichlorophenoxyacetic acid); 2.4.5 T (trichlorophenoxyacetic acid): these are herbicides that make up 40% or more of the total use of pesticides. They attack broadleaved plants, leaving cereals to grow

In the manufacture of 2.4.5 T, an impurity called dioxan is produced. One gramme of this can kill 5,000 people, and small quantities can cause cancer, a skin disorder called chloracne and abnormalities in unborn babies. We have two known examples of the havoc caused by this chemical. In Vietnam in the 1970s, the Americans used it to defoliate trees to spot camps, and consequent physical and mental defects in children born in the area were common. In 1976, at a factory in Serveso in Italy, there was a release of dioxan into the atmosphere. Despite the evacuation of the area, thousands suffered with chloracne, miscarriages, cancer and foetal abnormalities.

The effects of increasing urbanisation and population density on the environment and health

POPULATION TRENDS

The human population size was estimated to be 1,000 million in the year 1800, 1,500 million in 1900 and 2,500 million in 1950. The exponential increase was by now well under way, and by the year 1990 there were

5,300 million people. It is expected that by the year 2010, there could be 7,000 million, and over 8,000 million by 2020.

These latter figures are based on demographic trends – essentially, the expected birth and death rates. However, other factors which are difficult to predict will also come into play. Examples include the current Aids pandemic and possible improvements in the provision of health care, both of which will affect patterns of mortality. Since it is so difficult to predict population expansion precisely, low, medium and high variants are calculated. If the low variant were to actually happen, we could see a slight *decrease* in the rate of growth of the population after the first third of the next century.

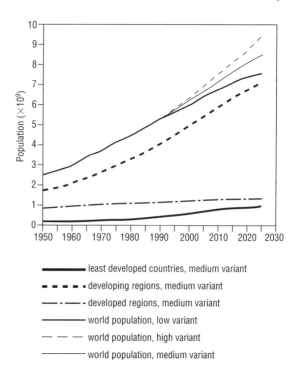

Figure 2.9 World population trends and projections, 1950–2025
Source: Our Planet, Our Health: Report of the WHO Commission on Health and the Environment, WHO, 1992; originally appeared in *World Population Prospects 1990*, United Nations, 1991 (document ST/SA/SER.A/120).

ACTIVITY 20

Look at Figure 2.9. Summarise the information shown in the graphs, and compare the details of the population predictions for the least-developed, developing and developed nations. Find out about possible reasons to explain the differences that you note in the development of the populations from the year 1950 to 2030. What is the difference between the low and high variants of the total-population prediction for the year 2020? Give four reasons to explain why we cannot be certain about future population growth.

URBANISATION

Urbanisation is caused by population movements from rural areas to usually-already-existing small towns. There has been a general trend in most countries over the last 40 years of rapid growth in the urban population, reflecting economic, social and political changes which are specific to each country.

ACTIVITY 21

Look at Table 2.5. Illustrate these trends graphically, and summarise the information shown in your own words. What reasons could you suggest to explain the trends? The projections for the year 2010 assume a continuation of trends deduced from the analysis of figures from the 1960s and 1970s. However, very recent evidence from already-urbanised countries in Europe and North America suggests that people are not moving to towns at the same rate as they used to. In addition, more people are moving to more rural areas and small towns. It seems, therefore, that urbanisation may be slowing down. Can you suggest a reason for this?

Table 2.5 Urbanisation trends and projections

	1950	1970	1990	2010
Proportion of population living in urban centres (%)				
World	30	37	45	56
Developing countries	17	25	37	52
Developed countries	54	67	73	78
Urban population (millions)				
World	730	1,350	2,380	4,070
Developing countries	280	650	1,510	3,050
Developed countries	450	700	870	1,020

Source: Our Planet, Our Health: Report of the WHO Commission on Health and the Environment, WHO, 1992; originally appeared in World Population Prospects 1990, United Nations, 1991 (document ST/SA/SER.A/120).

The fact that an increasing proportion of the world's population lives in urban areas has important implications for the environment and health. A nation's level of urbanisation and the pattern of distribution of towns and cities across the country affects the provision and distribution of resources like water and energy, and the supply of materials, like food, to sustain the population. Hence, transport systems, including road, rail and air systems, develop alongside urban growth. Industrialisation and urbanisation also usually develop in parallel.

Urban growth can bring great benefits in terms of health and the environment. Effective urbanisation policies could produce the following advantages:
- A concentration of production in certain areas brings cost advantages for waste disposal
- The cost of providing clean water and sanitation is cheaper and easier to accomplish and maintain than in less concentrated populations
- Education and health care can be provided more economically and to a higher standard for larger groups of people
- There is usually a more prosperous and productive economy in urban areas, and agricultural development can be stimulated and supported by the needs of the urban population

However, without effective policies, these potential benefits are not realised, so that substantial urban growth often brings many health and environmental problems, especially for poorer groups. An unhealthy environment may occur where there is a high density of population, and poverty prevents a good standard of living.

HEALTH AND HOUSING

The relationship between health and housing is very complex. People who live in housing which is in poor repair or is insanitary or is overcrowded often suffer from various forms of social and economic disadvantage and it is difficult to separate the effects of bad housing on health from the other factors related to poverty. However, poor housing which is damp, overcrowded and insanitary can lead to increases in the incidence of communicable and other diseases related to poor hygiene and lack of cleanliness. It has been shown that children who live in small flats have higher rates of respiratory infections than those who live in houses. In housing that is in bad condition, there may also be infestations with vermin and pests which spread disease. As well as physical disease, mental illnesses and emotional disturbances and other stress-related problems also increase amongst inhabitants of poor housing.

In inner-city areas, pollution from industry, noise and traffic fumes may cause an unhealthy environment. A lack of play space, gardens, shopping facilities, health centres and other amenities can add to the problems of bad housing. Child accidents are more prevalent in such areas. Low-income families are often forced to live in areas of 'environmental poverty'.

URBANISATION AND THE SPREAD OF DISEASE

In order to maintain health in urban conditions, a clean water supply and the efficient disposal of waste are essential to prevent the spread of disease. The following article on the increase in the rat population is just one example of what can happen when sewers are not kept clean enough and rats breed.

SURGE IN RAT INFESTATION LEADS TO HEALTH WARNING

... A survey ... of nearly half of Britain's local authorities last autumn found that rat infestation in homes had leapt by 39 per cent since 1979. In rural areas it had increased by almost half.

A rat is now estimated to be within 20 yards of every person, and rats are thought to outnumber Britain's human population.

The brown rat, *rattus norvegicus*, a relative of the kind which spread the Black Death in the 14th century, can bring dozens of infectious diseases to humans and animals, some potentially fatal. Rats have been blamed for food poisoning outbreaks and have spread a host of parasitic diseases, many through the creature's urine.

In theory, in one year of breeding, a single pair of rats and their offspring can produce 1,000 more. They eat virtually anything.

(The Observer, 2 October 1994)

This next article demonstrates the need for clean water in every household.

SLUM DISEASES RISE AS WATER SUPPLY IS CUT

Hepatitis and dysentery, diseases of Victorian slums, are spreading in Britain's inner cities as a direct result of privatised water companies disconnecting supplies ...

The principal anti-poverty officer at Birmingham City Council said: 'Outbreaks of hepatitis A occur when sewage cannot be washed away, when people cannot wash their hands after going to the toilet, and especially when there are children in the home. Disconnecting the water supply takes us back to the nineteenth century.'

Experts at the Department of Health are worried by the huge rise in dysentery and hepatitis cases since water privatisation ...

Last year, 21,000 households in England and Wales were disconnected, an increase of 177 per cent on 1991. Among the worst cities were Birmingham, Bristol, Liverpool and Sheffield, where densely populated communities were cut off for more than two weeks.

Since 1988, there has been a threefold increase in the number of dysentery cases in England and Wales, from 3,692 to 9,935 in 1992. Hepatitis has increased from 3,379 cases in 1987 to 9,020 in 1992.

Water prices throughout Britain have risen by an average of nearly 50 per cent in the past five years, but this has not been matched by increases in housing benefit or income support ...

The director of public health at Sandwell Health Authority has completed a study relating disconnections to hepatitis and dysentery outbreaks in his area, which covers about 300,000 people. He compared the postcodes of the people whose water was cut off with those of the dysentery and hepatitis victims. The result was statistically 'very significant'.

'There is less than a one in a thousand possibility of us arriving at that correlation by chance,' he said.

There is no sign of a general change in policy by water companies, although some, including North West Water, have become less 'trigger happy', resulting in fewer disconnections over the past few months.

(The Observer, 1993)

ACTIVITY 22

1 Read the above article, 'Slum diseases rise as water supply is cut.'

2 Using both information from this article and the information on 'environmental poverty', carry out further research to show the relationship between environmental health and urbanisation. Write a report on your findings.

HEALTH AND VEHICLE POLLUTION

(See also the section on general air pollution earlier in this chapter.) There is increasing evidence that the emissions from the ever-increasing numbers of vehicles in towns and cities are causing a serious threat to our health. Table 2.6 on p. 97 gives the latest information on the health effects of the various substances involved in vehicle emissions.

ACTIVITY 23

Air pollution from car exhausts
Read both the following extracts:

ONE IN THREE AT RISK FROM AIR POLLUTION

In January this year Friends of the Earth's survey showing poor air quality in parts of Britain was dismissed by a Government Minister as 'cheap and cheerful'. We measured nitrogen dioxide (NO_2) levels using relatively unsophisticated diffusion tubes. What a shock to find Government scientists using exactly the same technique for their own national survey of NO_2 levels, published in May!

The Government survey of NO_2 levels [*A survey of nitrogen dioxide concentrations in the United Kingdom using diffusion tubes: July to December 1991, LR 893 (AP), Warren Spring Laboratory, May 1992]* (NO_2 is a toxic pollutant which causes breathing difficulties) shows that 19 million people in Britain (about one in three) live in areas which exceed EC recommended levels. Concentrations have increased by 35 per cent over the last five years, consistent with a similar increase in motor vehicle emissions...

Friends of the Earth has shown that many sites where major road building has taken place have seen substantially increased levels of NO_2. Only drastic curbs on traffic growth, including cancellation of the Government's £20 billion road building programme, will address the growing risk to public health.

(Earth Matters, *Autumn 1992*)

AIR POLLUTION CURB URGED IN LONDON

Urgent action is needed to reduce air pollution in London and prevent more deaths and respiratory illness, the London Boroughs Association said yesterday after publishing its first air quality survey.

The association said its findings were in sharp contrast to results given by the Department of Environment which, it claimed, failed to keep the public informed of the full danger to health from air pollution.

John Gummer, the Environment Secretary, opening a London Boroughs Association conference on the report yesterday said the Government would be issuing a consultation document this year reviewing ways of dealing with the situation. But he appeared to rule out curtailing the use of private cars even at times when it was clear that air pollution had reached levels which were damaging public health...

Councillor Ronnie Barden, chairman of the LBA's environment committee said: 'The priority must be to persuade people out of their cars and on to buses and trains. Greater investment in public transport to make it more attractive and efficient is vital, along with other initiatives such as more bus priority measures, park and ride schemes and tougher parking controls.' ...

The association's survey found high levels of nitrogen dioxide in Barking, the City of London, Westminster and Hounslow, and levels of carbon dioxide which breached World Health Organisation guidelines at Southwark and Hounslow.

High levels of ozone pollution were found in Bexley and Bromley last June, while sulphur dioxide was higher in Barking, Dagenham and Bexley than in central London.

The air quality report showed that in the capital's worst recent case of pollution in December 1991 the problem could have been prevented if traffic had been cut 50 per cent ...

(The Guardian, 24 February 1994)

1 How many people in the UK live in areas where there are levels of nitrogen dioxide higher than those recommended by the EC?

2 By how much have emissions increased over the last five years? What has coincided with this increase?

3 Why will the introduction of catalytic converters for new cars not provide the intended reduction in nitrogen dioxide?

4 Who published the report on air quality in London?

5 What other gases were investigated besides nitrogen dioxide?

6 Summarise the findings of the report.

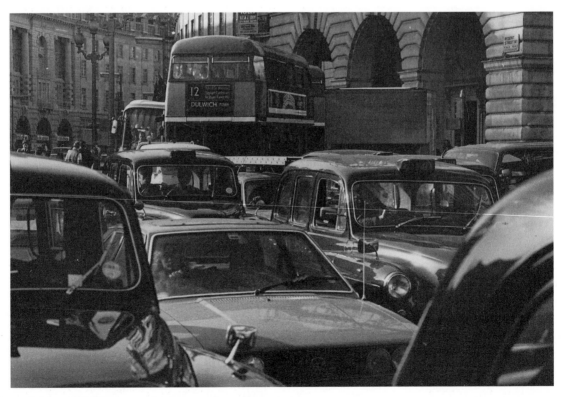

Figure 2.10 A health threat: the increase in traffic emissions

Table 2.6 The health effects of vehicle pollution

Pollutant	Source	Health effect
Nitrogen dioxide (NO_2)	One of the nitrogen oxides emitted in vehicle exhaust	May exacerbate asthma and possibly increase susceptibility to infections
Sulphur dioxide (SO_2)	Mostly produced by burning coal. Some SO_2 is emitted by diesel vehicles	May provoke wheezing and exacerbate asthma. It is also associated with chronic bronchitis
Particulates PM10, total suspended particulates, black smoke	Includes a wide range of solid and liquid particles in air. Those less than 10 µm in diameter (PM10) penetrate the lung fairly efficiently and are most hazardous to health. Diesel vehicles produce proportionally more particulates than petrol vehicles	Associated with a wide range of respiratory symptoms. Long-term exposure is associated with an increased risk of death from heart and lung disease. Particulates can carry carcinogenic materials into the lungs
Acid aerosols	Airborne acid formed from common pollutants including sulphur and nitrogen oxides	May exacerbate asthma and increase susceptibility to respiratory infection. May reduce lung function in those with asthma
Carbon monoxide (CO)	Comes mainly from petrol car exhaust	Lethal at high doses. At low doses, can impair concentration and neuro-behavioural function. Increases the likelihood of exercise-related heart pain in people with coronary heart disease. May present a risk to the foetus
Ozone (O_3)	Secondary pollutant produced from nitrogen oxides and volatile organic compounds in the air	Irritates the eyes and air passages. Increases the sensitivity of the airways to allergic triggers in people with asthma. May increase susceptibility to infection
Lead	Compound present in leaded petrol to help the engine run smoothly	Impairs the normal intellectual development and learning ability of children
Volatile organic compounds (VOCs)	A group of chemicals emitted from the evaporation of solvents and distribution of petrol fuel. Also present in vehicle exhaust	Benzene has given most cause for concern in this group of chemicals. It is a cancer-causing agent which can cause leukaemia at higher doses than are present in the normal environment
Polycyclic aromatic hydrocarbons (PAHs)	Produced by the incomplete combustion of fuel. PAHs become attached to particulates	Includes a complex range of chemicals, some of which are carcinogens. It is likely that exposure to PAHs in traffic exhaust poses a low cancer risk to the general population
Asbestos	May be present in brake pads and clutch linings, especially in heavy-duty vehicles. Asbestos fibres and dust are released into the atmosphere when vehicles brake	Asbestos can cause lung cancer and mesothelioma, cancer of the lung lining. The consequences of the low levels of exposure from braking vehicles are not known

Source: 'How vehicle pollution affects our health', Dr C. Read (ed), London Symposium of 20 May 1994, supported by the Ashden Trust.

ACTIVITY 24

This is an investigation into aspects of urbanisation and industrialisation in your own locality. You should divide into groups. Each group should take a different aspect of development and prepare an exhibition to display the findings.

Here are some examples of projects you could carry out:

1 Choose one particular industry in your locality. Investigate its development over the years and find out how it may have affected the environment, in terms both of new road and rail systems in the area, and of new levels of pollution.

2 Investigate the development of housing in your area. Take a historical perspective and try to find out how the existing patterns arose.

3 Investigate water supplies and sewage disposal in your area.

4 Has there been a major development in your area that may have led to a public inquiry? This could be a bypass or major road development, the expansion of an airport or the development of a town centre. Investigate any local debate on this development and find out about the arguments put forward by each side. The presentation could then take the form of a role play. You could nominate a representative for the developers and a representative for an opposing group. Each could put forward their case, and questions could be asked by members of the class. You will need to appoint a Chair of the Inquiry who will ensure fair play, and a vote could be taken to see who had won the debate.

Waste and pollution on land

RADIOACTIVE WASTE

Nuclear weapons and the use of nuclear fuels in power stations with thermal nuclear reactors are the main causes of concern about human contamination by radioactive materials. Table 2.7 shows the sources of

Table 2.7 Radiation absorbed by people in the UK in 1980

Source	Annual dose (µGy)	Percentage
Natural background	870.0	83.80
Medical	140.0	13.50
Nuclear fall-out	21.0	2.02
Miscellaneous	7.0	0.67
Radioactive waste	0.1	0.01

The unit Gy is a *gray*. 1 Gy = 1 joule of radiation energy absorbed by 1 kilogramme of body mass.

radiation absorbed by people in the UK in 1980. It can be seen that only a tiny amount is absorbed from radioactive waste. However, there is a great problem with the disposal of the ever-growing amount of nuclear waste. This comes from two sources, the spent cores from nuclear reactors and the waste products from the nuclear fuel uranium. These include strontium-90, which is radioactive and very persistent in the environment, and radioactive iodine and caesium.

We know about the effects of radiation from accidents in nuclear power plants, and from testing and using nuclear weapons. Waste strontium-90, iodine and caesium can be released into air or water as a result of accidents in nuclear power stations. This happened in the UK in 1957, at Sellafield, and there was a far worse accident in Chernobyl in the USSR in 1986. More than 200 people suffered radiation sickness, and 31 were killed. The radioactive content in the muscles of sheep was so high in Scotland, Cumbria and Wales after Chernobyl that slaughter was not permitted for two months. The

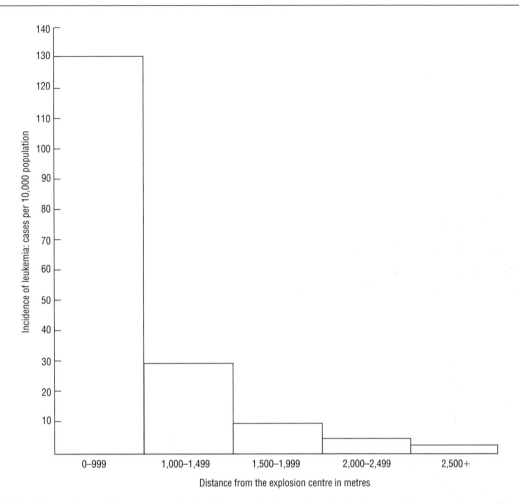

Figure 2.11   The relationship between the incidence of leukaemia and the distance from the centre of the
atomic explosion in Hiroshima
Source: Advanced Human Biology, J. Simpkins and J. I. Williams, Chapman and Hall, 1987.

radioactive wastes are carried in the air and
then absorbed into grass and from there into
cattle or sheep. Humans may also be
contaminated by eating the affected meat or
milk.

Radioactive iodine affects the thyroid, and
strontium-90 accumulates in bone adjacent to
the marrow where blood cells are made. A
nuclear bomb was dropped on Hiroshima and
Nagasaki in 1945, and strontium-90 was
amongst the radioactive materials released.
This radiation had very many effects,
including a high incidence of leukaemia. (See
Figure 2.11.)

Radioactive wastes from nuclear power
stations were dumped at sea before 1983.
Now they are stored in sealed containers and

placed in underground caverns. This is not a
satisfactory solution because of the further
amount of nuclear waste that will need
disposal in the future. Researchers are starting
to examine the rocks and movement of water
800 metres down with a view to creating a
very deep repository for nuclear waste. There
will not be a satisfactory place to dispose of
radioactive waste until the year 2010. In 1976
the Royal Commission on Environmental
Pollution warned, 'It would be irresponsible
and morally wrong to commit future
generations to the consequences of nuclear
power unless it has been demonstrated
beyond reasonable doubt that at least one
method exists for the safe isolation of these
wastes.'

ACTIVITY 25

1 List the advantages and disadvantages of using nuclear power stations to provide energy.

2 Where are the nuclear power stations in the UK, and where are the sites for the disposal of nuclear waste? Find out about existing and proposed ones.

3 Read the following *Guardian* report:

STUDY FINDS LIMITED SELLAFIELD CANCER LINK

In the widest and most detailed study so far, a government agency has found a statistical link between children with leukaemia and non-Hodgkin's lymphoma and radiation doses received by fathers who worked at the Sellafield nuclear plant in Cumbria.

However, the study published yesterday by the Health and Safety Executive also said that radiation alone does not explain the link.

The news comes two weeks after a High Court judge ruled that there was insufficient evidence to allow a suit by the families of two children whose fathers had worked at Sellafield. And a week ago two papers in the *British Medical Journal* suggested that a link between paternal exposure and childhood leukaemia was unlikely.

A 'cluster' of unexpected leukaemia incidence near the nuclear complex was first identified 10 years ago, and since then there has been a heated debate over its significance.

However, the latest study by the health executive does not resolve the confusion. It reported that a 'strong statistical association' appeared to exist only for children born to employees who lived in Seascale itself, and only for those who started work before 1965.

Many of Sellafield's workers live beyond the parish. 'For West Cumbria as a whole, we found little evidence to suggest a father's high pre-conception radiation dose increases the risk of leukaemia and lymphoma for

his children,' said Eddie Varney, the executive's deputy chief inspector of nuclear installations.

Later he added: 'We cannot find any single factor which satisfactorily explains what we have seen in West Cumbria. We can't find any causal links to workplace practices. All we have is statistical associations.' . . .

The research – the first to confirm findings three years ago by the late Professor Martin Gardner – covered not just cases of leukaemia in children born and diagnosed in West Cumbria, but in children born there and diagnosed elsewhere. The study also covered a wider timespan, and concerned itself with all other cancers.

Confusingly, the latest findings also appeared to support – but not confirm – another hypothesis, 'biological mixing', proposing that when settled communities are 'invaded' by people from outside there is likely to be a greater incidence of leukaemia.

'When you try to attach a cause,' said Mr Varney 'you run into difficulties. About 90 per cent of the Sellafield working population live outside Seascale, and a lot of those people have had very high radiation doses, and you don't see the same association.'

British Nuclear Fuels, which operates Sellafield, said in a statement yesterday that the executive had produced 'yet further evidence' that the father–child association 'does not work'.

Dr Patrick Green, of Friends of the Earth, said: 'Despite spending millions of pounds in a desperate attempt to get Sellafield off the hook, BNFL cannot explain away the radiation excess.' . . .

(The Guardian, *21 October 1993*)

Find out about the evidence that could suggest that there is a higher level of incidence of leukaemia in the Sellafield area. Is this evidence conclusive?

4 Write a report on all your above findings.

SOLID WASTES AND DEPOSITS

A vast quantity of industrial solid waste is produced – 400 tonnes every year – in the UK. Most of this is dumped in pits or heaps. *Spoil heaps* consist of waste material from activities like gravel extraction. These are unsightly but they do not present a direct threat to health. *Slag heaps* are the result of ore-digging and metal-refining activities, particularly from the mining of coal. These can contain toxic materials, like metals, which may be leached into water supplies. Copper, zinc and cadmium are examples of toxic waste from mining operations. Vegetation is difficult to grow, and slag heaps can become unstable. The Aberafan disaster in Wales in 1966 occurred when a slag heap became destabilised by heavy rain and engulfed a school and houses, killing 116 children and 28 adults.

Domestic rubbish is produced in millions of tonnes each year. It contains mostly plastics, organic material and paper. Disposal is vital as rubbish can be toxic and emit bad odours, and can become infested with flies and vermin. Moreover, bacteria will grow, and some of these could be pathogenic. Rubbish can be disposed of by infilling land sites which can be later reclaimed for agricultural or recreational purposes. Incineration is also possible. In Edmonton in North London, the heat produced in this way is used to generate electricity. Methane gas is released from domestic rubbish as the organic content is broken down by bacteria. This gas could also be used to make electricity, but most is currently released into the atmosphere, adding to the pollution in the air.

INDUSTRIAL TOXIC WASTE

There are many toxic materials produced as waste by industrial processes. These pose difficult problems for safe disposal: there are special regulated disposal sites and treatment plants around the country, but accidents and problems with transport are not uncommon.

The following are some toxic wastes:

- cyanides
- asbestos
- organic solvents
- acids
- alkalines
- metals
- oils
- tar
- paint sludge
- phenols

The polluting effects on the environment can be great. Plants and animals are affected both on land and in water as the toxic material may reach rivers and then the sea.

The poisonous effects on humans are various. Some examples include:

1 Mercury accumulates particularly in the kidney, liver and brain. Eventually, paralysis and death occur.
2 Aluminium poisoning can cause joint and muscle pains, headaches, diarrhoea, nausea, rashes and blisters. The incident that occurred in Camelford in 1988, when 20 tonnes of aluminium sulphate was accidentally poured into the town water supplies instead of a special tank for the storage of toxic chemicals, is still remembered since the residents are still suffering long-term effects.

TOXICITY ON TAP

Last July, tons of aluminium sulphate were dumped into a Cornish water supply. Residents began to complain of illnesses ranging from vomiting to lip blisters. But it took weeks for the full details to emerge, and incidents of aluminium pollution are still hitting the headlines.

(Guardian *headline, 14 June 1989*)

3 Asbestos fibres can be breathed in and can cause the destruction of lung tissues and cancer.

Toxic waste materials may also be flammable or explosive. Specialist treatment plants which render the toxic waste safe and incineration are both methods used to reduce contamination. However, some toxic waste is dumped without treatment. Sites for dumping include old mine shafts and marshy land. The contamination of underground water is a possible problem.

Hazardous waste and its disposal is also a matter of concern to the public:

UK'S TOXIC WASTE IMPORTS INCREASE BY 10,000 TONNES

About 44,000 tonnes of hazardous wastes were imported for disposal in Britain in 1990–91 – a third of which came from Switzerland, the nation with the foremost reputation for Eurocleanliness.

Official figures published by the Department of the Environment yesterday said the UK imported nearly 10,000 tonnes more waste in 1990–91 than in the year before. Nearly 4,000 tonnes of polychlorinated biphenyls (PCBs) came in; the biggest consignments of this were from Spain and Italy.

While imports increased, Britain was recycling less aluminium, lead, and scrap ferrous metal. In 1984, recycled scrap aluminium accounted for 20 per cent of annual consumption, but this fell to only 12 per cent by 1990. Similarly, we were recycling 9.6 million tonnes of ferrous metals in 1984, but only 8.19 million in 1990 . . .

(The Independent, 26 March 1992)

Table 2.8   Countries exporting hazardous waste into the UK, 1990/91

Country sending waste	Quantity (tonnes)
Switzerland	13,550
Belgium	9,229
Ireland	3,986
Netherlands	3,949
Italy	3,583
Austria	2,912
Sweden	1,595
Spain	1,194
Portugal	1,185
Germany	1,010
Others	1,762
Total	43,953

Source: The Independent, 26 March 1992.

WARNING ON TOXIC WASTE PERIL

The plight of a town stranded for a year with a lethal consignment of toxic waste because of legal loopholes has exposed a national risk to health – and a gap in the Government's Green Bill.

Legal wrangling over more than 500 tonnes of contaminated materials, received from the American chemicals giant FMC, has failed to get them moved from Wath upon Dearne, near Rotherham, South Yorkshire . . .

Mr Peter Hardy, Labour MP for Wentworth, said a whole series of loopholes had lumbered Wath with the waste. Friends of the Earth campaigner Blake Lee-Harwood said: 'The new Bill means that a Minister may act to stop an import of waste but he has no power once it is in this country to get shot of it.'

The waste, containing xylene and furan, is in sealed drums at the Wath recycling plant, guarded by two rottweilers and checked each day. British Rail has some of the waste in sealed drums at its depot.

(The Observer, 29 July 1990)

ASSESSMENT OPPORTUNITY

1 Write a report on an investigation into the harmful effects of human activity on the environment and health, which includes:
   - an explanation of three forms of pollution
   - a summary of the effects of the three forms of pollution
   - a summary of the impact of the intensification of agriculture
   - a summary of the consequences of urbanisation and population density

2 Write a summary which identifies, and provides examples of, damage to the environment and health from two different types of waste accumulation.

HUMAN ACTIVITIES DESIGNED TO REDUCE HARM TO THE ENVIRONMENT AND HEALTH

Specialist treatments reducing harm to the environment and health

CONTROL OF AIR POLLUTION

The legislation

The Environmental Protection Act 1990 and the Clean Air Act 1993 are the most important laws on the control of air pollution. The Health and Safety at Work Act 1974 also grants powers to impose restrictions on emissions from industrial premises. This law is mentioned later in the chapter, as is European law, which has had a major impact on the control of air pollution in Europe recently.

The central Inspectorate of Pollution enforces the Environmental Protection Act 1990 as it applies to major industries across the UK. It attempts to control air pollution caused by industrial processes. There is a list of noxious and offensive gases in the legislation that are specified as pollutants. These include over 3,000 industrial processes and about 2,000 major plants. The Inspectorate must be satisfied that an industrial process is operating using the best practicable means both for preventing the escape of noxious or offensive gases and for rendering gases harmless whenever possible. In practice, the inspectors check that approved anti-pollution equipment is installed and working effectively. There are minimum heights for industrial chimneys, and concentration levels for gases that are emitted are also specified. Unfortunately, although tall chimneys stop noxious gases from causing air pollution locally, they encourage the transport

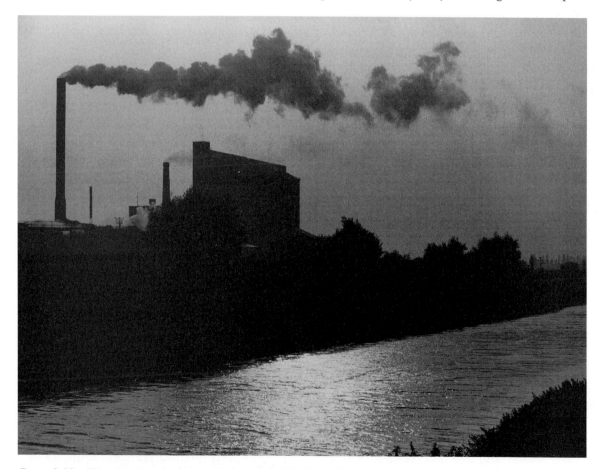

Figure 2.12   The visual environmental impact of tall industrial chimney stacks

of sulphur dioxide and other pollutants over long distances, causing regional hazes and acid rain.

The local authority, i.e. the district or borough council, is responsible for local air-pollution control, and it operates through special provisions made in the Environmental Protection Act 1990 and the Clean Air Act 1993. Much of the latter act is concerned with the prevention of pollution by smoke. It is an offence for levels of dark smoke to be emitted from industrial premises beyond those allowed in the regulations. Smoke-control areas can be designated. It was this latter provision, in the earlier Clean Air Act of 1956, which enabled London to be free of the smogs which were so common in the early 1950s. Only smokeless fuel can be burnt in the smoke-control areas. Grants can be paid to house-owners to enable them to convert boilers and fires to burn the right type of fuel. Environmental health officers employed by the local authority will carry out the enforcement of air-pollution legislation within their area.

There are also regulations about the sulphur and lead content of fuel used in motor vehicles, and about the sulphur content of oil fuel used in engines and furnaces. Further regulations relate to the level of asbestos in the air at premises where people are working. Legislation also prohibits burning straw or stubble in fields after a crop has been harvested.

CLEANING UP POWER STATIONS – AN EXPENSIVE BUSINESS

Power stations release about two-thirds of the sulphur dioxide given off in waste gases into the air in the UK. A process called 'flue-gas desulphurisation' (see Figure 2.13) can remove the sulphur dioxide from these waste gases by using limestone to neutralise the sulphur dioxide. Fitting the new equipment to do this would cost £200 million for a big power station, and £30 million annually just to run. This could add 10% to electricity bills.

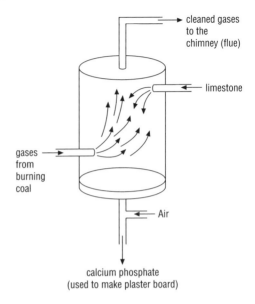

Figure 2.13   Flue-gas desulphurisation

Other serious air pollutants, oxides of nitrogen, are also released into the atmosphere from power stations. To convert 12 power stations to using the new burners to reduce this pollution would cost at least £170 million, but conversions *are* going ahead.

CUTTING DOWN POLLUTION FROM MOTOR VEHICLES

The burning of fuels in vehicles produces about 40% of the total oxides of nitrogen released into the air, as well as other air pollutants.

- Lean-burn engines have been designed which can cut down levels of nitrogen oxides in car exhausts by 75% at a cost of only about £60 for each car
- Catalytic converters can be fitted to cars. Since lead interferes with the conversion process, working cars with converters have to run on lead-free petrol. These converters cost over £500 per car, and usually have to be replaced after the car has travelled 50,000 miles.

SOLVING THE ACID-RAIN PROBLEM BY NEUTRALISING ACIDS

Sulphur dioxide in air pollution dissolves in rain and is converted into dilute sulphuric acid. This topic is discussed earlier in this chapter. It is a particular problem in Sweden, where over £25 million is spent each year 'liming' lakes. This involves adding limestone (calcium carbonate) – in powder form from an aircraft – which combines with the acid to neutralise it. This is cheaper than changing power stations to cut down sulphur-dioxide emission.

THE CONTROL OF WATER POLLUTION

The legislation

The Environmental Protection Act 1990 is the legislation which allows the control of water pollution from major industrial sources in conjunction with the work of the central Inspectorate of Pollution. In addition, there is the Water Resources Act 1991 which is a very important anti-pollution law. The National Rivers Authority was set up under this Act, and this body has responsibility for the protection and management of rivers and other waters, including coastal and ground waters. These are called 'controlled waters'.

The control of water pollution is one of the main activities of the National Rivers Authority, and there are river inspectors whose job it is to ensure that the quality of water is maintained to a high standard. They take samples of water regularly, and these are analysed to see if there are any polluting substances present. They will also investigate living organisms in the river to enable a judgement to be made about the degree of cleanliness of the water. It is an offence to allow any poisonous, noxious or polluting matter to enter controlled waters, and solid waste matter is included here. Certain trade effluents and effluents from sewage works are allowed to be discharged into rivers provided this is done under a special disposal licence that can be issued under the Environmental Protection Act 1990. Registers must be kept of all such consenting licences. There are various regulations linked to the Water Resources Act 1991, which relate to specific water-pollution problems. One example is a

regulation which allows areas to be designated as nitrate sensitive, and the entry of nitrates into the water in these areas can then be controlled by law. Earlier in this chapter, the problems of nitrates from fertilisers causing pollution in water were discussed.

Industrialists, farmers and others who cause pollution are given advice and warnings by the water inspectors. If they do not respond, a prosecution under the Water Resources Act 1991 will result.

WATER-SUPPLY AND SEWAGE SERVICES

The Water Industry Act 1991

Earlier in this chapter the problems of sewage pollution in rivers were discussed. In order to maintain clean rivers and to prevent the spread of disease, it is necessary to ensure that there is

- a source of clean water for domestic, industrial and agricultural purposes
- an effective sewage-disposal system

The main provisions relating to water-supply and sewerage services are contained in the Water Industry Act 1991.

A clean water supply

Companies who supply water are called 'water undertakers', and they have to conform to the rules in the Water Industries Act 1991 to make sure that the water is clean and pure. This Act states that it is the duty of a water undertaker to develop and maintain an efficient and economical system of water supply in its area. Water must be taken to premises requiring it, and mains and service pipes must be provided. Furthermore, water must be laid on constantly, in sufficient quantity and with enough pressure to reach every site. There are powers to prohibit the use of water for watering gardens or washing cars if a deficiency of water is threatened.

The water provided must be of good quality, wholesome and without contamination. There are regulations about the permitted levels of substances in the water. The fluoridation of water is permitted when a health authority has requested this as a measure to promote dental health. Water taken from a river, reservoir or underground aquifer undergoes treatment before it is pumped to users through mains and service pipes.

Regulations exist relating to payment and the powers to disconnect. There is a further discussion about the health effects of disconnecting water supplies in an earlier section in this chapter about social and economic influences on environmental health.

The various stages of water treatment involve the following elements of equipment:

1 *Primary grid*. This prevents large objects from the river entering the system.
2 *Settlement tank*. Water is pumped here to allow large particles and debris to drop out.
3 *Filter beds*. These vary in type. Some are *slow* sand filters which rely on a gelatinous film, which develops on the sand, which is produced by millions of protozoa and other micro-organisms which live on the sand. This filter will trap bacteria which provide food for the protozoa. *Rapid* sand filters are similar in principle, but the jelly is artificial and made from aluminium oxide.
4 *Contact tank*. This is where *chlorination* takes place. Any remaining bacteria are killed. The amount of chlorine added depends on the numbers of bacteria present, and may vary. The chlorine itself is destroyed as it kills the bacteria, and water companies must be careful not to add too much chlorine so that there is a surplus.
5 *Storage tanks*. The water is stored until required and then pumped to users through the mains supply.

SEWERAGE SERVICES

The Water Industry Act 1991 is also concerned with the provision of sewerage systems. In this Act, sewerage undertakers are required to maintain a system of public sewers and sewage-disposal works. There are regulations about the quality of sewage effluents which can be discharged into rivers. Provision is also made for the treatment of trade effluents from industry.

There are two types of sewage-treatment works. In all cases, however, the process starts with *screening*, which traps large objects, and a

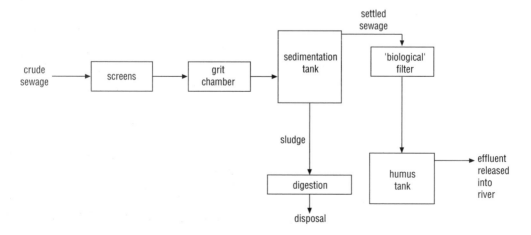

Figure 2.14 The biological filter method of sewage treatment

process which separates road grit from the sewage. The next stage is *sedimentation*, when solid matter settles out while the sewage stands in large tanks. The sedimented matter is called *sludge*, whilst the clearer liquid above it is called *settled sewage*.

Further treatment follows one of two courses. The simpler older method uses 'biological filters' (see Figure 2.14) where the settled sewage is sprinkled over *clinker*. Layers of bacteria and protozoa live on the clinker, and these feed on the organic matter suspended and dissolved in the settled sewage. The liquid is now safe to discharge into the river, after the humus has settled out. Most of the bacteria will have died during the latter processes as the organic material on which they feed is removed. However, there are still many bacteria present in sewage effluent.

Sludge from the sedimentation tank is transferred to a large tank for digestion. It is then disposed, in either dried or liquid form. Some is spread on land, or it may be deposited at sea.

More modern sewage works, on the other hand, use a method of sewage treatment known as the 'activated sludge' method. In this method, the liquid, following sedimentation, is pumped into long channels together with a small quantity of sludge containing a variety of bacteria and protozoa. Along the bottom of each channel is a perforated pipe, a diffuser, and air is bubbled into the sewage under pressure. This air has two functions. It agitates and mixes the sewage and it also maintains a high level of oxygen so that the aerobic micro-organisms present can thrive. These digest the organic material in the sewage very quickly, so this method of treatment allows a much faster processing of sewage than the biological filter process.

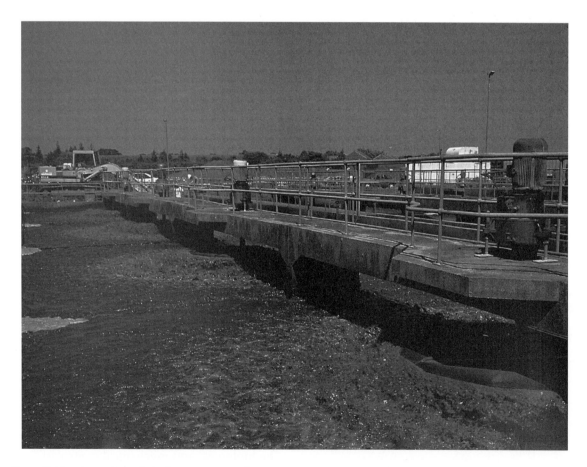

Figure 2.15 An activated-sludge treatment plant

The principles of this process are very similar to those in the biological filter method. In more modern sewage works, the problem of sludge disposal is partially solved by digesting it and using the methane produced to make electricity.

ACTIVITY 27

Plan a visit to your local sewage-treatment works. Which type of process is employed here, biological filter or activated sludge? Write a report on your visit. Especially note any precautions that are taken to test the quality of the effluent before it is released into the river. Does this sewage works deal with any trade or industrial waste?

Processes designed to conserve resources

RECYCLING

Many materials can be recycled and used again. Consumers can undertake the separation themselves and take their recyclable waste materials to the recycling centres provided by the local authority, or separation can take place in some modern disposal units.

Materials which can be easily recycled include:
- glass
- paper
- clothing
- cans and other metals

ACTIVITY 28

1 Investigate recycling arrangements in your area. You may find schemes to recycle glass, paper, clothing and cans. Contact your local council to find out more about how the schemes operate and how successful they are. What publicity is produced to ensure that the public knows about these schemes?

2 Investigate one industrial recycling scheme and produce a report. Choose one of the materials that is collected in your area. What happens to it after it is taken away from the recycling collection point?

ORGANIC FARMING

Since farming began, animal manure, compost from rotting vegetation and ashes from burnt vegetation have been used by farmers to keep soils healthy. In the eighteenth century, the idea of *crop rotation* was developed by Charles 'Turnip' Townshend. Different crops take different sorts and amounts of nutrients from the soil. If the same crops are grown in the same field year after year, the soil becomes exhausted. If crops are rotated, however, the soil has a chance to recover. Peas, beans and clover put nitrogen back into the soil. A typical four-crop rotation cycle would involve turnips, wheat, barley and clover.

In the last 40 years, farmers have turned to intensive farming methods, with the same crops grown in the same fields every year. Chemicals have been used as fertilisers and pesticides (the environmental effects of these have been discussed earlier in this chapter). Recently, there has been a growing concern about the use of chemicals, not only because of the environmental damage but also because it is claimed by some that pesticides remain in the crop plants, and since we then eat these plants, our own health is at risk.

Now, there is a renewed interest in completely organic farming methods. This approach uses only natural fertilisers such as animal manure. Pests are controlled either biologically, e.g. by encouraging ladybirds which eat greenfly, or mechanically, e.g. by protecting crops with netting. However, organic fertilisers work more slowly than chemical ones, and yields are less spectacular. The biological and mechanical control of pests is less effective than chemical control.

The scale of production is smaller, and organically produced crops can be more expensive to produce for the farmer, which means that the consumer pays more.

ACTIVITY 29

1 Explain the advantages of crop rotation. Can you think of any disadvantages?

2 Why do you think that crop rotation can help control plant pests and diseases as well as replenish soil nutrients?

3 Explain the advantages and disadvantages of 'chemical' farming.

4 What are the advantages and disadvantages of organic farming?

5 What points of view do you think the following people would have about organic farming:
  • European Community ministers with responsibility for reducing food surpluses
  • a family on low income
  • a family on high income
  • a wheat farmer?

Policies and legislation for reducing the harmful effects of urbanisation and industrialisation

HOUSING AND BUILDING

Aspects of health related to housing are considered earlier in this chapter. Policies are developed by each local authority to ensure that housing in the area is adequate. Legislation exists to provide a framework within which policies can be implemented. The housing and building legislation lays down standards to try to ensure good housing conditions. The structure of new buildings is controlled by very strict regulations, and there

are measures to rectify defects in older properties.

The conditions that form the basis for good housing, as outlined in the legislation, are as follows:
• The dwelling should be in a good state of repair and substantially free from damp
• Each room should be properly lit and ventilated
• There should be an adequate supply of wholesome water laid on inside the dwelling
• An adequate supply of hot water should be provided
• There should be an internal water-closet
• There should be a fixed bath or shower, preferably in a separate room
• A sink should be provided with suitable arrangements for the disposal of waste water
• There should be a proper drainage system
• Each room should have adequate points for electricity for lighting
• There should be adequate facilities for heating
• There should be satisfactory facilities for the storage, preparation and cooking of food
• There should be proper provision for the storage of fuel where appropriate

HOUSING LEGISLATION

There have been several recent Housing Acts; the most important one is the Housing Act 1985. There was also a separate Housing Associations Act, introduced in the same year; and the Local Government and Housing Act of 1989 introduced a new system of grants for improving housing.

The Acts are very wide ranging and give many powers to the local authority, which carries them out through the housing department.

The Housing Act 1985
Council housing

Under the 1985 Act, housing accommodation may be provided by the local authority and land may be purchased, compulsorily if necessary, to build dwellings. People who are homeless or who occupy insanitary, overcrowded homes or who have large families in unsatisfactory accommodation should be given preference in the allocation of council homes. Reasonable rents may be charged. The 1985 Act allowed local authorities to continue to sell council houses; and now the national stock of homes to rent from local authorities is severely depleted, since this provision first entered legislation in 1980. The sold homes have not been replaced by new buildings.

Homelessness

Local authorities have a responsibility to house homeless people. This first entered the statute book in a previous Housing Act of 1977, but it is now covered by the 1985 Act. Certain categories have priority; these include a pregnant woman, or a person with whom a pregnant woman resides, a person with whom dependent children reside and a person who is vulnerable on account of old age, mental illness, disability or other special reason. People who are made homeless through an emergency, like flood or fire, should also be housed.

Dealing with substandard housing

Under the Housing Act of 1985, local authorities are empowered to issue repair notices to owners of dwelling houses which are defective or unfit for human habitation. The owner is required to carry out repairs so that the dwelling is of a reasonable standard, and dates are set for the completion of work. This Act also enables local authorities to improve whole areas of housing by declaring housing action areas, general improvement areas and renewal areas. Central government funds can be made available. Slum clearance is also possible: local authorities can demolish buildings which are deemed to be unfit for human habitation or dangerous or injurious to health. Compulsory purchase orders are made, and the courts have considerable powers of enforcement in this respect. Entry

to premises for the purpose of valuation must be allowed, and any obstruction to the procedures leading to demolition is an offence.

Slum clearance has been a feature of housing policy for many years. Whilst slum clearances in cities such as Manchester certainly removed enormous numbers of unfit houses from our housing stock, and reduced pollution from burning coal, the high-rise flats that were often built to replace the slum houses were not without their own problems. The quality of building in the 1960s was not good, and the social effects of breaking up communities and putting people into blocks of flats had been underestimated.

Overcrowding

Overcrowding is prohibited under the 1985 Housing Act. Standards are laid down which define overcrowding:

1 when two children, over the age of 10 years and of opposite sexes, must sleep in the same room
2 when the room:person ratio exceeds one room:two people, two rooms:three people, three rooms:five people, four rooms:seven and a half people, or five rooms or more:10 people, with two then added for every room over five
3 when the floor-area:person ratio exceeds 110 square feet (10.2 square metres):two people.

(Children under one year are ignored for the purposes of assessing overcrowding.) These limits are recognised as being unrealistic.

An occupier or landlord who permits overcrowding commits an offence. The local authority can require the occupier of a dwelling to provide information as the numbers and sexes of people sleeping in the dwelling, and housing officers may enter a premises to investigate and measure rooms. If overcrowding is found, then a notice of abatement may be issued: this means that the overcrowding must cease within 14 days.

Application may be made to a county court if the notice is not carried out, and eventually the occupier can be turned out if they do not comply.

The same Act also deals with houses in multiple occupation. There are regulations which ensure that premises are suitable for the number of people living there, and powers exist to take offenders to court.

The Housing Associations Act 1985

This allowed housing associations to be set up and registered. A housing association may be broadly defined as a society, body of trustees or company which is established for the purpose of providing, constructing, improving or managing housing accommodation. It does not exist to make a profit. One of the advantages of being a registered housing association is that such an association then becomes eligible for grants. Local-authority assistance is sometimes available to help housing associations. The aim is to help people obtain housing through a scheme which is designed to replace simple renting from a local authority.

The Local Government and Housing Act 1989

There was a comprehensive system for grants for improving dwellings in place in many of the earlier Housing Acts. Nonetheless, the Local Government and Housing Act 1989 created an entirely new system for grants to be paid to private owners by the local authority. Resources are now only available for essential repair work and improvements where the need is greatest. There are also grants to enable disabled people to adapt their homes.

ACTIVITY 30

Carry out a survey of the different types of housing in the area where you live. Contact your local housing department to help you.

Are there any problem areas? The environmental health department will be able to help you as well.

BUILDING LEGISLATION

The Building Act 1984 is the latest Act which provides regulations covering the design and construction of buildings and the provision of services, fittings and equipment in them. The purpose of the regulations is stated as follows:

(a) to secure the health, safety, welfare and convenience of persons in or about the building;
(b) to conserve fuel and power;
(c) to prevent the waste, misuse or contamination of water.

There are sections of the Act relating to the preparation of sites, the suitability, durability and use of materials, and structural strength and stability. Fire precautions are covered, and resistance to moisture and damp is also given attention. There are rules relating to insulation, both to prevent heat loss and to prevent too much transmission of sound.

Many of the regulations relate to drainage and storage, and the treatment and removal of waste. This, together with the provision of clean water, is one of the most important aspects of a healthy environment (water services also, therefore, figure prominently in the legislation). In addition, heating, lighting and ventilation systems are all regulated. Finally, there must be safe access to the building.

Enforcement of the building regulations

Plans of all proposed buildings must be submitted to the local authority for approval before building can begin. Such plans may be rejected, for example, if a bathroom is not included with hot and cold water, or if there is not adequate space for food storage. Much attention is given to adequate provision for drainage, and to ensuring that proper arrangements exist for linking in to the sewerage system.

Building inspectors are employed by the local authority to work in the planning department. They inspect buildings both at different stages of their construction and on completion. It is an offence to contravene the provisions in the building regulations, and the local authority may require an owner to pull down or alter work carried out in contravention of the legislation. There is a right of appeal in a magistrates' court, and there may be reference to the secretary of state if there is a dispute.

ACTIVITY 31

Contact your local planning department and find out more about the processes of building regulation and inspection.

WASTE COLLECTION AND DISPOSAL

The Environmental Protection Act 1990 outlines the duty of the local authority to make arrangements for the safe disposal of waste. This 'waste disposal authority' may be a county council in country areas or a district council in towns. Waste from households and certain industrial and commercial premises is called 'controlled waste', and it must be collected. No charge should be made for the disposal of household waste provided it does not exceed 25 kilogrammes in weight or include garden waste, clinical waste – like syringes or dirty dressings – or dead pets. Charges can, however, be made for the disposal of other household rubbish.

Although most domestic and commercial waste is not very toxic, it can nonetheless only be disposed at licensed sites: it is an offence for anyone to dump waste at unlicensed sites. Often, local authorities use waste to infill gravel pits. There are many regulations relating to the type of site which can be used, so that common hazards like the leaching of contaminants into water supplies and methane production are reduced. One of the most useful ways of dealing with household waste is to *incinerate* it.

It is the duty of each waste-collection authority to investigate waste-recycling possibilities in their own areas. Recycling schemes are now common today, and this helps to cut down the amount of household waste to be disposed of, as well as to conserve useful materials. The legislation deals with all these aspects of household waste disposal. Figure 2.16 shows a landfill waste-disposal site. The waste will eventually be covered up and the land reclaimed.

ACTIVITY 32

Investigate the system used in your local authority to collect and dispose of your household waste. What happens to it? Write a short account of your findings.

There are very stringent regulations relating to the treatment, carriage and disposal of toxic and dangerous waste from industry. Special licensed sites exist for the disposal of such waste, including old mine shafts, marshy land and land-infill sites. The main problem is that this waste may enter water supplies. In some cases, however, it is possible to make the waste safe with special treatment before disposal. Environmental inspectors are employed both locally and by the central Pollution Inspectorate to carry out controls.

TRANSPORT

The local authority and Department of Transport are responsible for roads, and both British Rail – or rail companies if privatisation goes ahead – and the bus companies are responsible for public transport. The local authority plays a coordinating role in balancing transportation, planning and environmental issues in its area. Policies are adopted which seek to reduce congestion and pollution whilst improving the economy and

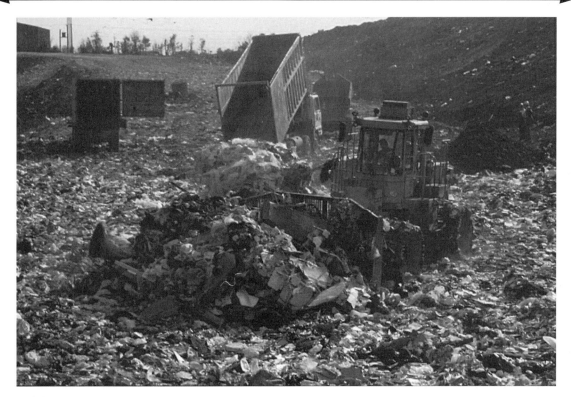

Figure 2.16 Waste disposal

quality of life for those who live, work and shop there. Some places rely on tourism, and have to try to make the area an even more attractive place to visit.

In the last few decades, the demand for transport within the UK has increased enormously – by 230% between 1952 and 1989. The Transport Act 1985 reduced the ability of local authorities to coordinate the provision of public-transport services, and a plethora of private bus operators led to increasingly patchy and uncoordinated local bus services. Also, there have been restrictions on British Rail's ability to invest in new infrastructure and rolling stock.

ACTIVITY 33

1 Figure 2.17 shows how types of transport have changed over the years.
(a) What does 'billion passenger kilometres' refer to?

(b) Summarise the information displayed in the graphs, commenting on the trends for each of the four types of transport. What has happened to the contribution of *public* transport to travel around the UK?
(c) List three ways in which the trends mentioned above damage both the environment and our health.

2 Write to the Department of Transport and find out about its national transport policies.

3 Investigate transport strategies in your local area. We have discussed the problems of cars in towns and cities earlier in this chapter. Have any special arrangements been introduced in your area designed to encourage people not to use their cars? (Examples could include free 'park and ride' schemes, bus lanes and cheap car parking near stations.)

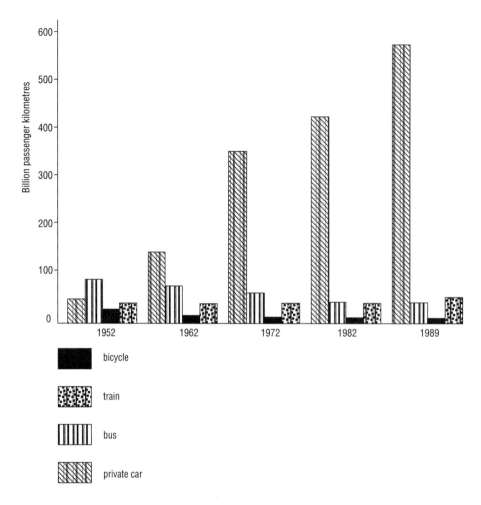

Figure 2.17   Passenger transport by mode in the UK

PROTECTIVE PRACTICES

The Health and Safety at Work Act 1974 is discussed earlier in this chapter. You will remember that safety policies must be adopted for the workplace and that employers are required by law to ensure the safety of employees at work. Employees, too, have responsibilities here.

Noise at work

An employer is required to make a noise assessment wherever an employee could have a personal daily exposure to 85 dB (decibels) or more. People must be told about the dangers and offered ear protectors. Where the noise is above 90 dB, employers must reduce these noise levels as far as possible and ensure

that ear protection is worn. Figure 2.18 shows a poster encouraging employees to take care of their hearing.

ACTIVITY 34

Investigate four further examples of protective practices, which may require the wearing of protective clothing. Read the section on procedures for controlling infection in a care setting before answering this. You may take your examples from your school or college, a hospital or other care setting, shops, leisure centres or catering outlets.

EMPLOYEES

Programmes are only likely to succeed in preventing hearing damage where there is co-operation between the employer and employee. To meet the requirements placed on you by the regulations you will need to:

Wear ear protection (ear plugs or ear muffs) provided to you whenever you are in places where the Second or Peak Action Levels might be reached, and every time you go into an area marked as an ear protection zone.

Use any other equipment the employer provides under the regulations. For example, if the machine is meant to have a silencer fitted — don't take it off.

Look after any equipment provided to you under the regulations.

Report any to your employer if you discover any defects in any of the equipment, report them to your employer.

Your employer should warn you when your exposure might reach the 85 dB(A) First Action Level and provide you with personal ear protectors if you want them. It is in your own interests to ask for them and to use them.

Your hearing might depend on it!

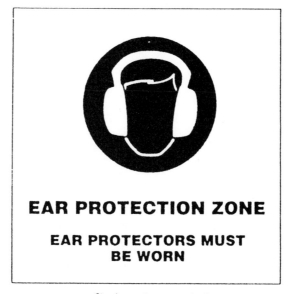

EAR PROTECTION ZONE

EAR PROTECTORS MUST BE WORN

Sign for marking ear protection zones

Figure 2.18   A poster on ear protection

Advice recommended for safeguarding individuals from harmful effects of the environment

There are many diseases around today against which individuals can take action to protect themselves. Chronic degenerative diseases on the increase include:

- heart disease
- cancers
- stroke
- arthritis

Infectious diseases on the increase include:

- *Campylobacter enteritis* – food poisoning
- *Helicobacter pylori gastritis* – duodenal ulcer
- human immunodeficiency diseases – HIV and Aids

It is now recognised that people's lifestyles and behaviour are causative factors in most of the diseases mentioned above. Important factors here are:

- diet
- exercise and maintaining mobility
- stress
- recreation and leisure activities
- smoking
- alcohol and substance abuse
- sexual behaviour
- housing and sanitation
- personal hygiene

Health education takes place on three levels. *Primary health education* is directed at healthy people and aims to *prevent* ill-health arising in the first place; for example, school children learn about basic hygiene, nutrition and road safety. *Secondary health education* is directed at people with a health problem or reversible condition; examples of this are screening apparently healthy people who may be at risk from developing a particular disease and encouraging both overweight people to change their dietary habits and smokers to give up smoking. *Tertiary health education* includes rehabilitation programmes.

SOME FACTS ON CANCER

- Smoking causes 30% of all cancer deaths, including 30,000 deaths from lung cancer
- Excess alcohol consumption is linked to 3% of all cancers
- Diet is possibly related to 35% of all cancers. Some fruits and vegetables may be preventative
- Skin cancer is the second most common cancer in the UK, linked to too much ultraviolet light from sunshine
- The UK has the highest death rate from breast cancer in the world, with 16,000 women dying each year
- 2,000 women in the UK die each year from cervical cancer
- Testicular cancer is the commonest cancer in the UK in men aged 20–34, with 1,000 new cases reported each year

REDUCING THE RISKS OF CORONARY HEART DISEASE

- Cut out smoking
- Take regular exercise – a brisk walk for 20 minutes each day will improve circulation
- Drink alcohol sensibly – consider a pint of beer or two glasses of wine as a maximum for each day
- Eat healthily
- Avoid stress

ACTIVITY 35

Work in pairs. Produce a health-education fact sheet designed for distribution to members of the general public. You may take a particular disease, or just promote a healthy lifestyle.

The content of your fact sheet should include the following:

- the nature of the risks involved
- possible causes of the relevant diseases
- ideas for minimising risks

Ideas for your health-education leaflet might include:

- tobacco

- diet
- exercise
- sexual behaviour
- sexually transmitted diseases
- certain cancers
- stress
- road safety
- dental health
- immunisation
- personal hygiene
- heart disease
- HIV/Aids
- high blood pressure

Strategies to improve the environment

The environmental approach has made great contributions to public health in the past – for instance, the provision of clean drinking water and protection from sewage and other contamination. Nowadays, an environmental approach is often called 'intersectoral' policy or action because the health sector works with another sector, such as transport, agriculture or housing, to remove or reduce health-damaging policies and promote those that are health-enhancing. The World Health Organization has been encouraging the adoption of an intersectoral approach for about 15 years.

The relevant UK legislation has been discussed earlier in this chapter. European legislation and policies are now having a strong influence.

The European influence

CONTROL OF POLLUTION AND ENVIRONMENTAL HEALTH

The European Community (EC) was founded in 1957 when various European countries signed the Treaty of Rome. One of the fundamental principles in the Treaty was a commitment to improve the living and working conditions of people in Europe. The environmental policies that have been developed have the following aims:

- to keep pollution to a minimum and where possible eliminate it altogether
- to maintain the ecological balance of the environment
- to avoid the exploitation of natural resources
- to pursue economic development within defined quality standards for living
- to plan urban development with environmental issues in mind
- to participate in finding international solutions to environmental problems
- to contribute towards protecting human health

The EC works towards achieving these aims through a combination of legislative measures and provision of funding for environmental research. Over 100 laws relating to environmental issues have been implemented so far. EC member states can be given *directives* through European legislation which are binding as to the results to be achieved. Often, the method that is used to achieve the required outcome is left to the member country to decide, but sometimes *regulations* are also provided which lay down very detailed and specific rules which relate to the implementation of the directives.

It is important that European countries work together on environmental issues in order to control pollution: acid rain and pollution of the North Sea are two examples of where a collaborative approach is required to solve the problem, since pollution travels. In order to reduce pollution and introduce 'environmentally friendly' products, there is a great financial cost to industry when new production processes become necessary. However, if all countries are investing at the same level in clean technologies, there are no unfair advantages in the importing and exporting of goods, and all are contributing equally to a better environment. One example is shown in the car industry where the

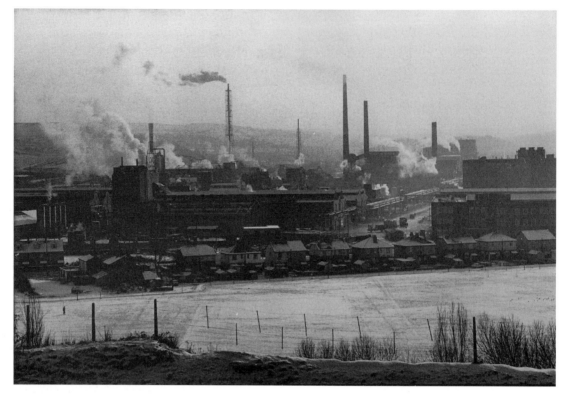

Figure 2.19 Air pollution has been blamed for the increase in respiratory diseases over the last decade

harmonisation of exhaust emissions will mean that eventually one standard will apply to the production of exhaust systems in all parts of Europe.

AIR POLLUTION

Britain is committed to a European climate-change treaty agreed in 1992 to tackle the threat of global warming. We are pledged to stabilise annual emissions of carbon dioxide at their 1990 level by the year 2000. The article below shows that we may have achieved this already without any special laws or policies. However, our future levels of emissions will depend on economic growth and the cost of fuel.

BRITAIN'S CARBON DIOXIDE EMISSIONS FALL BY 3%

Britain's emissions of carbon dioxide, the pollutant that poses the greatest threat of man-made climate change, dropped by 3 per cent last year owing to declining consumption of coal, oil and gas . . .

Britain is committed, under last year's climate change treaty, to stabilise annual emissions of CO_2 at their 1990 level by 2000. Last year's drop, due mainly to the recession, mild weather and a switch from coal-fired to nuclear electricity, shows there is a chance that Britain could hit the target by accident without bringing in any new policies or taxes.

In 1990, emissions stood at 160 million tons and they rose marginally to 161 million in 1991, according to government estimates. These are the most recent Whitehall figures, but it is possible to estimate how much CO_2 was produced last year from fossil fuel consumption figures, which are kept much more up-to-date. Almost all of the CO_2 that is emitted is produced as a result of burning coal, oil and gas.

Last year, emissions fell to 156 million tons, well below the stabilisation target. Government experts project that if energy prices are high and economic growth is low through the 1990s then emissions will have fallen substantially by 2000.

But if energy prices remain low and economic growth is high then the projection is for a 12 per cent increase in emissions by the end of the century – unless new policies are introduced in order to meet Britain's treaty commitment.

Environment experts pointed out that the target for advanced industrial nations to stabilise emissions by 2000 was only agreed because it was reasonably easy to achieve.

Stewart Boyle, Greenpeace's energy director, said: 'It's an extremely modest target. If we are going to avoid fundamentally altering climate while coping with the needs of the Third World then countries like Britain are eventually going to have to curb their emissions by 80 per cent or more.' . . .

(The Independent, 23 March 1993)

HEALTH AND SAFETY AT WORK

In 1989 the European Commission adopted a Community Charter of Fundamental Social Rights known as the 'Social Charter'. This is a formal declaration committing member states to the implementation of certain social rights. The UK was the only one of the 12 member states not to sign, although it does play its part in negotiations on social proposals. Health and safety at work is one of the five areas of social rights that make up the Action Programme to implement the 'Social Charter'. The Charter states that every worker must enjoy satisfactory health and safety conditions in the working environment.

The following aspects of health and safety at work are included in the Action Programme:

• Training and information must be available
• Workers must be consulted about and participate in risk analysis
• Steps must be taken to reduce or eliminate risks

A recent example of European-inspired legislation in the UK is the new health and safety law applying to working with VDU screens.

ACTIVITY 36

Read the following article:

NEW COMPENSATION LAW IS SIGHT FOR SORE EYES

Employees working with computers and word processors who suffer eye problems or headaches which they believe are caused by screen work will, from January 1, be able to claim from their employer the cost of professional eye tests and any special glasses or lenses prescribed as necessary for working with the equipment.

Employers will be able to protect themselves against the cost of employee claims by taking out a new insurance plan launched this week by the National Dental Plan stable. This will cover the cost of eye test fees, reimburse the cost of lenses prescribed by an optician up to £100 a year, and provide a £35 allowance towards the cost of spectacle frames chosen each year.

The cover will cost employers an annual premium of £35 to £55 per employee, depending on the age of the workforce and their concentration on screen work.

The new EC-prompted regulations will require employers to evaluate staff computer work-stations to determine whether they are likely to cause health and safety problems. Any risks must then be reduced. Under the new laws employees will have the right to regular breaks from screen work. In some cases this will mean employers having to change an employee's work practices to reduce their exposure to continual word processor or computer-type work.

Before starting display screen work, staff will be entitled to a professional eye test and then further tests at regular intervals or at any time during their employment if they feel they are suffering eye problems or headaches which could be due to screen work. Employers will have to meet the cost of the tests and any corrective appliances, such as special spectacles, required for work with the equipment...

Employers will also have to provide health safety training and information for users of display screen work-stations...

(The Guardian, 12 December 1992)

1 Summarise what employers will now have to provide for employees who are working at display-screen work stations.

2 How will employers be able to protect themselves against employees' claims?

3 What risks will be reduced as a result of compliance with the new law?

LOCAL AUTHORITY ACTION

Local authorities are required to produce a 'Local Plan' which looks forward over the next 10 to 15 years. This includes policies for housing, factories, shops and offices, the retention of green spaces and historic buildings. It supports development with consideration for the environment, and is mainly concerned with land use and transportation. Litter and waste pollution and recycling are also considered.

ACTIVITY 37

1 Contact the planning department of your local authority and find out about your local plan. If possible, invite a planning officer to your class to discuss the plan. Write a report to summarise the main features.

2 Find out if your local authority has a 'Green Charter'.

EDUCATIONAL PRESSURE GROUPS

There are many educational pressure groups: Friends of the Earth and Greenpeace are two of the most well-known ones. Publicising environmental issues and running campaigns to develop public awareness are their main function. As well as aiming to influence governments, these groups encourage individuals to take their own green action:

• write to MPs, manufacturers and water authorities
• save energy
• cut your car emissions by going more slowly, using unleaded petrol and having your car tuned regularly. The annual MOT now tests emissions
• avoid aerosols
• use fewer harmful household chemicals like detergents
• use public transport or bicycles whenever possible

ACTIVITY 38

1 Divide into small groups, and let each group find out about the activities of one educational pressure group. Prepare a presentation for your class.

2 Monitor the media, and note how environmental issues are reported.

ENERGY POLICIES

The use of non-renewable energy resources, such as fossil fuels, is considered earlier in this chapter. Read through the section on air pollution again.

ACTIVITY 39

Find out about alternative energy sources; nuclear power, wind power and solar power are examples. Prepare an exhibition to show how these could be used to provide energy. Have they been adopted to any great extent? Are there any government policies in the UK or the rest of the world to promote their use?

ASSESSMENT OPPORTUNITY

1 Report on a detailed investigation into human activities designed to reduce harm to the environment and health, which includes:
   - an examination of two specialist treatments
   - a description of one process designed to conserve resources
   - an explanation of three policies for reducing the harmful effects of urbanisation and industrialisation
   - an identification of one strategy for improving the environment

2 Write summary notes explaining advice recommended to safeguard individuals from harmful effects of the environment.

3 Write summary notes on the remaining processes for conserving resources, and on the remaining strategies for improving the environment.

REFERENCES AND RESOURCES

Alcock, P. A. (1986), *Food Hygiene – a Study Guide*, Stanley Thornes Ltd.

CANS Trust, *Citizens Advice Notes Service*, cumulative edition to 1993, London: CANS Trust.

Gee, D., *Health and Safety at Work: a Guide to Hazards and How to Avoid Them*, Cass, B. (ed), London: Thames Television.

Elsom, D. (1987), *Atmospheric Pollution*, Oxford: Blackwell.

Health and Safety Commission (1988), Control of Substances Hazardous to Health Regulations 1988 – Approved Code of Practice, Norwich: HMSO.

Health and Safety Executive (1989), *Health and Safety Law: What You Should Know*, Norwich: HMSO.

Health and Safety Executive (1992), Manual Handling Operations Regulations 1992 – Guidance on Regulations, Norwich: HMSO.

Health and Safety Executive (1989), *Noise at Work*, Norwich: HMSO.

Helman, C. G. (1990), *Culture, Health and Illness*, 2nd edn, Oxford: Butterworth-Heinemann.

Stretch, A. and Southgate, H. (1991), *Food Hygiene, Health and Safety*, London: Pitman Publishing.

Taylor, C. and Press, A. (1991), *Europe and The Environment*, the Industrial Society.

Trickett, J. (1992), *The Prevention of Food Poisoning*, 3rd edn, Cheltenham: Stanley Thornes.

Williams, K. (1991), *A Practical Approach to Caring*, London: Pitman Publishing.

World Health Organization (1992), *Our Planet, Our Health: Report of the WHO Commission on Health and Environment*, Geneva: WHO.

USEFUL ADDRESSES

Friends of the Earth
26–28 Underwood Street
London N1 7JQ

Greenpeace UK
Canonbury Villas
London N1 2PN
Tel. no.: 0171 354 5100

Health and Safety Commission
Rose Court
2 Southwark Bridge
London SE1 9HS
Tel. no.: 0171 717 6000

Health and Safety Executive
Baynards House
1 Chepstow Place
Westbourne Grove
London W2 4TF

HMSO Books Publication Centre
PO Box 276
London SW8 5DT

Institution of Environmental Health Officers
Chadwick House

Rushworth Street
London SE1 0QT

United Kingdom Atomic Energy Authority
11 Charles II Street
London SW1Y 4QP

3

INFLUENCES ON HEALTH AND DISEASE

AN ANALYSIS OF RESEARCH INTO PATTERNS OF DISEASE

The first element of this Unit will give you a basic introduction to *epidemiology*, which can be defined as 'the study of the distribution and determinants of health-related states or events in specified populations, and the application of this study to the control of health problems'. This definition emphasises that epidemiology is concerned not only with disease but also with more positive health states and with ways of improving health.

Methods used to determine patterns of disease

An important aspect of the work carried out by epidemiologists is the study of *patterns of* disease. In other words, both the *incidence* (frequency of occurrence) and the *distribution* (on a local, national or global scale) are investigated. There are a variety of methods which may be used in this research.

DESCRIPTIVE STUDIES

Descriptive studies give a simple description of the health status of a community, and are based either on routinely available data or on data obtained from surveys. They can describe the pattern of a disease by person (e.g. age, sex or ethnicity), by time period or by place. Descriptive studies can be used to generate hypotheses about the outbreak and transmission of a disease.

Table 3.1 presents the results from a descriptive study of hepatitis B in children in central Tunisia, and shows that the prevalence of this disease increases with age.

ANALYTICAL STUDIES

Whereas a descriptive study is limited simply to a description of the occurrence of a disease in a population, an analytical study goes further by looking at *relationships between health status and other variables* – for example, it may be noted that people with a particular disease are more likely to be smokers. Analytical studies identify factors associated with either disease or health, but do not *prove* that these factors are causing a state of either disease or health (see the section on correlation in Thomson et al. 1995, Chapter 8, pp. 407–9). For example, in the case mentioned above it may be that smokers are likely to take less exercise than non-smokers, and that it is that lack of exercise that is causing the disease.

Table 3.1 The prevalence of hepatitis-B markers in the blood of children in central Tunisia, by age

Age group (years)	Prevalence of hepatitis B markers (%)
1–3	7
4–6	16
7–9	21
10–12	24

Source: Said et al. (1985), 'Seroepidemiology of hepatitis B in a population of children in central Tunisia', *International Journal of Epidemiology*, vol. 14, no. 2, pp. 313–17.

ACTIVITY 1

Figure 3.1 shows the relationship found in an analytical study between the occurrence of skin melanoma and latitude. What hypotheses could this data generate?

EXPERIMENTAL STUDIES

Experimental studies follow on from analytical studies, and are carefully designed *to prove an association between a given factor and the occurrence of a disease.* Because the health of people are at risk, there are ethical constraints on the epidemiologist, which other scientists do not have. For example, no patient should be denied appropriate treatment as a result of participation in an experiment, and the treatment tested must be acceptable in the light of current knowledge.

An example of an experimental study is the work done by Mola et al. (1995). A group of patients in Bangladesh with acute watery diarrhoea were randomly given either a glucose-based oral rehydration solution, or a rice-based oral rehydration solution. The study showed the rice-based solution to be more effective.

ACTIVITY 2

Read the account of the occurrence of spina bifida below. Identify the information which comes from:

(a) descriptive studies
(b) analytical studies
(c) experimental studies.

Spina bifida is a disorder in which the spinal cord and backbone of the developing foetus do not form correctly. It has been estimated that in the UK in the late 1980s, it occurred in just under 200 births per year. It is much more common in some areas than others. For example, it is twice as common in Northern

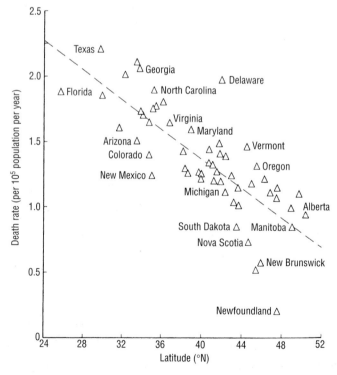

Figure 3.1   The relationship of skin melanoma cancer to latitude in the USA and Canada
Source: Elwood et al. (1974), 'Relationship of melanoma and other skin cancer mortality to latitude and ultraviolet radiation in the United States and Canada', *International Journal of Epidemiology*, 3, 325–32; Environmental Data Report, UNEP 1989, the United Nations Environment Programme.

Ireland as it is in London; and in some areas it is more common in less wealthy families. The babies of mothers who smoke do not seem more prone to having spina bifida. Furthermore, it seems that mothers who have a good, well-balanced diet are less likely to have an affected baby than mothers with a poor diet. If a mother gives birth to an affected baby, her next baby stands a 5% chance of having the disorder. A group of women who were given folic-acid supplements had a lower incidence of babies with spina bifida than a group of women who were given placebos.

THE PURPOSE OF RESEARCH INTO PATTERNS OF DISEASE

The main purposes of epidemiological studies are to reduce the incidence of disease and to assist with strategic health planning.

Reducing the incidence of disease

Before you read further, jot down what you must find out about a disease to reduce its incidence. Probably, your list will include the following:

1 *The cause of the illness.* For example, is there a *pathogen* (a disease-causing organism)? Can it be identified? Is it caused by something present in the diet, or by a dietary deficiency?
2 *The method of transmission.* If a disease is caused by a pathogen, how is it spread? Is it passed on by direct contact or droplets, or is it food- or water-borne? Are there vectors involved?
3 *Identifying at-risk populations.* Which populations are likely to develop the disease? Are socioeconomic factors involved? Are people of one sex, or from a particular age group, particularly susceptible?
4 *Prevention.* Once the three points above have

been understood, steps can be taken towards preventing people from catching the disease. For example, people could avoid contact with infected individuals if the disease is caused by an easily transmitted pathogen, or alter their diet if a dietary factor is responsible.
5 *Cure.* If people can be cured, not only will they be relieved of the symptoms, but this may help to reduce the spread of the disease. Chemicals and pharmaceuticals will be trialled to find if they are effective, and at what doses.
6 *Control of the disease/illness.* It is unlikely that a disease will be completely eradicated (although there are exceptions to this, such as smallpox), so it is important that a disease be kept at the lowest level possible in the populations within which it occurs. Vaccination and health-education programmes are examples of strategies which may be employed (see the 'Public health' section below).

ACTIVITY 3

Find out about the history of the research into *one* of the following diseases:
- Aids
- lung cancer (caused by smoking)
- cholera
- scurvy
- smallpox

Write an account of how the cause, transmission, at-risk populations, prevention and cure (if any) were discovered.

Assisting with strategic health planning

Research into patterns of disease is essential for the long-term planning of health care.

PUBLIC HEALTH

This area is concerned with assessing needs

and trends in the health and disease patterns of *populations* as distinct from individuals. Formerly known as community or social medicine, it includes epidemiology, health promotion, health-service planning and the evaluation and control of communicable diseases and environmental hazards. The following list (taken from Timmreck 1994) gives the seven main uses of epidemiology in public health:

1 *To study the history of disease.*
   • Epidemiology studies the trends of a disease for the prediction of trends
   • The results of epidemiological studies are useful in planning for health services and public health
2 *Community diagnosis.*
   • What are the diseases, conditions, injuries, disorders, disabilities or defects causing illness, health problems or death in a community or region?
3 *To look at risks of individuals as they affect groups or populations.*
   • What are the risk factors, problems, behaviours that affect groups?
   • Groups are studied by doing risk-factor assessments and health-appraisal approaches, e.g. health risk, appraisal, health screening, medical exams, disease assessments etc.
4 *Assessment, evaluation and research.*
   • How well do public health and health services meet the problems and needs of the population or group?
   • Effectiveness; efficiency; quality; quantity; access; availability of services to treat, control or prevent disease, injury, disability or death are studied
5 *Completing the clinical picture.*
   • Identification and diagnostic processes to establish that a condition exists or that a person has a specific disease
   • Cause–effect relationships are determined, e.g. strep throat can cause rheumatic fever
6 *The identification of syndromes.*
   • Helps to establish and set criteria to define syndromes, some examples being: Downs, fetal alcohol, sudden death in infants etc.
7 *To determine the causes and sources of disease.*
   • Epidemiological findings allow for the control, prevention and elimination of the causes of disease, conditions, injury, disability or death

HEALTH PROMOTION

Once the cause and spread of a disease have been understood, and at-risk populations identified (see above), a health-promotion programme can be designed.

ACTIVITY 4

Find educational material produced to help prevent the spread of human immunodeficiency virus (HIV). Which sectors of the population is this information aimed at? On what epidemiological evidence is this based? (In other words, what data can you find to show that these groups are particularly at risk?)

THE EVALUATION OF HEALTH PROGRAMMES

To find out whether a health programme has been effective or not, it is essential that epidemiological information be collected. For example, look at Figure 3.36 which comes under 'immunisation programmes' later in this chapter, and you will see that information has been collected which demonstrates the effectiveness of a measles-immunisation programme. Another example is the information which has been gathered on the drop in cases of Sudden Infant Death Syndrome (cot death) following a health-promotion campaign encouraging parents to put their baby to sleep on its side or back.

ACTIVITY 5

Find other examples of epidemiological information which show whether a particular health programme has been effective.

SOURCES OF INFORMATION FOR DETERMINING PATTERNS OF DISEASE

There is a wide range of sources of information available for students and health professionals. (See the list of addresses at the end of the chapter from which the information described below can be obtained.)

Government statistics

The Office of Population Censuses and Surveys (OPCS) produces national, regional and local annual medical and population tables published in separate topic-oriented volumes on: family statistics, deaths, morbidity (disease, injury, disability), population estimates and projections, births, cancer, communicable diseases, congenital malformations, demographic reviews, general household surveys, the workforce, longitudinal studies, marriage and divorce, abortion statistics, migration, local-authority vital statistics and electoral statistics. The information gathered by the OPCS comes from a variety of sources:

1 *Registration.* Records of births, deaths and marriages are collected in this way. At birth, the only information collected about a baby is its name, sex, place and date of birth (other information refers to the baby's parents). In death registration, more information is gathered. The age and occupation of the dead person and where they lived are recorded, as well as the cause of death. This information usually comes from a death certificate completed by a doctor.

2 *Surveys of the population.* The census is the only survey which samples every member of the population. This survey is completed every 10 years in the UK. The head of the household is asked for information about everyone in the house on one particular day. Usually, however, only a representative sample of the population is taken. For example, the annual General Household Survey collects data from a number of families who fill in an extensive questionnaire. The annual Health Survey for England, which was first conducted in 1991, involves both an interview, which includes a self-assessment of general health as well as questions about lifestyle, and a medical examination in which blood pressure and body size (height, weight, waist and hip) are measured and a blood sample is taken.

3 *Special notification.* For example, data is gathered from certificates for sickness and notifiable diseases, and from hospital records of patients.

Reports

The Department of Health produces the following reports which give national, regional and local information:

- *The Health Service in England* (annual report)
- *On the State of the Public Health* (the annual report of the Chief Medical Officer of the Department of Health)
- *Health and Personal Social Services Statistics for England*

Non-governmental organisations such as cancer societies and heart foundations also publish useful statistics and reports.

World Health Organization statistics

Various World Health Organization (WHO) publications contain useful epidemiological information, for example *World Health Statistics Quarterly* and the *Bulletin of the World Health Organization* which is published bi-monthly.

Further information on these and other WHO publications can be obtained from the address shown at the end of this chapter.

Epidemiological studies

There are a number of journals with a focus on epidemiological studies, such as the *International Journal of Epidemiology* and the *Journal of Epidemiology and Community Health* (see the list of useful addresses at the end of this chapter for details). Mainstream medical and health journals also publish an increasing number of articles with an epidemiological content.

THE EXAMINATION OF SPECIFIC DISEASES AT A LOCAL, NATIONAL AND WORLDWIDE LEVEL

ACTIVITY 6

If you are working as part of a group of students, you may wish to choose one of the diseases listed below, read the information given, complete the relevant activities and then give a presentation to the remainder of the group to enable your findings to be shared.

Skin cancer

Variations in the incidence and distribution of skin cancer can be seen on a worldwide level. In Caucasian populations, it is one of the most common cancers. Worldwide, about 10,000 people die from skin cancer each year. During the last few decades the global incidence of melanoma (one of the most serious cancers with respect to fatal outcomes) has steadily been increasing. Figures to demonstrate this can be found in the United Nations Environment Programme's (UNEP's) *Environmental Data Report* which is compiled biennially. These figures also show the variation from one country to another. In Australia, for example, age-standardised death rates from melanoma in both sexes have risen by a factor of over 5 in the past 50 years. In other countries, melanoma rates are rising at the rate of 3–7% per year.

Epidemiological studies have demonstrated a link between skin melanoma and exposure to ultraviolet radiation. In Australia, North America and most European countries, an inverse relationship exists between melanoma incidence and latitude (see again Figure 3.1).

Within countries, there are *regional* variations in the incidence of skin cancer. For example, it has been shown that the death rate from this disease is significantly higher in the *south* of the UK – a reversal of the usual pattern for cancer deaths.

ACTIVITY 7

Find figures to produce tables or maps to illustrate the variation in the incidence of skin cancers from country to country; and from region to region within the UK. Can you find any variation between the incidence in males and in females? Which occupations do you think may be associated with an increased risk of skin cancer?

Lung cancer

Lung cancer also shows considerable variations in both space and time. Table 3.2

Table 3.2   The incidence of lung cancer worldwide around 1980 (crude rate per 10^5 of the population)

	Male	Female
Africa	3.1	0.8
America	40.7	15.6
Asia	10.0	3.7
Europe	76.4	13.7
Australia/New Zealand	61.6	15.9
Developed regions	65.3	16.3
Developing regions	9.2	3.1
World	23.0	6.6

Source: Environmental Data Report, UNEP 1989, the United Nations Environment Programme.

shows that the incidence is higher in developed than in developing countries. Globally, lung cancer has shown a progressive increase since 1975 (about 0.5% per year for the world as a whole). However, in some groups it is now decreasing.

ACTIVITY 8

1 Study Figure 3.2, and identify the groups in which mortality from lung cancer is decreasing.

2 Find figures to show the regional variations in the incidence of lung cancer within the UK.

3 Would you predict that the incidence of lung cancer is higher in rural or urban areas?

Coronary heart disease

Coronary heart disease is a major cause of death in both developed and developing countries. However, mortality rates for this disease are decreasing in the former (see Figure 3.3) and increasing in the latter (see Figure 3.4). The WHO coordinated a major international collaborative study called Project MONICA (Multilateral Monitoring of Trends and Determinants in Cardiovascular Disease)

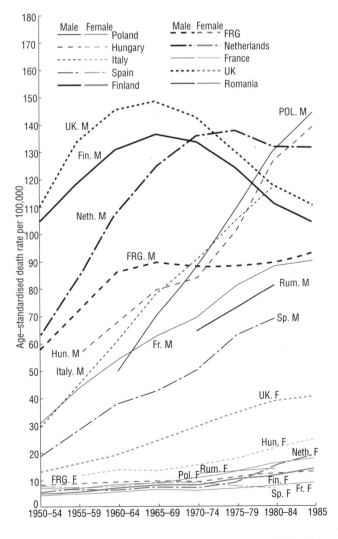

Figure 3.2 Trends in mortality from lung cancer in the European region, 1950–85
Source: WHO, *The World Environment 1972–1992*, the United Nations Environment Programme.

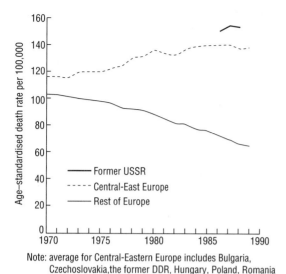

Note: average for Central-Eastern Europe includes Bulgaria, Czechoslovakia, the former DDR, Hungary, Poland, Romania and former Yugoslavia

Figure 3.3 Subregional trends in cardiovascular mortality in the age range 0–64 years, 1970–90
Source: WHO, *The World Environment 1972–1992,* the United Nations Environment Programme.

Table 3.3 Age-standardised mortality rates (per 100,000) in the 30–69-year age group, for coronary heart disease

	Coronary heart disease	
	Men	Women
Northern Ireland	406	130
Scotland	398	142
Finland	390	79
Czechoslovakia	346	101
England and Wales	318	94
New Zealand	296	94
Australia	247	76
United States of America	235	80
Poland	230	54
Greece	135	33
Portugal	104	32
France	94	20
Japan	38	13

Reproduced, by permission of WHO, from: Uemura, K and Pisa, Z, Trends in cardiovascular disease mortality in industrialized countries since 1950, *World Health Statistics Quarterly,* 1988, **41** (3/4), 155–78.

which, over a 10-year period (1984–93), measured trends in cardiovascular events, focusing partly on fatal and non-fatal heart attacks. Table 3.3, which shows the large variations in mortality rates for coronary heart disease over a number of countries, also demonstrates the great difference between the incidence in men and women.

Research has shown that within a locality, there is a far higher mortality rate from

coronary heart disease amongst people from the lower social classes. Even when the figures are adjusted to make allowances for other factors which increase risk, such as smoking and high levels of cholesterol and blood sugar, there is still an excess mortality, in the lowest grades, of almost 40%.

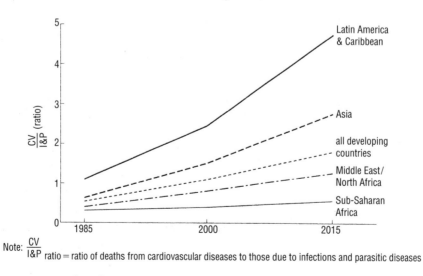

Note: $\frac{CV}{I\&P}$ ratio = ratio of deaths from cardiovascular diseases to those due to infections and parasitic diseases

Figure 3.4 The emergence of cardiovascular diseases in the cause-of-death structure in developing countries, 1985–2015
Source: WHO, *The World Environment 1972–1992,* the United Nations Environment Programme.

Table 3.4 Standardised mortality ratios (SMRs) for coronary heart disease by regional health authority (RHA) in England and Wales, 1989, and by health board in Scotland, 1980–85

England and Wales, RHA	SMR	Scotland, health board	SMR
Oxford	83	Lothian	92
South-east Thames	84	Borders	92
East Anglia	85	Grampian	93
North-west Thames	85	The Islands	94
North-east Thames	87	Tayside	96
Wessex	88	Highland	98
South Western	99	Forth Valley	98
West Midlands	106	Greater Glasgow	100
Wales	107	Fife	102
Trent	108	Dumfries and Galloway	105
Mersey	114	Ayr and Arran	108
Yorkshire	114	Argyle and Clyde	108
North Western	121	Lanarkshire	113
Northern	123		

Source: Thomson et al. 1995.

ACTIVITY 9

Look at Table 3.4 and describe the main trends in the regional differences in the incidence of coronary heart disease within the UK.

Tuberculosis

There has been an overall decline in the number of cases of, and therefore deaths from, tuberculosis (TB) over the last few decades, both globally (see Figure 3.5) and within the UK (see Figure 3.6). However, it is possible that there could now be a resurgence, partly related to the Aids epidemic. For example, in Africa, TB has already become the leading cause of death in adults with HIV.

ACTIVITY 10

Find figures to show the variation in the incidence of TB between:

(a) different countries
(b) different regions of the UK.

HIV infection

Figure 3.7 shows the global distribution of cumulative adult HIV infections. At least 80% of cases of Aids/HIV are in the developing

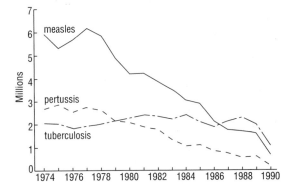

Figure 3.5 Global annual reported cases of pertussis, tuberculosis and measles, 1974–90 (provisional date only for 1990)
Source: WHO, *The World Environment 1972–1992,* the United Nations Environment Programme.

world, but the disease is still showing an alarming increase in both developed and developing countries (see Figure 3.8).

There are pronounced differences in the incidence of the disease in different regions of the UK. For example, between 1982 and 1992, over 70% of all diagnoses of Aids occurred in one of the four regional health authorities covering London and the South East, a proportion far in excess of the population covered by these health authorities. (An explanation for this may be that some of these people moved to London from other areas of the UK to obtain treatment, and perhaps also to get more help from support organisations.)

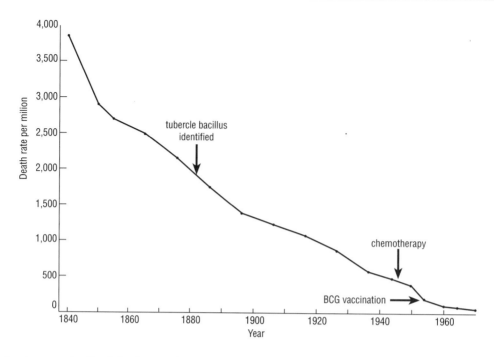

Figure 3.6   Age-standardised death rates from tuberculosis in England and Wales, 1840–1968
Source: Beaglehole et al. 1993; originally appeared in *The Role of Medicine: Dream Mirage or Nemesis?*,
T. McKeown, Nuffield Provincial Hospitals Trust, 1976.

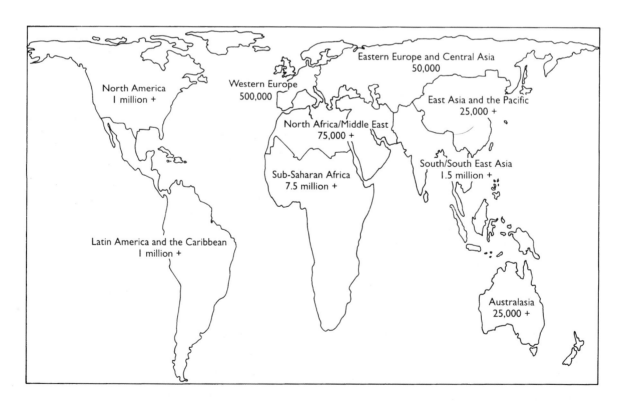

Figure 3.7   Estimated cumulative adult HIV infections, end 1992
Source: Thomson et al., 1995.

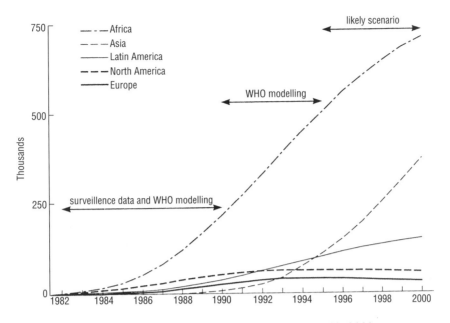

Figure 3.8   An estimated and projected incidence of Aids by region, 1982–2000
SSource: WHO, *The World Environment 1972–1992*, the United Nations Environment Programme.

ACTIVITY 11

1 Study Figure 3.7. Draw a bar graph or pie chart to show the distribution of HIV infections.

2 Aids is a *pandemic* disease. What does this mean?

3 Find out about the male–female differences in the incidence of HIV/Aids.

Malaria

The global total of malaria cases has been relatively stable over the last decade (about 270 million people are infected with the disease). However, the problems with this disease are largely local, with important epidemic outbreaks – 'hot spots' – contributing to the high incidence of illness and death in specific situations (see Figure 3.9).

It might be thought that in the UK malaria is not a problem, but in 1992 the Public Health Laboratory Service warned that with global warming, malaria could become a

hazard in blood transfusion, and urged a surveillance of mosquito populations around international airports. In the past, there have been cases of people in the vicinity of UK airports becoming infected with malaria from mosquitoes that had escaped from 'planes. There have also been brief epidemics, notably after the Second World War as servicemen returned with the parasite.

ACTIVITY 12

On a map of the world, shade in those countries to which a visit necessitates the use of drugs for the prevention of malaria.

Salmonella food poisoning

Read the section 'Bacterial food poisoning' on pp. 142–145 below, and you will note that outbreaks of salmonella food poisoning are of a very local nature. Many cases of food poisoning go unreported, but the symptoms associated with salmonella are serious, and therefore likely to be reported.

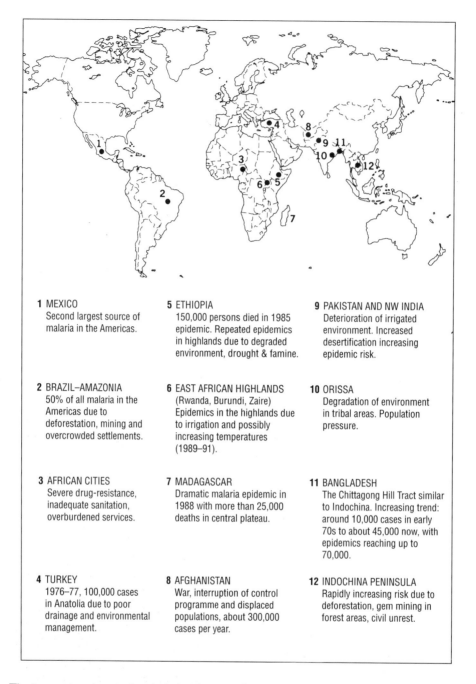

1 MEXICO
Second largest source of
malaria in the Americas.

2 BRAZIL–AMAZONIA
50% of all malaria in the
Americas due to
deforestation, mining and
overcrowded settlements.

3 AFRICAN CITIES
Severe drug-resistance,
inadequate sanitation,
overburdened services.

4 TURKEY
1976–77, 100,000 cases
in Anatolia due to poor
drainage and environmental
management.

5 ETHIOPIA
150,000 persons died in 1985
epidemic. Repeated epidemics
in highlands due to degraded
environment, drought & famine.

6 EAST AFRICAN HIGHLANDS
(Rwanda, Burundi, Zaire)
Epidemics in the highlands due
to irrigation and possibly
increasing temperatures
(1989–91).

7 MADAGASCAR
Dramatic malaria epidemic in
1988 with more than 25,000
deaths in central plateau.

8 AFGHANISTAN
War, interruption of control
programme and displaced
populations, about 300,000
cases per year.

9 PAKISTAN AND NW INDIA
Deterioration of irrigated
environment. Increased
desertification increasing
epidemic risk.

10 ORISSA
Degradation of environment
in tribal areas. Population
pressure.

11 BANGLADESH
The Chittagong Hill Tract similar
to Indochina. Increasing trend:
around 10,000 cases in early
70s to about 45,000 now, with
epidemics reaching up to
70,000.

12 INDOCHINA PENINSULA
Rapidly increasing risk due to
deforestation, gem mining in
forest areas, civil unrest.

Figure 3.9   The increasing threat of malaria incidence in frontier areas of development
Source: WHO, *The World Environment 1972–1992*, the United Nations Environment Programme.

ACTIVITY 13

Find out about recent outbreaks of
salmonella in your area. What was the
source of the contamination? How many
people were affected?

Cholera

See the 'Diarrhoeal diseases' section on p.142
below for examples of both cholera epidemics
and endemic cholera. More than 95% of cases
are reported from Asia and Africa, and trends
for these regions are shown in Figure 3.10.

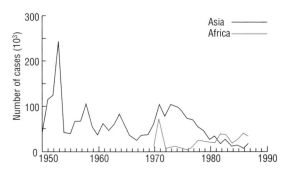

Figure 3.10 Cholera cases reported to the World Health Organization since 1950
Source: WHO, *Environmental Data Report, UNEP 1989,* the United Nations Environment Programme.

ACTIVITY 14

1 Cholera is no longer present in the UK, but the research by John Snow in the 1850s on an outbreak in London was one of the most important contributions to epidemiology. Find an account of his work and read it to see how his methodology is still of use today.

2 What is meant by the terms:
 (a) epidemic
 (b) endemic?

THE RANGE OF INFLUENCES ON PATTERNS OF DISEASE

There are obviously a large number of factors which influence both the incidence and distribution of diseases. Some of these influences are dealt with in the section below on the role of socioeconomic factors, so this should be read in conjunction with the following information.

Developed countries compared with undeveloped countries

The causes of death differ dramatically between developed and undeveloped (or developing)

countries. Infectious and parasitic diseases are by far the leading cause of death in undeveloped countries, while cardiovascular diseases are the leading cause of death in developed countries (see Figure 3.11).

In undeveloped countries, the commonest diseases are water related: 80% of all illness is attributed to unsafe and inadequate water supplies, and half the hospital beds are occupied by people with water-related illnesses. Diarrhoeal disease is the leading cause of infant and childhood deaths. Diseases for which the immunisation programme has expanded – for example, poliomyelitis, tetanus, measles and tuberculosis – are now declining. HIV infection and Aids, however, is showing an alarming increase, particularly in sub-Saharan Africa.

In all countries, nutrition and health are closely related. In poorer regions of undeveloped countries, undernutrition is a major factor in increasing vulnerability to infectious and parasitic diseases. By contrast, in developed countries, obesity and high intakes of saturated animal fats are believed to be linked to the high incidence of cardiovascular disease.

ACTIVITY 15

1 Find out about the different criteria which may be used to classify a country as 'developed' or 'undeveloped', 'developing' or 'Third World'.
 On a map of the world, indicate which countries are considered to be developed and which undeveloped.
2 Cancer rates within developed and undeveloped countries differ, as Figure 3.12 shows. Explain these differences for
 (a) lung cancer
 (b) cancer of the cervix.

Temperate zones compared with tropical zones

Many of the so-called 'tropical diseases' have a

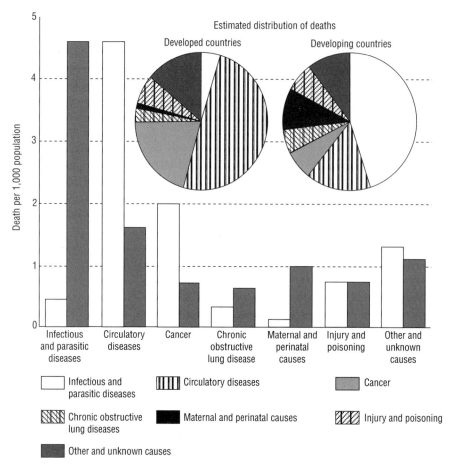

Figure 3.11 Causes of death in developed countries (left-hand bars and pie diagram) and developing countries (right-hand bars and pie diagram) 1985
Source: WHO, *The World Environment 1972–1992*, the United Nations Environment Programme.

higher incidence in tropical areas compared with temperate areas because of increased poverty rather than differences in climate. However, it is also true that some of the *vectors* and *pathogens* (disease-causing agents) involved can only survive in warmer conditions. For this reason, some scientists believe that the greenhouse effect could trigger new epidemics of tropical diseases in regions which are presently free of them (see Table 3.5).

ACTIVITY 16

Which diseases and illnesses do you think may have a higher incidence in temperate countries than in tropical countries?

Environmental factors

The climate (as seen above) is one example of an environmental factor which has an influence on the incidence and distribution of diseases, but there are many other environmental factors which have such an effect. Some of these are listed below.

THE SETTING

There is a description above of how the different settings of either a developed or undeveloped country affect the types of disease which are prevalent. The pattern of disease distribution can also, however, be affected by whether the setting is *urban* or *rural*. It has been demonstrated that, both globally and within the UK, there is a higher death rate in an urban environment than in a rural

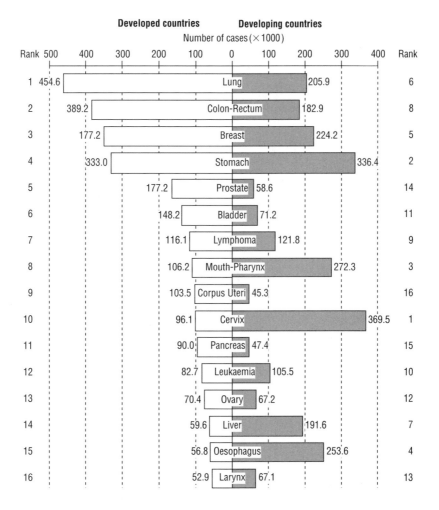

Figure 3.12 The number of new cancer cases by type in developed and undeveloped countries, 1980
Source: Parkin et al., 1988, *The World Environment 1972–1992*, the United Nations Environment Programme.

Table 3.5 Climatic change: the potential effects on disease

	Distribution	Prevalence of infection	At risk of infection	Climate change spread risk
Malaria	100 countries	170 million	2,100 million	Highly likely
Schistosomiasis (Snail fever)	74 countries	200 million	600 million	Very likely
Lymphatic filariasis (Elephantiasis)	Global, except for Europe	90.2 million	900 million	Likely
Leishmaniasis (Oriental sore)	80 countries	12 million	350 million	Unpredictable
Dracunculiasis (Guinea-worm disease	Sub-Saharan Africa, India, Pakistan	Under 3 million	140 million	Unlikely
Onchocerciasis (River blindness)	Africa and Latin America	17.5 million	85.5 million	Likely
African trypanosomiasis (Sleeping sickness)	36 countries in Sub-Saharan Africa	25,000 new cases a year	50 million	Likely

Source: WHO, *The World Environment 1972–1992*, the United Nations Environment Programme.

one. The reasons for this vary. It is thought that the increased level of *pollution* (see below) associated with towns may be responsible, but there are also other factors, such as the higher prevalence of smoking in these areas, which may have an effect.

THE GEOGRAPHICAL LOCATION

Many geographical factors influence patterns of disease. For example, if a disease is spread by a vector, there may be specific features that the vector will require. The mosquito which spreads malaria, for example, has to have access to a body of water for the insect to breed.

The *geological structure* may also have an effect on health. In parts of the UK in which houses are built over granite, there are high levels of radon gas which can cause lung cancer.

POLLUTION

Both at work and in the wider environment, pollution is a factor which is linked to health. In the past two decades, there has been an improvement in air quality in the urban environment of developed countries but a decline in the urban environment of undeveloped countries, and an increase in ozone levels in rural areas. Pollution by fertilisers, pesticides and industrial waste is a problem throughout the world (see pp. 75–90).

Sometimes it may be very difficult to prove a link between an environmental factor and disease. For example, in the UK it has been established that deaths from cardiovascular disease are partly associated with 'soft' water (water containing low concentrations of calcium salts). However, it is not known whether there is any causal significance in this. There is much controversy over whether there is a higher level of diseases such as leukaemia in communities living around a nuclear power station.

ACTIVITY 17

Look back at the patterns of both the distribution and incidence of the diseases mentioned in the above sections on specific diseases (i.e. skin cancer, lung cancer, coronary heart disease, tuberculosis, HIV infection, malaria, salmonella food poisoning and cholera). Now explain these patterns on the basis of environmental and geographical factors. (NB: this Activity can form the basis of the report for the 'Evidence indicators' assignment below.)

ASSESSMENT OPPORTUNITY

1 Prepare and give a *presentation* of research analysis on patterns of disease which:
* describes the patterns of *three* specific diseases, one of which should occur worldwide
* describes the sources and methods which have been used to gather the information
* summarises the way this research could be used in reducing the incidence of disease and assisting with strategic health planning

2 Produce a *report* which explains how patterns of disease are influenced by environmental and geographical factors at local, national and worldwide levels.

CAUSES AND CONTROLLING FACTORS IN HEALTH AND DISEASE

What is health?

The World Health Organization defines health as 'a state of complete physical, mental and social well-being and not merely the absence of disease or infirmity'.

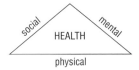

Figure 3.13 The three aspects of health

A person can be described as healthy provided the three sides – social, mental, physical – of the triangle (see Figure 3.13) remain intact. If the natural equilibrium is damaged, then a state of ill-health (albeit often only temporary) results.

Causes of disease and illness

Diseases and illnesses may be classified according to their cause. The following categories are often used:

INFECTIOUS

Infectious diseases are the leading cause of global mortality and debility, accounting for approximately one-third of all deaths and more than two-thirds of child deaths. Together with malnutrition, infectious diseases are largely responsible for the differential in infant mortality rates and life-expectancies between developed and developing countries (UNEP 1989).

Infectious diseases are caused by *pathogens*. These organisms are *parasites*, i.e. they are dependent on a live host for food and shelter. *Ectoparasites* live on the skin, while *endoparasites* are internal. Types of parasites are:

* viruses
* bacteria
* fungi
* protozoa
* worms (platyheliminthes, nematodes)

VIRUSES

Viruses are, on average, about 50 times smaller than bacteria. They cannot be seen with a light microscope, and can only reproduce inside the living cell of a host. Viruses have a very simple, non-cellular structure. They contain a core of DNA or RNA surrounded by a protein coat.

ACTIVITY 18

1 The tapeworm and the liver fluke are parasites. What other examples can you think of?

2 Viruses are considered to be on the border between living and non-living. Which characteristics of living organisms do they possess, and which do they not possess?

3 List any viral diseases you can think of. How are these diseases spread?

The influenza virus

Four strains are known: A, B, C and D. Strains C and D are stable, whereas variants of strain A are very common, and strain B is rare. Influenza epidemics break out frequently, affecting large numbers of people in a particular place. Sometimes the outbreaks are *pandemic*: they spread across continents. A serious pandemic outbreak occurred in 1918, when 20 million people died worldwide. This was caused by an A strain. Another strain of the A virus caused a pandemic in 1957–8; this was known as Asian 'flu. A similar outbreak happened in 1968, infecting about a quarter of the population in the UK, and killing 1,000 people. Nationwide epidemics of influenza caused by the A strain occur every two to three years, while B strains have a four- to six-year cycle.

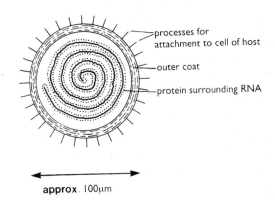

Figure 3.14 An influenza virus
Source: Thomson et al., 1995.

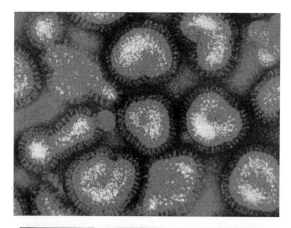

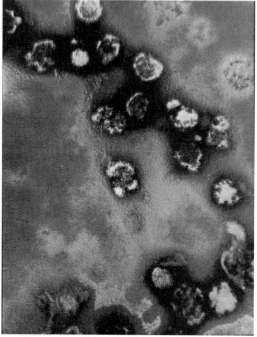

Figure 3.15 Photomicrographs of disease-causing viruses: (a) influenza and (b) rubella

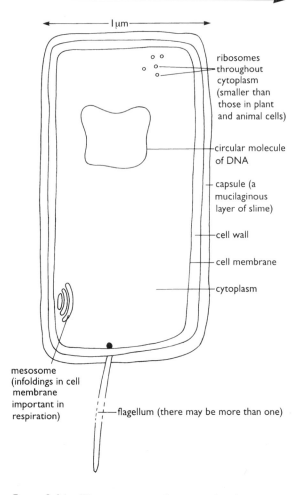

├ 1 μm ┤

ribosomes throughout cytoplasm (smaller than those in plant and animal cells)

circular molecule of DNA

capsule (a mucilaginous layer of slime)

cell wall

cell membrane

cytoplasm

mesosome (infoldings in cell membrane important in respiration)

flagellum (there may be more than one)

Figure 3.16   The structure of a generalised bacterium
Source: Thomson et al., 1995.

BACTERIA

Bacteria are the smallest organisms which have a cellular structure (see Figure 3.16). They can be found in many environments, including in and on humans.

ACTIVITY 19

1 Study Figure 3.16. Construct a table to compare the structure of this cell with that of a generalised human cell.

2 If a single bacterium is placed into a fresh medium, and divisions take place every 20 minutes, how many bacteria will there be after 10 hours? You may be surprised by the answer!

The virus enters the respiratory tract in droplets, and attacks the epithelial cells lining the air passages. There is an incubation period of two to three days. Then the symptoms appear. The temperature rises to 40 °C on the first day, and this is accompanied by shivering, headache, sore throat and nasal congestion. Aches in limbs are common. After three to four days the temperature will fall, but a cough may develop due to damage of the trachea and bronchioles. Sometimes pathogenic bacteria invade the damaged air passages and cause bronchitis or pneumonia.

Shape	Example	Disease caused	Shape	Example	Disease caused
spherical (cocci) single			**rod-shaped (baccilli)** single	Escherichia coli	gut symbiont
chains	Streptococcus pyrogens	scarlet fever	chains	Bacillus anthracis	anthrax
clumps	Staphylococcus aureus	boils Pneumonia	flagellate	Salmonella typhi	typhoid fever
pairs in a capsule	Diplococcus pneumoniae	Pneumonia	**spiral-shaped (spirillum)**	Treponemia pallidum	syphilis
pairs	Neisseria gonorrhoea	gonorrhoea	**comma- shaped (vibro)**	Vibrio cholerae	cholera

Figure 3.17   Forms of bacteria
Source: Thomson et al., 1995.

Figure 3.17 shows the four main bacterial shapes.

If conditions (e.g. temperature, nutrient availability, pH (acidity) and oxygen availability) are suitable, bacteria reproduce by dividing into two identical daughter cells (binary fission). This may happen every 20 minutes, which means huge numbers may be formed.

ACTIVITY 20

Experiment to investigate the effect of temperature on bacterial growth.

You will need five petri dishes of nutrient agar.

1 Leave the petri dishes uncovered in the laboratory for about 30 minutes.

2 Replace the lids and treat as follows:
   Plate 1:   Leave at room temperature (20–25 °C)
   Plate 2:   Leave in a refrigerator (3–5 °C)
   Plate 3:   Leave in the freezing compartment of a refrigerator (below 0 °C)
   Plate 4:   Leave in an incubator (37 °C)

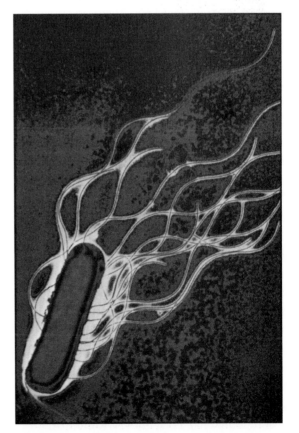

Figure 3.18   A photomicrograph of disease-causing bacteria

Plate 5:   Heat in a hot oven or place in
           a pressure cooker for 15
           minutes (121 °C+) and then
           at room temperature
           (20–25 °C)
Label each plate.

3 After two to three days, tape the two
  halves of each plate together for safety
  reasons, and then examine. Make a table
  to show your observations.

4 To dispose of the plates safely, place in a
  disposable autoclave bag and autoclave
  for 15 minutes.

• At what temperature did bacteria grow
  quickest?
• What implications do your results have
  for food storage?

DIARRHOEAL DISEASES

Cholera affected many Latin American countries
in 1991, the first such epidemic in the region this
century. It had been assumed that improvements
in water, sanitation, sewage treatment and food
safety had eliminated this disease just as it had in
Europe and North America in the late
nineteenth and early twentieth century, when
large-scale cholera epidemics in major cities had
helped spur major investment in improving water
supplies and installing sewers.

   The epidemic first appeared in Peru in January
1991, and by the end of the year more than
276,000 cases and 2,664 deaths from cholera had
been reported. At the same time, 39,154 cases
and 606 deaths had been reported in Ecuador,
and cases were also reported in other Latin
American countries, plus 24 imported cases in
the USA.

   Cholera remains a serious problem in many
African and Asian countries. It is endemic in India
and Indonesia and has been reported in Iraq,
although the number of cases and number of
deaths at mid-July 1991 were relatively low; for
all of Asia 6,700 cases were reported, with 68
deaths. Cholera was also reported in many

African countries. In 1991 a total of 134,953
cases were reported in 19 of these countries,
with 12,618 deaths. The actual numbers of cases
of cholera will be substantially higher than the
number reported in these countries, since no
figures are available from other countries in the
region known to have been hit by the epidemic.

*(World Health Organization, provisional figures,
1991, in* Our Planet, Our Health, *WHO 1992)*

Cholera is one of the more severe diarrhoeal
diseases. Five million lives, mainly those of
children, are lost each year through diarrhoea.
Most of these deaths result from acute
dehydration, and can be prevented by
treatment with oral rehydration salts (ORS).
In 1986, an estimated 59% of the population
had access to ORS, and it is estimated that this
may have prevented some 700,000 diarrhoea-
related deaths (UNEP 1992).

ACTIVITY 21

Study the extract from the WHO
publication on cholera.
• What type of micro-organism causes
  cholera?
• How is it spread?

ACTIVITY 22

What can be concluded from Figure 3.19,
which records the distribution of
rehydration salts in 1982–86?

BACTERIAL FOOD POISONING

Serious diseases such as cholera, typhoid and
dysentery may be caused by contaminated
food or water. They have very specific
symptoms, and a long incubation period.
They are very dangerous, and can be
described as food poisoning, but they are
most commonly referred to by their actual
names. The term 'food poisoning' is used to
describe acute attacks of an explosive nature.

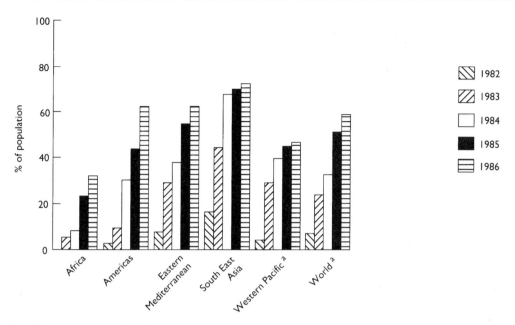

Figure 3.19   The proportion of world populations with access to oral rehydration salts, by WHO region, 1982–86
Source: Martinez et al. (1988), 'Control of diarrhoeal diseases', *World Health Statistics Quarterly*, vol. 41, no. 2, pp. 74–81.

Abdominal pain, diarrhoea and vomiting are associated with food-poisoning episodes, and these symptoms usually arise between two and thirty-six hours after eating contaminated food.

Food-poisoning bacteria divide very rapidly in conditions which are favourable to their growth. These include a warm temperature, humidity and a good food supply. Most bacteria usually require oxygen, but some, on the other hand, can only multiply when oxygen is absent: this latter condition is described as 'anaerobic'. The bacterium *Clostridium welchii* (*perfringens*) is a common cause of food poisoning. This is a bacterial organism which is also the most common cause of *gas gangrene* (the breakdown of skin and muscle tissue by toxins and gas production). The organism is resistant to heat, and may survive in pre-cooked foods, such as stews and pies, which are not correctly stored.

Some food-poisoning bacteria produce heat-resistant spores. These form when conditions are unfavourable for growth. They survive heat treatment, then start to grow again when favourable conditions return. Some food-poisoning organisms produce

toxins, which can be very dangerous, for example *Clostridium botulinum*.

In order to investigate food poisoning, typhoid and cholera, carry out the class research exercise described below.

ACTIVITY 23

Divide your class into five groups. Each group should investigate a different food-poisoning organism(s) and will produce a display and a short presentation. Use the information provided and other sources obtained from the library or other centre.

Group 1   salmonella organisms
Group 2   *Staphylococci*
              Streptococci
Group 3   *Clostridium welchii* (*perfringens*)
Group 4   typhoid
              cholera
Group 5   listeria
              Bacillus cereus
              hepatitis-A

You should consider the following aspects:

1 General characteristics of the organism.
Different types.

2 Toxins produced?
Spore-bearing?

3 How is the organism spread?
Type of food involved?

4 What are the symptoms of the attack?
How long do they take to appear?
How long do they last?

5 Precautions and treatment.

6 Any other features of interest.
How common?
Recent outbreaks? Investigate these.

Study Table 3.6 and then read the following case studies. Answer the questions that relate to each case study.

Case Study 1: the steak and kidney pie

A person suffered from severe food poisoning for 24 hours, the symptoms arising 10 hours after eating a steak and kidney pie.

1 What organism caused the bout of illness?
2 Discuss the possible origin of the organism and factors which may have led to the

contamination of the pie with enough bacteria to cause an infection.

Case Study 2: the duck egg mousse

Several people in a hotel suffered from food poisoning for a week after eating mousse made with duck eggs.

1 What was the likely cause of the illness?
2 Discuss factors which could have lead to the outbreak.

Case Study 3: the shepherd's pie

An outbreak of food poisoning occurred among schoolchildren after eating shepherd's pie made in the school. A cook was later found to have a very septic finger.

1 What could have been the organism which caused the outbreak?
2 How could the bacteria have entered the pie?

Case Study 4: Scout camp

The following is an account of a food-poisoning outbreak at a Scout camp.

Some meat pies were bought during the first day to be eaten that evening. By the next morning, 21 of the 27 Scouts at the camp showed symptoms of headaches, fever, vomiting and abdominal pain. Many of these Scouts were ill for the first week of the camp.

Table 3.6 Food-poisoning organisms

Causative organism	Foods usually implicated	Incubation period	Duration of illness
Salmonella	Cooked meats, meat, poultry, eggs, warmed up meat pies, ice cream, shellfish	12–24 hours	1–8 days
Clostridium welchii (perfringens)	Joints and poultry reheated, large joints, gravy, stews, meat pies	8–18 hours	12–24 hours
Staphylococci	Custard, reheated meat, ice cream, poorly canned food	2–6 hours	6–24 days
Clostridium botulinum	Poorly processed food, meat paste, fish	24–72 hours	Death in 8 days or a prolonged illness

Source: Thomson et al., 1994.

Latrines were dug for sanitation but rain flooded them for several days. Water for the camp was obtained from a nearby stream. For the whole three-week period of the camp, there were always further invalids suffering from the same symptoms as the first Scouts that were ill.

1 Identify the organism that caused the illness.
2 What conclusions can be drawn about the spread of the disease from one person to another from the evidence in the case history outlined above?
3 Why are meat pies more likely to cause food poisoning than lamb chops?

Case Study 5: school canteen
In a school canteen, large joints of beef (6–8 lb) were boiled for two hours in a large modern boiler. After removal from the boiler, the joints remained covered in the kitchen overnight, left to cool down. This meat was served for lunch the next day (9–12 hours later). Large numbers of children were subsequently ill with abdominal pain and diarrhoea. Some meat was left over; when tested it was found to contain the sporing bacterium *Clostridium welchii*.

1 Suggest how the meat became contaminated.
2 What factors in the treatment of the meat could have led to enough bacteria cells to cause an outbreak of food poisoning to be present in the meat?

Case Study 6: salmonellosis from imitation cream
For many years, outbreaks of salmonellosis were traced to imitation cream. Yet, when the cream arrived at the bakery in cans from the manufacturer, it was quite clean and bacteriologically safe. All food in the bakery was tested, and the only material found to be contaminated was imported bulk egg from China. This was found to contain salmonella organisms which were the same as those isolated from the faeces of patients with salmonellosis. Yet this egg product was not used in the manufacture of imitation cream.

How do you account for the fact that the imitation cream contained salmonella?

Case Study 7: typhoid outbreak – Aberdeen 1964
Over a three-week period, 400 people in Aberdeen caught typhoid. The investigation by the public health inspector and his staff tracked down the origin of the outbreak as follows.

All typhoid sufferers had eaten cold cooked meat which had been purchased from the same small supermarket in Aberdeen. The investigation was hampered by the fact that typhoid has a two-week incubation period, and that the sufferers had eaten two types of cold meat. There was not one type of meat which was immediately suspect. The origins of all cold meats involved were traced. Some corned beef from a certain cannery in the Argentine became suspect. This cannery had been traced as a source of contaminated ox-tongue which caused a smaller outbreak of typhoid in Britain in 1954. It was discovered then that the water from the river De La Plata was used for cooling cans of the tongue. The river had untreated sewage discharged into it and contained typhoid bacilli of the same type that caused the outbreak in the UK. It was postulated in 1954 that there must have been a tiny hole in the tongue can and that a few bacilli entered during the cooling process. After this event, the water was chlorinated before being used for cooling, but it was established that, in 1963, this chlorination plant had broken and that again untreated water was used for cooling. So it was thought possible that the corned beef suspected of causing the 1964 outbreak in Aberdeen was canned during the period when untreated water was used again. Typhoid bacilli caused no swelling of the can, no discoloration or bad odour, and no unfavourable taste.

However, this explanation did not account for the fact that not all typhoid sufferers had eaten corned beef. So, attention was now turned to the hygiene of the supermarket. It was found that the can-opener, slicer machine, pedestals for window displays, price tickets and trays used for storage overnight were common to all cold meats. Although the washing of these, and shelves, was carried out, no disinfectant was used, and the clothes and scrubbing brushes were not thoroughly cleaned each day. So, for a matter of weeks, the typhoid organisms were lingering and were being spread around the shop. All cold meats became infected eventually, being contaminated by a single can of corned beef.

1 Name two factors which hampered the investigation. Explain why.
2 Why was the corned beef not immediately suspect?
3 Why was it eventually suspect? Explain how the experience of the previous typhoid outbreak contributed to an understanding of the 1964 outbreak.
4 Draw a 'flow' diagram to show the passage of the typhoid bacillus from the river De La Plata to an Aberdeen resident.
5 List four factors concerning the hygiene of the shop, and show how they contributed to the outbreak.

FUNGI

Fungi are a third group of micro-organisms that can cause disease. However, unlike bacteria, they are far more likely to infect plants than animals, and few are human parasites.

ACTIVITY 24

Ringworm and athlete's foot are two common fungal skin infections. For each of these, find out the symptoms, how it is treated and how it is spread. Suggest ways in which the spread can be prevented.

PROTOZOA

Protozoa are single-celled animals, some of which are parasitic. Many diseases are caused by these parasites, particularly in developing countries. The protozoan *Plasmodium*, which

causes malaria, is probably responsible for more human deaths in the tropics than any other organism. It is estimated that about 100 million cases of malaria occur in the world each year (WHO 1987).

It has been estimated that in tropical Africa alone, malaria accounts for approximately 750,000 deaths each year, mainly among young children. In some developing areas, up to 5% of children under the age of five die from malaria each year (UNICEF 1986). In a number of areas the situation has been becoming worse since the late 1970s. This is largely due to the growing resistance of the mosquito vector to insecticides, and of *Plasmodium* parasites to anti-malarial drugs.

The simplified life cycle of *Plasmodium*

When the *Plasmodium* first enters the human, it goes to the liver where it feeds and reproduces for about two weeks. During this time the person will start to feel ill, and there will be a rise in body temperature. A fever then develops as the parasite leaves the liver and enters the bloodstream. The fever subsides as each parasite enters a red blood cell. A few days later the fever returns as the red blood cells burst, releasing many more parasites, and their waste products, into the blood.

When the female mosquito feeds on the blood of an infected person, the protozoa enters her blood. The parasite undergoes sexual reproduction in the stomach of the mosquito, and the offspring make their way to the salivary glands. When the mosquito feeds again, the parasites are injected into the new host.

ACTIVITY 25

1 Draw a flow diagram to illustrate the life cycle of *Plasmodium* described in the text.

2 Can you suggest methods to help prevent malaria which could be used at different stages of the life cycle?

3 Find out what effect sickle-cell anaemia has on the susceptibility of the sufferer to malaria.

4 What other diseases are caused by protozoa?

5 What other parasites utilise an insect vector?

It is often known as an *economic disease* as it makes people too weak to work. Can you find other examples of serious economic diseases?

PLATYHELMINTHES

Two groups of platyhelminthes (flatworm) are parasitic: the tapeworms and the flukes.

The *pork tapeworm* and the organism that causes *bilharzia*, *Schistosoma*, are two well-known parasitic platyhelminthes. Their life cycles are shown in Figures 3.20 and 3.21.

ACTIVITY 26

1 Study the life cycles of the pork tapeworm and *Schistosoma* (Figures 3.20, 3.21). Suggest possible methods of disease control for each.

2 Bilharzia affects over a quarter of a million people in developing countries.

NEMATODES

Nematodes are elongated, round 'worms' with pointed ends. They are found in very large numbers in a wide range of habitats. It is estimated that the 10,000 known species represent only about 2% of their full number. Most are free-living, although it is the parasitic ones that are the best known.

A well-known example of a disease caused by nematodes is *river blindness* or *onchocerciasis*. It is estimated that more than 17 million people are infected by this disease, mainly in west and central Africa. The severity of onchocerciasis is usually greatest in rural settlements located close to rapidly flowing rivers and streams which are the breeding sites of the blackfly, the vector of the disease. Blindness rates as high as 10% have been reported in many endemic areas. Without sight, hundreds of thousands of people lose the ability to fend for themselves and die prematurely (see Figure 3.22).

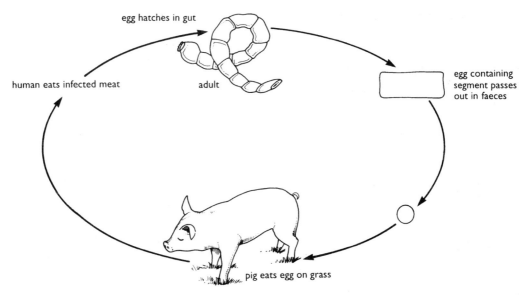

egg hatches in gut

human eats infected meat   adult   egg containing segment passes out in faeces

pig eats egg on grass

Figure 3.20   The life cycle of a pork tapeworm
Source: Thomson et al., 1995.

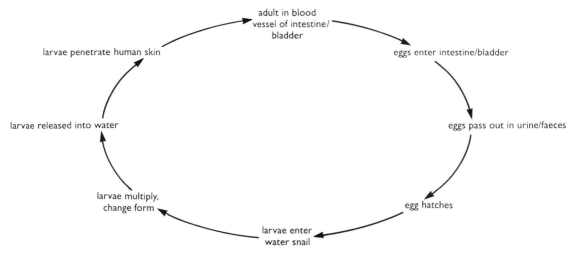

Figure 3.21 The life cycle of *Schistosoma*
Source: Thomson et al., 1995.

In recent years, as a result of the control of the larvae of blackflies by the release of biodegradable insecticides into rivers, the disease has been eradicated in some areas. Remarkable achievements have also been achieved in the treatment of river blindness with drugs.

ACTIVITY 27

From Table 3.7 calculate the percentage of the total population:

(a)   at risk of infection of onchocerciasis;
(b)   infected;
(c)   blind as a result of the disease.

NB: the figures in the table are likely to be an underestimate.

DEGENERATIVE

These are caused by the effect of wear and tear on the human body. Refer back to Thomson et al. 1995, Chapter 3, and you will find a description of how the body systems deteriorate with time, eventually leading to death. Diseases that these deteriorations can lead to include the following:

Atheroma

Atheroma are fatty deposits on the inner lining of an artery that can cause atherosclerosis. Atheroma are discrete plaques containing a mixture of low-density lipoproteins, decaying muscle cells, fibrous tissue, clumps of blood platelets, cholesterol and sometimes calcium.

Atherosclerosis

This is a disease of the arterial wall in which the inner layer thickens, causing a narrowing

Table 3.7   Onchocerciasis morbidity: the estimated numbers of persons at risk, infected and blind, in 1993

Region	Total population (10^3)	Population at risk of infection (10^3)	Number infected (10^3)	Number blind as a result of onchocerciasis (10^3)
Africa	360,500	118,100	17,486	267.2
Eastern Mediterranean (Sudan, Yemen)	38,300	2,681	650	10
Americas	308,800	4,700	140	0.75

Source: Onchocerciasis and its control: report of a WHO Expert Committee on Onchocerciasis Control. Geneva, World Health Organization, 1995 (WHO Technical Series, No. 852)

The bite spreads parasitic worms. They breed under your skin and produce hordes of microscopic worms called micro-filariae which infest your body for years. You itch, you get skin problems, you become debilitated.

Then the microfilariae invade your eyes.

And you slowly become blind.

It's called River Blindness, "the disease at the end of the track". You'll find it in a host of fast-flowing rivers in West and Central Africa.

And there you will find most of the victims – the million or so who have already lost their sight and the seven-teen million who have the symptoms and are at risk of blindness; their sight could be saved – quickly and easily.

The price of river blindness.

Consider what happens if you lose your sight in a poor African country. No disability benefit, no regular medical facilities, little prospect of remedial work.

There is just your family living at the harshest subsistence level. You become a burden on them. You will need to be led from place to place. You can do little to contribute to their welfare.

For this is the particular agony of River Blindness. It takes years to gestate. When blindness strikes, you are likely to be in your thirties or forties. You are likely to be the family breadwinner. Without you, the family will lose their hard-won self-sufficiency and become dependent on the charity of neighbours.

And it is all avoidable.

THE BLACK SIMULIUM FLY

Ivermectin: it works, it's cheap, it's available.

Merck, Sharp and Dohme have developed a drug to halt River Blindness. It is a simple-to-take white tablet called ivermectin and it has been thoroughly tested in Africa. It not only prevents blindness but it tackles the painful symptoms as well. There are no serious side effects.

The manufacturers have generously agreed to supply ivermectin free. Sight Savers is committed to distributing it in Nigeria, Ghana, Mali, Uganda and Sierra Leone. We intend to expand the programme to include Guinea and Senegal.

If this sounds easy, it isn't. Sight Savers works worldwide and River Blindness is just one part of our work. So, a distrib-ution programme on this scale will strain our resources to the utmost – we will need all the help we can get.

Then again, you have to allow for the reality of medical work in poor countries. In some of those countries there are village health workers or committees who we can train to distribute ivermectin. In others we are relying on nurses who go from village to village. We shall be very reliant on local people, village chiefs in particular, to guide much of this programme.

And there are transport problems. The dry flatlands of Mali make a 50cc motor cycle a reasonable means of travel; in the hilly, forest regions of Sierra Leone, we'll need a tougher 125cc machine. A lot of

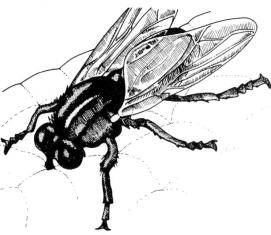

IT BITES YOU

ivermectin will be distributed by simple bicycle.

And the programme will go on for years. In each community at risk, ivermectin will have to be distributed annually for at least ten years to break the transmission cycle of the disease. Our aim worldwide is to ensure that, within twenty five years, nobody will lose their sight through River Blindness.

A massive campaign, then. But how can we look at that small white pill and at the terrifying statistics of River Blindness and at the harrowing stories of its effects... how can we know all these things and do nothing about it?

How much can you help us?

The whole world is full of claims on your generosity and the problems of the Third World will never go away in our lifetimes. But our River Blindness campaign is a hard-headed, practical and immediate chance to do something to prevent one evil once and for all.

It may help to think of your donation in very literal terms.

For it takes just £25 to protect twenty five people against River Blindness for a whole year.

£70 buys one of those bicycles for a medical assistant.

And £400 sponsors a training course for health workers.

But, whatever you can afford to send us, you will know of the scourge of River Blindness. There are not many things you can do that can achieve so much, so profoundly, so quickly.

Thank you for whatever you can do.

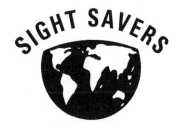

Sight Savers, FREEPOST, Haywards Heath, West Sussex RH16 3ZA Reg. Charity No. 207544

Figure 3.22 An advertisement publicising treatment for river blindness
Source: Sight Savers.

of the channel, thus damaging blood flow. This is often called 'hardening of the arteries'. The narrowing is due to the development of *atheroma*. Contributing factors include high blood pressure, carbon monoxide in cigarettes and a high cholesterol level.

Arthritis

The term arthritis refers to many different diseases. Osteoarthritis is the most common degenerative form of the disease. It results from a combination of ageing, irritation of the joints and wear and abrasion, and is a progressive, non-inflammatory disorder of moveable joints, particularly the load-bearing ones. The cartilage of the joint slowly degenerates, and as the bone ends become exposed, small bumps are formed on them. These restrict joint movement.

Rheumatism

This refers to any painful state of the supporting structures of the body – its bones, ligaments, joints, tendons or muscles. Arthritis is a form of rheumatism.

Alzheimer's disease

This is a disabling neurological disorder that affects 5% of the population over 65. Its causes are unknown, its effects are irreversible and it has no cure. The disease kills over 120,000 people each year, making it the fourth leading cause of the death of the elderly after heart disease, cancer and stroke. Victims of this disorder have difficulty in remembering recent events. Next, they become confused and forgetful. Disorientation grows, and memories of past events disappear. There may be episodes of hallucinations, paranoia or violent changes in mood. Eventually, they lose their ability to read, write, talk, eat, walk or take care of themselves. A person with Alzheimer's disease usually dies of some complication that effects bed-ridden patients, such as pneumonia. Hypotheses suggest that the disease may be caused by the inheritance of faulty genes, an abnormal accumulation of protein in the brain, or environmental toxins such as aluminium.

Osteoporosis

This disorder is characterised by a decrease in bone mass and an increased susceptibility to fractures. It primarily affects middle-aged and elderly women. The decrease in the amounts of sex hormones that accompanies the menopause results in a decrease in the formation of new bone. Osteoporosis affects the entire skeleton, but especially the spine, hips and legs. The disorder is responsible for shrinkage of the backbone and height loss, hunched backs, hip fractures and considerable pain. Calcium or vitamin-D deficiency, the loss of muscle mass and inactivity have been blamed for the condition.

ACTIVITY 28

1 Research the methods of treatment for each of the above-mentioned diseases.

2 Can you think of further examples of degenerative diseases?

OCCUPATIONAL

There is some overlap in the classification of diseases as occupational or environmental (see below). Occupational diseases are those caused by a hazardous working environment, and examples include those listed below.

Repetitive strain injury (RSI)

This is a newly discovered hazard caused by the repetitive movement of part of the body. The strain is felt in the joints and muscles – hence, 'tennis elbow'. Typists, assembly-line workers and musicians may all experience pain and stiffness in the affected joints and muscles.

Symptoms usually disappear with rest, but can have long term effects.

Noise

Although noise is not restricted to the workplace, noise levels in factories are

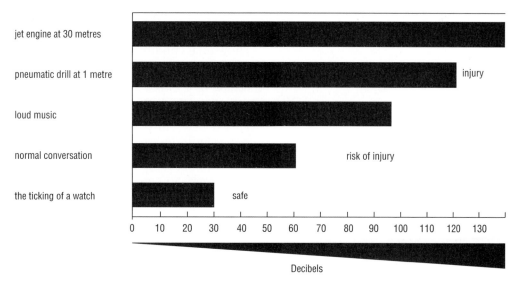

Figure 3.23 Comparative noise levels
Source: Thomson et al., 1995.

generally higher than elsewhere because of the large numbers of moving parts and their concentration in a limited space. A high level of noise can result in both physical symptoms, such as tinnitus (ringing in the ears), and psychological symptoms. Any noise above 90 decibels may cause damage (see Figure 3.23). A great number of developed countries have now adopted noise-limiting standards. Where exposure cannot be avoided (e.g. when workers use pneumatic drills), ear protection should be worn.

Cancer
See the 'Environmental' category below.

Dermatitis
Skin infections can result from working with chemicals, such as those used in hairdressing, or in enzymic washing powders.

Arthritis
See the 'Degenerative' category above.

Back injury
Sixty million working days are lost per year due to back pain. This can be caused by bad posture whilst sitting at a desk or whilst lifting heavy objects. A recent government report recommended that sufferers should choose manipulative therapy – such as osteopathy – as a first line of treatment. This

is largely because osteopathy has been found to be more effective than the old-fashioned approach of pain killers and bed rest.

ACTIVITY 29

1 Find out about the Health and Safety at Work Act 1974.

2 When you are working in a health or social care setting, ask to see how accidents are reported and dealt with by staff.

GENETIC

These conditions arise from the genotype of the individual. They are hereditary conditions, and may be caused by dominant or recessive genes, or by chromosome abnormalities. Examples of hereditary disorders are:

- haemophilia
- Down's syndrome
- cystic fibrosis
- Huntington's chorea
- achondroplasia
- retinal aplasia
- phenylketouria

- muscular dystrophy
- cretinism
- albinoism
- sickle-cell anaemia
- red/green colour blindness
- Klinefelter's syndrome
- Turner's syndrome

ACTIVITY 30

Select one of the following diseases:
- haemophilia
- Down's syndrome
- cystic fibrosis
- Huntington's chorea

Gather information, and give an oral presentation (including visual aids) to the rest of your group. Include an explanation of the genetics; the signs and symptoms; the treatment; and the prognosis. Make notes from other people's presentations on the other three diseases.

Definition of terms

1 *Congenital*. This term means 'present at birth'. A congenital abnormality may be inherited (i.e. passed down) from the parents; it may have occurred at the time of birth, or it may have occurred as the result of injury or infection in the womb. Congenital abnormalities are often called *birth defects*.
2 *Hereditary*. This term is used to describe the transmission of traits and disorders through *genetic* mechanisms. A disorder may be hereditary *and* congenital, but many hereditary diseases are not present at birth, e.g. Huntington's chorea and Friedreich's ataxia.
3 *Acquired*. Diseases and disorders which are neither congenital nor inherited are termed *acquired*. These are caused by external factors, e.g. infection, accidental injury or poisoning.

MENTAL

Some mental disorders are congenital. These are disorders that are recognised at birth and may be inherited or caused by an environmental factor. An example of a congenital condition is Down's syndrome. Other mental disorders are described as *neuroses* or *psychoses*. A neurosis is a mental illness in which insight is retained but there is a particular way of behaving or thinking that causes suffering. The symptoms may include a severe emotional state such as an *anxiety* state or *depression*. Sometimes the symptoms involve distressing behaviour, as in *phobias* (abnormal intense and irrational fears – see Activity 31 below) or obsessions. Other neuroses may be recognised by physical states, for example hysteria or hypochondria. A psychosis is a much more severe type of mental illness. The sufferer loses contact with reality, and delusions and hallucinations often occur. Thought processes are usually altered. *Manic depression* and *schizoprenia* are the most commonly occurring psychoses.

ACTIVITY 31

1 Find out about the symptoms and treatment of the following disorders:
- anxiety
- depression
- schizophrenia

2 Phobias can be treated in the following three ways:
- Systematic desensitisation: the client and the therapist draw up a list of frightening situations and put them in order. For example: most frightening – a spider crawling up your skin; least frightening – a spider seen on a TV programme. The client is then trained in relaxation, and if they can remain relaxed through the least frightening situation, they will move up to a slightly more frightening situation. The process is repeated up the scale.
- Implosion therapy or 'flooding': here the client faces the thing they are most frightened of, perhaps is put in a room

with some spiders. This provokes a strong emergency reaction, but the client cannot flee. Arousal cannot last indefinitely at its maximum level. After a while it will die down, and the client will feel calmer and more able to face the thing that frightens them.

• Modelling: here the client watches someone dealing confidently with the frightening object – for instance, lifting a spider out of the bath, showing it to children, putting it gently outside. This works best if the model is like the client (similar stage of life, same sex).

Discuss the advantages and disadvantages of each method, and decide which you think would be most effective.

ENVIRONMENTAL

These are diseases caused by a harmful environment. Some of those caused by a harmful working environment have already been covered under the 'Occupational' category above.

Cancer

The term cancer is applied to a group of *neoplastic* (literally meaning 'new growth') diseases in which normal body cells are changed into *malignant* ones.

Normally, the cells of tissues are regularly replaced by new growth, which stops when old cells have been replaced. In cancer, this cell growth is *unregulated*. The cells continue to grow even after the repair of damaged tissue is complete. The malignant cells multiply and invade neighbouring tissues, thereby destroying the normal cells and taking their place. If the *lymphatic vessels* are invaded, the malignant cells are carried away in the lymph until their progress is halted by the filtering effect of the lymph glands. Here, they may be deposited and cause a *secondary* tumour (also called a *metastasis*).

Statistically, 1 in 4 of all infants born in the UK will develop cancer at some time in their lives, and it is the second major cause of death.

There are over 150 types of cancer in humans, but they fall into two main groups:
• Sarcomas affect *connective* tissue, i.e. bones and muscles. They tend to grow very rapidly and are very destructive
• Carcinomas affect *epithelial* tissue and make up the great majority of the *glandular* cancers, e.g. thyroid, pancreas and prostate. Also, cancers of the breast, stomach, uterus, skin and tongue.

A *carcinogen* is any substance that causes cancer.

Biological factors and heredity play some part in the incidence of cancer, but, although it is known that there is permanent alteration in the DNA of the cell involved, it is not clear why some people succumb to a cancer and others do not. Research is still trying to discover the role of *viruses* in causing cancer. It is estimated that 70% of all cancers are caused by *environmental* factors:
• *cigarette smoking including passive smoking*: this is directly related to approximately 90% of all cancers of the lung
• *industrial pollutants* such as asbestos, benzene, solvents and insecticides
• *radiation from the sun*: people with outdoor occupations in sunny climates are at increased risk of skin disease, e.g. skin cancer
• *ionising radiation*: X-rays and radiation from nuclear waste may cause cancer (particularly leukaemia) if levels of exposure are not controlled. Controlled radiation, or radiotherapy, is, however, useful in the treatment of some cancers.

ACTIVITY 32

Find out the incidence of:

1 cancer of the lung and bronchus;
2 cancer of the breast;
3 cancer of the stomach;
4 cancer of the skin;

in:

(a) the UK,

(b) Japan,

(c) USA,

(d) Australia.

Prepare bar graphs or pie charts to display your findings, and try to account for the variations found.

Lead

Children are particularly susceptible to lead poisoning due to several factors such as their small ratio of volume-to-body surface area, their high metabolic rate and oxygen consumption, and their different body composition. Even very low levels of lead in the blood adversely affect cognitive development and behaviour, with potentially long-term effects; and higher levels result in damage to the kidneys, liver and reproductive system. Growth is impaired and blood synthesis is interfered with. Much of the lead contamination comes from industrial processes and traffic.

Silicosis

This is caused by particles of silica from rock or stone. The inhaled particles are trapped in nodules in the alveoli, and the lungs become fibrous and distorted. This reduces the surface area for gas exchange.

Asbestosis

This is caused by the inhalation of particles of asbestos. The lower part of the lung becomes fibrous, and lung cancer can result.

QUESTION

What symptoms are caused by inefficient gas exchange?

DIETARY

In the Third World, dietary diseases tend to be linked to the deficiency of elements in the diet, such as protein or vitamins. In developed countries, however, the following dietary diseases are the most common:

Obesity

Obesity can be linked to heart disease, strokes, diabetes, raised blood pressure, some cancers, gout and arthritis.

ACTIVITY 33

Read the following article:

OBESITY COSTS EARLY DEATH AND £200M

Obese people are costing the National Health Service some £200 million a year and shortening their lives, says a report out today.

Around 13 per cent of men and 15 per cent of women are obese according to government figures, and 38 per cent of men and 26 per cent of women – 20 million adults – are overweight.

The Office of Health Economics, a health research organisation funded by the pharmaceutical industry, says that obesity is one of the most important preventable causes of ill health. The direct treatment costs are around £30 million, but obesity is a major contributor to heart disease, strokes, diabetes, raised blood pressure, some cancers, gout and arthritis, adding £165 million to the bill.

The risk of death for the obese at 45 is three times that of a person of desirable weight. The risk is 12-fold for the severely obese aged 25–35. The office refers to 'body mass index' calculated by dividing the weight in kilos by the height in metres squared.

A BMI of 20–25 is desirable, between 25–30 is overweight, between 30–40 is obese, and over 40 severely obese. A man of 1.83 cm (6 ft) with a weight of 82.55 kg (13 stone) has a BMI of 24.65, desirable.

The Government is aiming to reduce the number of obese men by a quarter by 2005, and the number of obese women by a third.

Obesity, as measured by a BMI over 30, has increased by 50 per cent among men and by 25 per cent among women since 1986–87. The office calculates that more than 700,000 people consult their GPs each year and the cost of these visits in GP time is around £14 million. One per cent are sent for further investigations or to hospital as outpatients, costing £850,000 ...

(The Guardian, 18 July 1994)

1 Use the information given to calculate your BMI.

2 What type of diet and exercise regime would you recommend to an obese person?

Anorexia

Anorexia nervosa is a recognised eating disorder. Between 1 in 100 and 1 in 250 women are likely to be affected; sufferers are most frequently found among the higher social classes in the developed world. The disorder is occasionally, but rarely, seen in men (only 10% of sufferers are men).

Anorexia nervosa is characterised by severe weight loss, the wilful avoidance of food and an intense fear of being fat. It is popularly, but wrongly, called the 'slimmer's disease'.
Features of the disorder are:
- weight loss
- overactivity and obsessive exercising
- tiredness and weakness
- *lanugo* (baby-like hair on the body; the thinning of hair on the head)
- extreme choosiness over food

The criteria for diagnosis established by the American Psychiatric Association can be described as follows:
- an intense fear of becoming obese which does not diminish as weight loss progresses

- a disturbance of body image, e.g. claiming to feel fat when emaciated
- weight loss: of at least 25% of original pre-illness body weight; or, if under 18 years of age, weight loss from the original pre-illness body weight plus projected weight gain expected from growth charts, which may be combined to make at least 25%
- a refusal to maintain body weight over a minimal normal weight for age and height
- there is no physical illness that would account for the weight loss

The causes of anorexia nervosa are much debated. The following are some theories:
- Dieting is seen by sufferers as a way of controlling their lives
- Sufferers do not wish to grow up and are trying to keep their childhood shapes. In part, this may be influenced by the media obsession with achieving the 'perfect' (i.e. slim) body, and also by the desire to defer the turbulence of adolescence
- Some specialists see it as a true phobia about putting on weight
- Feminist writers have suggested that the condition may be related to a new role for women within society
- The development of eating disorders may be seen as the avoidance of adult sexual feelings and behaviours
- The individual is over-involved in their own family so that when they enter adolescence, there is a confrontation between the peer group and the family
- Some specialists believe that the real cause is depression, a personality disorder or, rarely, schizophrenia
- Some doctors point to both the hormonal changes related to weight loss and the absence of menstruation, and regard anorexia nervosa as a physical illness that is caused by a disorder of the hypothalamus (part of the brain concerned with hunger, thirst and sexual development)

Hospital treatment is often necessary to help the sufferer return to a normal weight. Treatment is usually a combination of:

- a controlled refeeding programme, sometimes via a naso-gastric tube in severe cases
- individual psychotherapy
- family therapy

Occasionally, drug abuse and alcohol abuse also occur, and these require specific treatment. Drug treatment may be needed if there is a depressive or other illness.

Psychotherapy may be needed for months or even years after the sufferer has achieved a more normal weight. Relapses are common whenever there is the slightest stress.

About 50% of all patients treated for anorexia nervosa in a hospital continue to have symptoms for many years; 5–10% later die from starvation or suicide.

Cardiovascular disease
Quick facts
- People with high blood pressure (see the 'Obesity' section above) are three times more likely to have a heart attack
- People with high blood pressure who also have raised cholesterol levels are nine times more likely to have a heart attack
- People with high blood pressure who also have raised cholesterol levels and who also smoke have a risk 16 times higher than average

Cholesterol is an essential part of all of our cells, and two-thirds of the approximately 150 grammes of it in each of us is made in our own bodies. The danger of cardiovascular disease arises when the amount of cholesterol-containing foods in our diet, such as dairy products, is too high. This leads to raised cholesterol levels in the blood and the deposit of cholesterol on the walls of the arteries, which can cause atherosclerosis (see the 'Degenerative' section above).

A diet which leads to obesity and thus brings about an increased blood pressure can also lead to cardiovascular disease, as can a diet containing high levels of salt.

ACTIVITY 34

1 Cholesterol-testing kits can be purchased from chemist shops. These are not suitable for use in schools or colleges as they involve taking a sample of blood, but you could use one at home to test your cholesterol level.
2 Plan a week's menu for a person on a low-cholesterol diet.

Food allergies

A true allergy involves the production of *antibodies* (see p. 164 below), so although adverse reactions to food are common, food allergies are rare. In children, the foods most commonly causing an allergic reaction are cows' milk, egg (usually white only), wheat, chocolate, shell fish, nuts (especially peanuts) and citrus fruits. Food-allergic symptoms usually become less frequent as the child gets older. The signs and symptoms vary. In extreme cases, people can collapse and die. Any of the body systems may be affected, and because this includes the neurological system, the symptoms may be psychological rather than physical.

Allergies to food additives such as the colouring agent *tartrazine* have been blamed for many disorders, including eczema, asthma and hyperactivity.

ACTIVITY 35

Find a person who has a food intolerance, interview them and write a case study which includes details of:

(a) the foods that cause this intolerance;
(b) the signs and symptoms of the intolerance;
(c) the treatment of these signs and symptoms.

SELF-INFLICTED

In some ways the dietary diseases could be considered as self-inflicted, but there are other illnesses which are even more deserving of this label, such as those caused by smoking, drinking and drug and solvent abuse.

Smoking

An estimated 110,000 people die in the UK each year directly from smoking-related illnesses. Meanwhile, tobacco companies spend an estimated £12 million each year sponsoring sports, such as motor racing, which would be hardest hit by a ban forbidding the display of brand logos. In addition to the diseases lung and coronary artery disease, many other diseases and health problems are caused or complicated by smoking, including:

- cancer of the mouth, lip, larynx, oesophagus, lung, pancreas, cervix, stomach, bladder and kidney (the direct evidence that cigarette smoking causes cancer of the lung is clear: fewer than 10% of lung cancers occur in non-smokers)
- emphysema
- stroke (CVA or cerebro vascular accident)
- leukaemia
- chronic lung disease – bronchitis and COLD (chronic obstructive lung disease)
- fertility problems
- early menopause
- cataracts
- male impotence
- sickle-cell anaemia
- stomach ulcers

There are also diseases and health problems associated with *passive smoking*, i.e. inhaling the smoke from other people's cigarettes. *Mainstream smoke* is that delivered directly to the smoker by inhalation. It tends to be filtered, whereas the *sidestream smoke* emitted into the atmosphere from the burning end of a cigarette is unfiltered and contains a higher proportion of *carcinogens* (cancer-producing substances) than mainstream smoke. Diseases caused are:

- lung cancer
- bronchitis
- heart disease
- low birth weight
- respiratory disease in children

Quick facts

- 33% of the adult population of the UK are smokers
- Almost one in three of all school-leavers are regular smokers
- Out of 1,000 smokers who die each year, one will be murdered, six will die on the roads and 250 will die from smoking-related disease
- On average, babies whose mothers are smokers weigh 200 g less at birth than the babies of non-smokers
- Out of every 10 smokers, six say they would like to give up; they also say they need the support of a health professional
- Giving up smoking reduces the risk of premature death: the risks return to those of a non-smoker within 5–10 years

ACTIVITY 36

Set up a 'No Smoking' campaign in college.
- Obtain posters from the local health-promotion unit, or make some using the 'Quick facts' section
- Choose a prominent site to display posters and fact sheets
- Obtain several *peak flow meters*. Learn how to use them and to instruct others in their use. (NB: follow the rules of hygiene)
- Ask each volunteer if they smoke and offer them a chance to test their own peak flow
- Record results from smokers and non-smokers on separate charts
- At the end of the session, analyse the results and present them on a poster

For a fuller discussion on smoking, see Thomson et al. 1995, Chapter 7, pp. 368–72.

Drugs (including alcohol and solvents)

A drug is any chemical substance which changes the function of one or more body organs or alters the process of a disease. Drugs may be:

- prescribed medicines
- over-the-counter remedies
- alcohol, tobacco and caffeine
- illegal drugs

Drug abuse is the use of a drug for a purpose other than that for which it is usually prescribed.

Drug dependence is the compulsion to continue taking a drug, either to produce the desired effects that result from taking it, or to prevent the ill-effects that occur when it is withdrawn. There are two types of drug dependence:

- psychological
- physical

Four main groups of drugs are commonly abused:

1 stimulants ('uppers'), including caffeine, cocaine, crack and nicotine;
2 depressants ('downers'), including alcohol, sleeping tablets or hypnotics, tranquillisers and solvents;
3 psychedelics or hallucinogens, including LSD, cannabis and ecstasy;
4 narcotics, including heroin, morphine, pethidine, methadone, codeine and opium.

Why do people take drugs?

Obviously no one knows for certain why people abuse drugs, but some of the reasons might include:

1 relief from worry or depression;
2 rebellion;
3 curiosity;
4 fear of missing out/losing face;
5 boredom and frustration;
6 the desire for attention from others;
7 pleasure;
8 a search for self-knowledge.

For a full and detailed discussion on drugs, refer to Thomson et al. 1995, Chapter 7, pp. 372–78.

ACTIVITY 37

1 Draw up a chart showing the 'pleasant' and 'unpleasant' effects of ecstasy, heroin, amphetamines and cocaine.

2 Choose one of the following drugs and research it:
- alcohol
- tobacco
- cocaine
- heroin

Include as much up-to-date information as you can; use your library's resources centre. The project should cover:
- What is the drug, and what are its effects?
- Who uses the drug and why?
- How can health promoters change the patterns of drug abuse?

ACTIVITY 38

Can you think of any other illnesses or diseases which could be thought of as self-inflicted? What methods of prevention could be applied?

MODES OF TRANSMISSION OF DISEASES

1 *Droplet infection.* Respiratory infections in particular are usually spread by droplet infection. Sneezing, coughing or even talking can result in a spray of droplets containing viruses or bacteria (see Figure 3.24). These can then be inhaled by other people.
2 *Direct physical contact (contagious).* Relatively few diseases are spread through direct physical contact with an infected person. Examples include sexually transmitted diseases; the

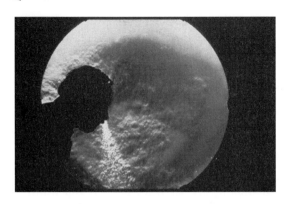

Figure 3.24 A photograph of a sneeze

tropical disease *yaws*; *trachoma* (a common eye disease); the common wart; and herpes simplex, which causes 'cold sores'.

3 *Vectors.* An organism that transmits a pathogen is known as a *vector*. It may actually contain the pathogen, which then multiplies within it – for example, the flea as the vector of the endemic typhus bacteria; or it may carry the pathogen on the outside of its body – for example, a house fly might transfer cholera from faeces to food where it may be ingested.

4 *Airborne.* If an agar plate is left open to the air, within a few days fungi and bacteria will be seen growing. This is because fungal spores and bacteria settle on the plate from the air. In this way, pathogens can infect their host, for example through wounds or the respiratory pathway.

5 *Food-borne.* Salmonella and botulism are examples of true food-borne diseases. Pathogens found in faeces (e.g. cholera, typhoid and dysentery) may also be transmitted to another host via food (see the 'Bacterial food poisoning' section under the 'Infections' category above).

6 *Water-borne.* Many of the bacteria which are food-borne can also be water-borne, for example typhoid fever. This is most common where sanitation is poor and water purification is inadequate. Faeces of the infected individuals contain the pathogenic bacilli. If there are inadequate means of sewage disposal, the water supplies become contaminated, and healthy individuals drinking the water acquire the disease. In 1937 there were 43 deaths and over 300 cases of typhoid fever in Croydon, in the south of England, arising from contaminated drinking water.

Table 3.8 shows how the major infectious diseases are transmitted.

Table 3.8   The classification of major infectious diseases by mode of transmission

Airbone respiratory diseases	Intestinal discharge diseases (includes water- and food-borne)	Open sores or lesion diseases (direct contact)	Vector-borne diseases	Droplet spread diseases
Chicken pox	Amoebic dysentery	Aids	African sleeping sickness	Anthrax
Common colds	Bacterial dysentery	Anthrax	Encephalitis	Chicken pox
Diphtheria	(shigellosis)	Erysipelas	Lyme disease	Common colds
Influenza	(staphylococcal)	Gonorrhea	Malaria	Diphtheria
Measles	Cholera	Scarlet fever	Rocky Mountain	Influenza
Meningitis	Giardiasis	Small pox	spotted fever	Meningitis
Pneumonia	Hookworm	Syphilis	Tularemia	Poliomyelitis
Poliomyelitis	Poliomyelitis	Tuberculosis	Typhus fever	Rubella
Rubella	Salmonellosis	Tularemia	Yellow fever	Scarlet fever
Scarlet fever	Typhoid fever			Streptococcal
Small pox	Hepatitis			throat
Throat infections				infections
Tuberculosis				Tuberculosis
Whooping cough				

Source: Timmreck 1994.

7 *Hereditary.* If you look back at the section above on genetic diseases (see pp. 151–152), you will see that these are transmitted in an entirely different way from the six methods mentioned above. This is because there is no pathogen involved. Genetics is an extremely complicated and extensive area, and it is not possible within the scope of this book to cover it. Very simply, individuals can acquire a 'faulty' gene, from one or both parents, which means that a particular protein cannot be made correctly. This can have disastrous effects: for example, sickle cell anaemia. Other examples are given in the genetic-diseases section above.

ACTIVITY 39

1 Recommend precautions to prevent the transmission of diseases by each of the methods outlined in the text.

2 Divide the following list into bacterial or viral diseases, and for each of them, find out by which of the methods listed in the text the pathogen is spread:

influenza; tetanus, common cold; diphtheria; mumps; tuberculosis (TB); whooping cough; measles; Aids; gonorrhoea; syphilis; polio; typhus; German measles; yellow fever; rabies; chicken pox, yaws.

THE CONTROL AND PREVENTION OF DISEASE AND ILLNESS

Natural methods

These are the mechanisms which the body itself deploys in an effort to control and prevent disease. They begin with the prevention of invasion.

BARRIERS TO INVASION

The skin

The skin covers the body and provides a physical barrier that protects underlying tissue from physical abrasion, bacterial invasion, dehydration and ultraviolet radiation.

See Figure 3.25 which shows the human skin structure. The epidermis contains *keratin*, a waterproofing protein which serves as an effective barrier against bacteria. The ability of the skin to detect temperature, touch, pressure and pain also helps in the avoidance of physical damage, and hence of the entry of bacteria.

Mucous membranes

A mucous membrane lines the body cavity that opens directly to the exterior. Mucous membranes also line the digestive, respiratory, excretory and reproductive tracts. These membranes secrete mucus which prevents the cavities from drying out and traps dust particles and microbes. In the respiratory tract, cilia sweep these particles away (see Figure 3.26).

Chemical barriers

Many of the body fluids produced on the exterior of the body contain antimicrobial substances. For example:
- *tears* produce a bactericidal enzyme
- *sebum*, an oily fluid produced by the sebaceous glands in the skin, inhibits the growth of certain bacteria

The hydrochloric acid produced in the stomach lowers the pH to 2. This is acidic enough to kill off many potentially harmful bacteria. The natural pH of the skin, which is between 3 and 5, is also acidic enough to discourage the growth of many of the microbes with which it comes into contact.

REPAIR MECHANISMS

Even though the skin is such an effective barrier to micro-organisms, it is still essential that any damage be rapidly repaired. Repair consists of the following stages:

(a)

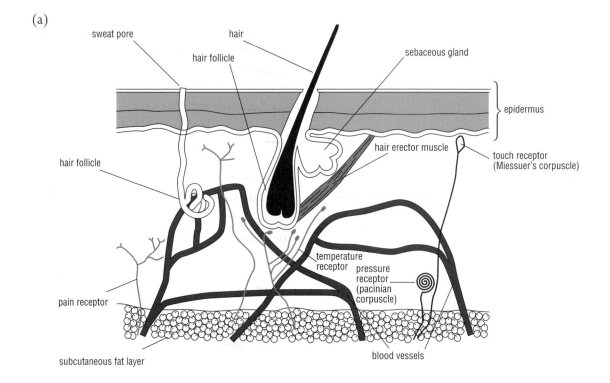

(b)

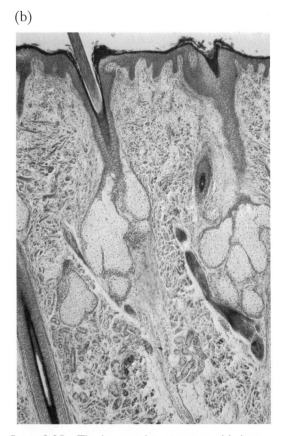

Figure 3.25 The human skin structure: (a) diagram of transverse section; (b) micrograph of transverse section
Source: (a) Thomson et al., 1995.

- clotting
- an inflammatory response
- phagocytosis
- the production of scar tissue
- the creation of a new skin surface
- the scab sloughing off

Clotting

A clot forms for two main reasons:
- to prevent further blood loss
- to block the entry of micro-organisms

Because blood circulation is pressurised, speed is vital in dealing with any leaks. Within the first few seconds of bleeding, the platelets react (see Figure 3.27). They stick to the damaged tissues and send out biochemical messages to soluble clotting proteins in the plasma. This causes them to change into solid gel-like and fibrous clots (see Figure 3.28).

If a clot forms in undamaged blood vessels, it can have very serious consequences. To prevent clots accidentally forming when they are not needed, the clotting process takes place through a highly complex series of reactions dependent on at least 12 clotting factors (see Figure 3.29).

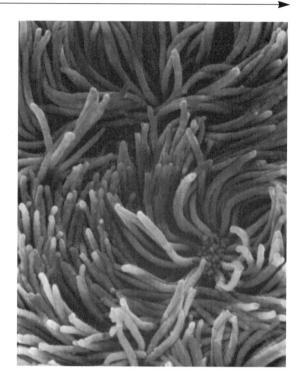

Figure 3.26 A cross-section of the tracheal epithelium in the respiratory tract

ACTIVITY 40

1 Find an account of the steps involved in blood clotting and use this to complete Figure 3.29 to show a simplified account of the process. The terms you will need to insert in the appropriate blank spaces are:
- thromboplastin
- fibrin
- blood cells
- platelets
- fibrinogen
- thrombin
- fibrin fibres

You will also need to identify the vitamin involved.

2 Find out:
- What is the condition caused by the formation of unnecessary blood clots?
- What factors make people particularly susceptible to this condition?
- How is this condition treated?
- What is the genetically inherited condition in which clotting is inadequate?

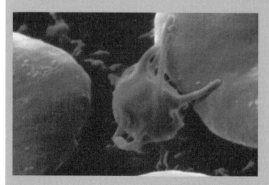

Figure 3.27 An activated platelet

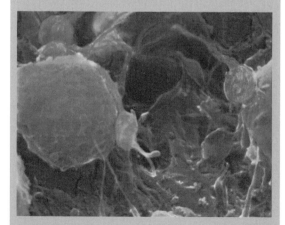

Figure 3.28 A red blood cell enmeshed in fibrin in a blood clot

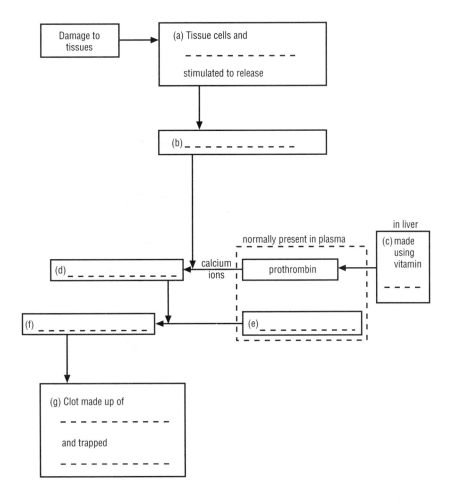

Damage to tissues

(a) Tissue cells and

– – – – – – – – – –

stimulated to release

(b) – – – – – – – – – –

normally present in plasma

in liver

(c) made using vitamin

– – – –

(d) – – – – – – – – – –

calcium ions

prothrombin

(f) – – – – – – – – –

(e) – – – – – – – – – –

(g) Clot made up of

– – – – – – – – – –

and trapped

– – – – – – – – – –

Figure 3.29   The main stages in the clotting of blood

- Why are males more susceptible to this disease than females?
- How is this condition treated?

Inflammatory response

The inflammatory response is both protective and defensive. It attempts to neutralise and destroy toxic agents and to prevent their spread, and is characterised by the tissue that surrounds a wound becoming *red, swollen, hot* and *painful*. Think, for example, of the response to a rusty nail scratching the skin, or to a sore throat caused by bacteria. Figure 3.30 shows the main steps involved in the inflammatory response. The immune response and phagocytosis mentioned are explained below.

In all but the mildest inflammations, *pus formation* occurs. Pus contains living and non-living white blood cells and debris from other dead tissue. If it does not drain it becomes an *abscess*, and if inflamed tissue is shed several times an *ulcer* forms.

Phagocytosis

Phagocytosis is a non-specific form of resistance against micro-organisms or other foreign particles of matter. It involves the ingestion and destruction of these by *phagocytes*. The white blood cells, *neutrophils*, are a type of phagocyte. In response to chemicals released by damaged cells, they may leave the blood vessels and migrate to the site of the infection (see the 'Inflammatory response' section above). Non-migratory or *fixed*

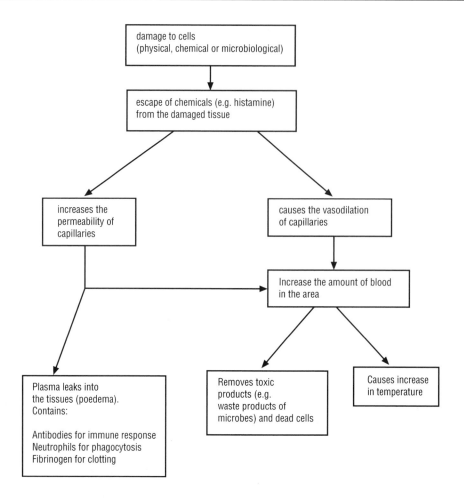

Figure 3.30 The main stages of the inflammatory response

phagocytes are found in many organs, for example liver, lungs, brain, spleen and lymph nodes.

Both types of phagocyte function in the same way, with the first step involving attachment of the bacteria and the second step involving its ingestion (see Figure 3.31).

COPING WITH INVADING PATHOGENS

If pathogens overcome the barriers described above and invade the body, there are various coping mechanisms which can be used to eliminate them, or at least prevent harmful symptoms they may cause.

The immune system process

Antibodies are protein molecules produced by white blood cells known as *lymphocytes*. They are produced in response to *antigens* – proteins or polysaccharides that coat foreign material such as bacteria. Antibodies are produced which are each specific to a single antigen. The production of antibodies is not restricted to the blood: they also occur on mucus surfaces – for example in the respiratory system – and in the alimentary canal.

There are two types of lymphocyte, the T and B *cells*, which develop in different ways and have different functions.

- T cells have membranes in which there are receptors for antigens. When one of these

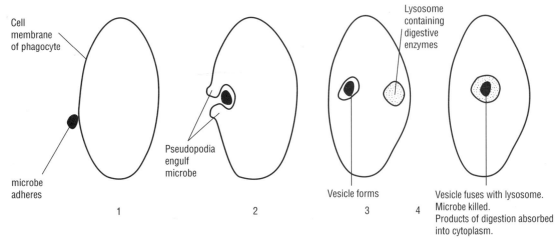

Figure 3.31 The mechanism of phagocytosis
Source: Thomson et al., 1995.

cells recognises a complementary antigen, it attaches itself to it and destroys it

- B cells recognise antigens in a similar way to T cells, but respond differently. They are stimulated to produce many *plasma cells*, each of which synthesises and liberates identical antibodies at a rate of nearly 2,000 molecules per second

There are many different ways in which antibodies prevent the replication and harmful effects of micro-organisms. These include:

- causing the foreign particles to stick together
- neutralising the toxins produced by the pathogen
- breaking down foreign material
- stimulating phagocytosis (see above)

As well as forming antibody-producing plasma cells, the B lymphocytes also produce

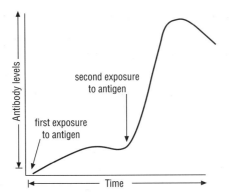

Figure 3.32 The primary and secondary response to an antigen
Source: Thomson et al., 1995.

memory cells. These enable an individual who has been exposed to an antigen once to respond more promptly and rigorously in a subsequent encounter (see Figure 3.32). This is called the *secondary response*, and is what gives an individual *immunity* to a disease which they have already encountered.

Artificial methods

IMMUNITY AND VACCINATION

The immune response can be artificially induced by *vaccination*. When the vaccine is introduced into the bloodstream, the antigens it contains stimulate the production of antibodies without causing the disease itself.

There are a number of different types of vaccine:

- *Living attenuated micro-organisms.* These are living pathogens which multiply but have been weakened, e.g. by heating or by culturing them outside the human body, so that they are unable to cause the symptoms of the disease. Examples include the vaccines against measles, tuberculosis, poliomyelitis and rubella (German measles)
- *Dead micro-organisms.* Although harmless, these still induce antibody production. Examples include vaccines against typhoid, influenza and whooping cough

- *Toxoids.* In some cases (e.g. diphtheria and tetanus) the toxin alone will cause antibody production. The toxin can be made harmless (e.g. with formaldehyde) and used as a vaccine
- *Extracted antigens.* The antigens can be taken from the pathogens and used as a vaccine. For example, the influenza vaccine can be prepared in this way
- *Artificial antigens.* The genes responsible for antigen production in a pathogen can be transferred to a non-pathogen. This harmless organism can be grown in a fermenter where it will produce the antigen which can be harvested and used in a vaccine

All the above methods produce what is known as *active* immunity because they cause the individual to synthesise their own antibodies. *Passive* immunity involves the acquisition or synthesis of antibodies. These can be acquired artificially. Antibodies from other mammals, e.g. horses, are injected in the form of a *serum.* For example, tetanus and diphtheria can be prevented in this way.

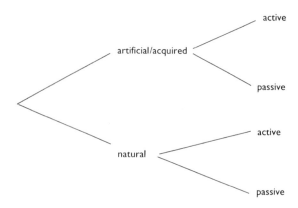

Figure 3.33　A summary of types of immune status

ACTIVITY 41

- Which type of immunity acts most immediately, active or passive?
- Which type of immunity would be the longest-lasting, active or passive?
- Suggest a situation in which passive immunisation would be more useful than active immunisation
- These examples of active and passive immunity are *artificial* or *acquired.* The *natural* immunity described earlier in this chapter can also be *active* or *passive.* Natural active immunity is the synthesis of antibodies by an individual in response to antigens acquired by natural infection. In natural passive immunity, the individual *acquires* antibodies. Where might these antibodies come from? (Clue: think about a baby.)

Immunisation programmes
The progress made in the control and prevention of infectious diseases has been the result of a number of factors, including improvements in water supply and sanitation, personal hygiene and nutritional status. However, the development of vaccines and immunisation programmes has been the most important factor in the prevention of many infectious diseases.

There is still a long way to go. Each year in developing countries, almost four million children die, and a similar number are permanently disabled from six of the most common childhood diseases: pertussis (whooping cough), diphtheria, measles, poliomyelitis, tuberculosis and tetanus. Of these deaths, nearly two million are from measles, 800,000 from neonatal tetanus, 600,000 from pertussis and 30,000 from tuberculosis. It is estimated that 250,000 cases of poliomyelitis occur annually (UNEP 1990). There are effective vaccines against each of these diseases, but the immunisation levels, although improving, are still not adequate in many parts of the world (see Figure 3.34).

In the UK, as in most countries, immunisation coverage is continuing to rise (see Figure 3.35). The national target for childhood immunisation is 90%, and this has been reached for all infections except pertussis (whooping cough). It has been proposed that the targets should be increased to 95% by 1995.

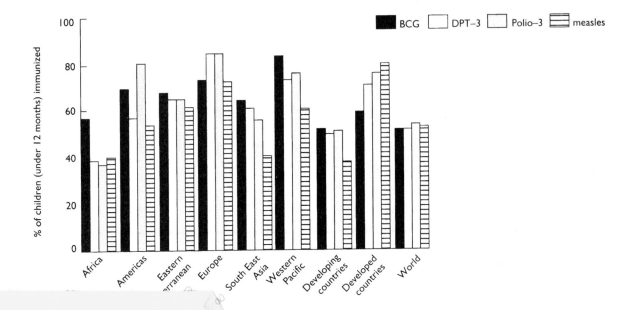

by WHO region and level of development, in 1987
EP 1989, the United Nations Environment Programme.

e has
the relevant
e, in 1991
sles cases
(see Figure
(mumps,
introduced.
rubella has

dropped, both for children and for pregnant women. There has been a corresponding drop in rubella-associated terminations of pregnancy and cases of congenital rubella.

The number of notifications of mumps has fallen to even lower levels than those for measles and rubella. It is likely that mumps will shortly disappear, as a result of the very high uptake of the MMR vaccine.

land in to
Rosemary.

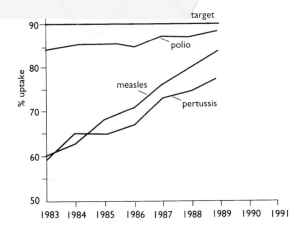

Figure 3.35   The immunisation uptake rate, England, 1983–91
Source: Crown copyright. Reproduced with the permission of the Controller of Her Majesty's Stationery Office.

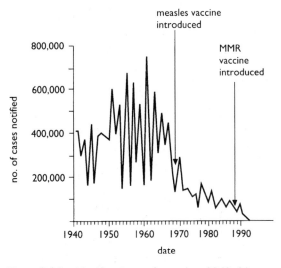

Figure 3.36   Notifications of measles, 1940–91
Source: Crown copyright. Reproduced with the permission of the Controller of Her Majesty's Stationery Office.

ACTIVITY 42

1 How does rubella harm the developing foetus?

2 Role-play the following situation. In advance, gather together and prepare appropriate materials to help you.

You are a health visitor in an antenatal clinic. A mother with a 3-week-old baby comes to you for vaccination advice. Explain what the likely immunisation schedule will be for her child. She tells you that she has heard that vaccines contain viruses, and so is worried that they may endanger her baby. Spend about 10 minutes responding to this, using simple visual aids to help you with your explanation.

3 Give an oral, visual or written presentation of an investigation into one named pathogen for which a vaccine is available. Your investigation should include the effect of the pathogen on the body, and the body's response. Investigate the effectiveness of the vaccine through the analysis of statistics, either globally or in one country.

THE USE OF CHEMICALS AND PHARMACEUTICAL COMPOUNDS

An effective vaccination programme can protect a person from many diseases caused by bacteria or viruses. If, however, an infection does develop, there are various ways in which chemical intervention can be used either to rid the body of the pathogen or to cure the symptoms of a disease.

Antimicrobial drugs

Antimicrobial substances must be toxic to pathogenic microbes but non-toxic to the host. Some chemotherapeutic substances are *narrow-spectrum* and affect only a few pathogens, whereas others are *broad-spectrum* and attack a wider range. Some substances are *bacteriostatic* drugs (i.e. they prevent bacteria from growing and multiplying); others are *bactericidal* (i.e. they kill the bacteria).

The ways in which they are effective are as follows:
- the inhibition of DNA synthesis (e.g. sulphonamides)
- the inhibition of cell wall synthesis (e.g. penicillin)
- the lysis of cell membranes (e.g. nystatin)
- the inhibition of protein synthesis (e.g. streptomycin, chloramphenicol and tetracylines)

Common antimicrobial drugs include the following:
- *Penicillin*: broad-spectrum and effective against most bacteria. Staphylococci are resistant to penicillin, and erythromycin is used against these
- *Cephalosporins*: broad-spectrum and used as an alternative to penicillin if resistance is encountered
- *Chloramphenicol*: used in the treatment of meningitis and typhoid
- *Griseofulvin and nystatin*: used to treat fungal infections; the former for ringworm and athlete's foot, and the latter for oral and vaginal thrush
- *Streptomycin*: a broad-spectrum antibiotic used mainly to treat tuberculosis
- *Tetracyclines*: broad-spectrum, used in the treatment of gonorrhoea
- *Sulphonamides*: used for treating infections of the urinary tract. Also useful in treating malaria

ACTIVITY 43

Find out about the discovery and present-day synthesis of antibiotics.

Replacement therapies

The symptoms of some diseases are caused by the lack of a vital component in the body, either through loss (for example, plasma from a burns victim) or because of a deficiency in synthesis (for example, of a particular hormone). In some cases it is possible to replace these important factors and thus prevent harmful symptoms.

ACTIVITY 44

1 Find out about the symptoms caused by the deficiency of a particular hormone, for example, insulin, growth hormone, thyroxine, sex hormones.

2 What factors may cause the deficiency?

3 How is the hormone replaced?

Many deficiencies of vital components are caused by a faulty gene (*gene mutation*). This means the correct protein will not be made. Rather than replacing the protein, recent research suggests that the *faulty gene itself* can be replaced. This is known as *gene therapy*. For example, cystic fibrosis, the most common inherited disease, is caused by a gene which produces a defective protein. Researchers are now putting the normal gene into fat droplets which are then introduced into patients' lungs. In the lung cells these genes will produce the correct protein. This is not a cure, but it is hoped that it will provide patients with decades of illness-free time.

Strategies

HYGIENE

Once the methods by which parasites spread have been understood, it is often possible to prevent disease. For example, *personal hygiene, food hygiene, a clean water supply* and efficient *sewage disposal* are all important in the maintenance of a healthy population. The first step in the process of providing a clean water supply is the treatment of sewage; and the treatment of water by chlorination before it is taken to homes is a precaution against bacterial contamination (see pp. 106–108).

ACTIVITY 45

1 Find out how a sewage-treatment works functions. Discover and explain the role of the following processes in sewage treatment:
   • initial screens and disintegrator
   • grit tanks
   • sedimentation tank
   • biological filters
   • humus settling tanks
   Sometimes an 'activated sludge' process is employed. How does this work?
   Draw a flow diagram to illustrate sewage treatment.
   Visit your local sewage-treatment works if possible.

2 Water is treated before it is piped out to homes. Find out how it is purified. Consider the following processes, and draw a flow diagram to illustrate them:
   • primary grid
   • settling reservoir
   • filter beds (primary and secondary)
   • chlorination plant
   • pumping house

3 Find out about water-borne diseases. Which of these have been eradicated in the UK by the treatment of sewage and the provision of a clean water supply? Which are still prevalent in other parts of the world?

4 Look back at the section above on 'Bacterial food poisoning' (see above). List the precautions to prevent infection which should be taken when handling and storing food.

5 What hygienic practices are regularly carried out in the home (not including food hygiene)? How do they help prevent the spread of disease?

CONTACT TRACING

The aim of health professionals involved in contact tracing is to find key people who have been in contact with patients suffering from certain diseases. Once traced, these people can then be tested for the disease, given prophylactic treatment (to prevent the disease occurring), and advice on how to limit the spread of the disease. If a disease is classed as *notifiable*, then once a case is suspected or diagnosed by the GP, it has to be reported to the Department of Public Health (see p. 59).

(For a fuller discussion, refer to Thomson et al. 1995, Chapter 6, pp. 352–3.)

ACTIVITY 46

What particular problems do you think may occur with contact tracing involving a sexually transmitted disease (STD)?

COPING STRATEGIES

Some diseases cannot be cured. However, there will usually be a number of things which can be done at least to alleviate the signs and symptoms or to delay the progression of a disease. For example, drugs, physiotherapy, occupational therapy, 'alternative' therapies or changes to diet may help.

There are a number of self-help groups to give people practical and moral support with coping with such diseases. Increasingly, there are also technical and manual aids to enable people with illnesses and disabilities to live as full a life as possible (See Chapter 3, 'Promoting individual independence and autonomy' in the other 'Optional Unit' book Holden et al., *Further Studies in Social Care*, 1996, Hodder & Stoughton).

ACTIVITY 47

Choose one of the following diseases, find out its progression, signs and symptoms, and then list the coping strategies which could be employed:
- Alzheimer's disease
- Parkinson's disease
- cystic fibrosis
- Aids/HIV infection

LIFESTYLE CHOICES

It is now recognised that people's lifestyles and behaviour are causative factors in many diseases. Important factors are:
- diet
- exercise and maintaining mobility
- stress
- recreation/leisure activities
- smoking
- alcohol and substance abuse
- sexual behaviour
- housing and sanitation

Self-empowerment

Throughout life we are faced with decisions regarding our lifestyle and behaviour. Self-empowerment, or genuine informed decision-making, starts with parental and family influences and ideally should be developed through formal education.

ACTIVITY 48

1 List some reasons why people may not adopt a healthier lifestyle. Consider: foods which constitute a healthy diet; smoking; alcohol; exercise.

2 Collect some advertisements for alcohol, cigarettes and 'fast' or 'junk' food, and discuss their effectiveness. What are the advertisers promoting? Which social groups are they targeting?

Health education is a method of self-empowerment, i.e. it enables people to take more control over their own health, and over the factors which affect their health. *Health promotion* is a term used to include all aspects of health education, but placing greater emphasis on changes in health policy and on *positive health* as opposed to the rather negative *prevention of ill-health*.

The nursing profession has evolved over the last two decades into a research-based profession; care plans and nursing procedures are continually modified to take account of the latest research findings. Health promoters need access to all kinds of health information before they can identify the needs, goals and methods appropriate to their task.

ACTIVITY 49

1 Who are the health promoters in society?

2 How much should society interfere with the freedom of the individual, e.g. smoking at work, the sale of alcohol at concerts etc.?

3 How effective do you think the shock-horror tactics were of the campaigns popular in the 1970s and 1980s, e.g. pictures of cancerous lungs and photos of emaciated drug addicts? Discuss the campaigns memorable to you and the reasons for their success.

During the latter part of the twentieth century, the shift of emphasis has moved from cure to prevention.

THE ROLE OF SOCIOECONOMIC FACTORS AFFECTING HEALTH AND DISEASE

Income, expenditure and health

(For a fuller discussion, plus suggested Activities, see Thomson et al. 1995, Chapter 4, pp. 251–3.)

With politicians arguing that the amount of money which can be spent on health and social care services for people is limited, pressing questions on the relationship between health and social and economic circumstances have become a prominent element in public and political debates. For example:

• What are the choices, or lack of them, which arise for individuals and families in relation to their health as a result of the income and other *economic resources* (savings, winnings, inheritance etc.) available to them?

• Can people be said to be contributing to their own ill-health by choosing to spend their money on an unhealthy lifestyle, by making the wrong choices in their diet and by showing a defeatist and passive response to difficult life situations?

• Alternatively, how might people's health be affected by social and economic factors outside their control?

• Even if there were total agreement upon what a healthy lifestyle was, would everyone be equally able to choose to follow it?

• What impact could differing levels of income and economic resources have on people's lifestyles, their resulting health and their ability to cope with life-event threats?

Government health-education campaigns have generally targeted the individual and their lifestyle, exhorting us to exercise more frequently, eat less fat, avoid dangerous drugs and so on: in other words, implying that good health is to a very great extent within the grasp of anyone.

In the UK, the right of everyone to health care is increasingly being questioned, raising ethical dilemmas for medical and social workers about who should be treated or helped.

Differences in income, economic resources and wealth

A wide range of official reports covering both the general distribution of income, of personal wealth and of work and earnings, and the regional distribution of income all confirm that the gap between the rich and the poor in the UK is growing wider.

In their book *Income, Poverty and Wealth*, Thomas Stark and Giles Wright use official statistics and the results of government surveys to show how, throughout the 1980s, the share of disposable income taken by the top 10% of the population has steadily risen while the poorest fifth of all households suffered a fall in their average income between 1987 and 1989. This trend was confirmed by a Labour Commission on Social Justice report in July 1993 which suggests that nearly two-thirds of the population has an income below the family average of £250 a week and that extremes of income are wider than at any time since 1886.

There are also marked and widening regional differences in average household income. Greater London in the late 1980s was the most prosperous region, with average incomes 26% above the national average. At the other end of the scale, the least well-off regions – namely Northern Ireland and Wales – had average incomes only 73% and 82% respectively of the national average.

Personal wealth remains concentrated among the richest 10% of the population.

Poverty

(For a fuller discussion, see Thomson et al. 1995, Chapter 4, pp. 258–9.)

There is no official definition of poverty. Two poverty lines drawn from official and quasi-official data are commonly used:
- Income Support level
- 50% of average income after housing costs

In her book *Poverty: the Facts*, Carey Oppenheim suggests that:

- Using either poverty line, between 11 million and 12 million people in the UK were living in poverty in 1988/9
- In 1988/9, 4.4 million people were living below the level of the government's 'safety net' of Income Support. A principal reason for this was the low take-up of benefits. According to government figures, 1 in 4 of those eligible for Income Support do not claim it, and around 1 in 2 do not claim Family Credit to which they are entitled
- Certain groups face especially high risks of poverty: 50% of lone-parent families, 42% of single pensioners, 69% of families where the breadwinner(s) are unemployed and 26% of families with an adult in part-time work lived in poverty (defined as below 50% of average income after housing costs) in 1988/9. There are no poverty figures broken down by ethnic origin, but Afro-Caribbeans and Asians have much higher rates of unemployment

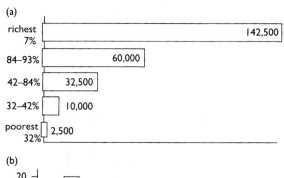

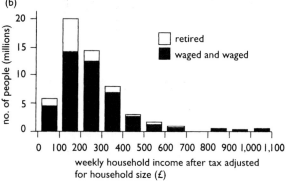

Figure 3.37 Wealth and income distribution in the UK

Source: The Guardian, 20 July 1993; wealth statistics from the Inland Revenue, income-distribution statistics from the Institute for Public Policy Research.

and are more likely to have low wages or to rely on inadequate benefits

- Between 1979 and 1988/9, the composition of the poorest 10% of the population changed: pensioners fell from 31% to 14% of the poorest 10%; families with children grew from 50% to 54%; and single people without children more than doubled from 10% to 22%

ACTIVITY 50

Examine the points made about those in poverty.

1 Work out what proportion of the total population of the UK is below the 'poverty line'.

2 Suggest reasons why the take-up of benefits is low.

3 Why do certain groups face a higher risk of poverty than others?

4 What factors could account for the changing composition of the poorest 10%?

(For a full discussion of the relationship between levels of income and economic resources and health, see Thomson et al. 1995, Chapter 4, pp. 259–61.)

Trends in income, class and health

(For a fuller discussion, plus further Activities, see Thomson et al. 1995, Chapter 4, pp. 261–2.)

- At almost every age, people in the poorer social classes have higher rates of illness and death than people in wealthier social classes
- A study by Smith et al. 1990, reported in the *British Medical Journal*, argued that the disparity in death rates between the social

classes is widening, and that as changes in income distribution continue to occur, such disparities can be expected to increase. Good health and longevity are most directly related to levels of affluence

- Blaxter (1990), analysing data from the Health and Lifestyles Survey, has found that the apparent strong association between social class and health was primarily one of income and health. Other studies have shown how changes in income levels can correlate with changes in health. This may explain how social class differences in health can widen, despite rises in absolute income and living standards. Around the year 1950, the proportion of the population living in relative poverty was at its lowest level since 1921, with only 8% of the population living in relative poverty. By 1987 the number of people living in poverty had risen to 28% of the population. With overall rises in living standards over the century, death rates for the poor have not fallen as fast as death rates for the rich. Being healthy seems, then, to require a level of income which allows families to enjoy similar living standards to and participate in a similar way to families with higher incomes (adapted from Blackburn 1991)

ACTIVITY 51

Read the two articles below, and write a list of recommendations you would make to the government to help solve the national and global health problems described.

THE UNEQUAL STRUGGLE

Since the influential Black Report was published in 1980, the international evidence has grown to such an extent that it is now indisputable that social and economic circumstances dominate the distribution and overall standards of health in modern populations. Statistics everywhere reveal that death rates at most ages are two or three times greater in disadvantaged than in affluent social classes. Most of the main causes of death contribute to these differences and together they reduce the life expectancy of the least privileged by some eight years in Britain. As with premature death, disability and illness are most common among disadvantaged groups.

Some of the things that affect health, such as age, sex and genetic make-up, cannot be changed by individual choice or public policy. The causes of ill health include

- the physical environment: housing, working conditions and air pollution
- social and economic influences: income and wealth, levels of unemployment, the quality of the social environment and social support
- behavioural factors and barriers to adopting a healthier personal lifestyle
- access to appropriate and effective health and social services

(The Guardian, 26 April 1995)

'FIFTH OF WORLD'S PEOPLE LIVE IN POVERTY'

Poverty is the leading cause of premature death and ill-health across the planet and the gaps between rich and poor are widening, not closing, the World Health Organization warns today.

In one of the most outspoken reports it has produced, the WHO says that more than one-fifth of the 5.6 billion people in the world live in extreme poverty, almost a third of the world's children are undernourished, and half the global population lacks regular access to essential drugs ...

It points out that 12.2 million children under five die every year, in many cases for lack of treatments costing 13p or less. If the children enjoyed the standard of living found in western countries, some 95 per cent would survive.

The WHO says that poverty is the main reason why babies are not vaccinated, why clean water and sanitation are not provided, why curative drugs and other treatments are not available, and why more than half a million mothers a year die in childbirth. More than a million children a year are still dying of measles, when the vaccine to save them costs 9p each. More than half a million babies die of tetanus, in many cases because instruments as simple as a clean razor blade are not available to cut the umbilical cord.

The report points out that in the poorest countries, life expectancy is a little above 40 years, while in the richest it approaches 80. Half a lifetime's difference separates countries which can be spanned by a short air journey.

In some countries, the amount available to be spent on health per person over a year is just £2.50 ...

(The Guardian, 2 May 1995)

Unemployment and health

(For a fuller discussion and an Activity, see Thomson et al. 1995, Chapter 4, pp. 262–3.)

Most research shows beyond doubt that there is an association between unemployment and ill-health. Mortality rates, rates of long-standing illness, rates of disability and rates of psychological disturbance have all been shown to be higher among the unemployed than among those with jobs. A higher risk of suicide and diseases such as stomach ulcers have also been traced in part to the effect of unemployment.

Ill-health may occur as a result of:

- the threat of job loss
- the actual event
- the state of being out of work

Housing and health

People who live in unhealthy homes usually suffer from other forms of social and economic disadvantage, so it becomes difficult to disentangle the effect of housing conditions on health from other factors (see

p. 93). Moreover, there may be links between housing conditions and health not necessarily connected to poverty. For example, it has been suggested that the trend towards centrally heated homes with fitted carpets has increased the likelihood of allergies resulting from 'dust mites'.

Nevertheless, the strong relationship between health and housing can be related to four aspects of that housing:

• the geographical location – where people live
• patterns of tenure
• the poor layout and design of homes
• the costs of fuel and other essential services

For a full discussion of these four aspects, see Thomson et al. 1995, Chapter 4, pp. 263–5.

ACTIVITY 52

Read the article below. What strategies would you recommend to reduce the incidence of TB?

SHARP RISE IN TB AMONG THE POOR

The incidence of tuberculosis rose by more than one-third in the poorest one-tenth of the population in England and Wales between 1988 and 1992, according to a study that blames poor living conditions and over-crowding for the increase, writes Liz Hunt.

Overall, the number of TB cases nationally was up 12 per cent but the increase affected only the poorest areas of both countries.

The study shows that the increase in some areas affected white people, West Indians, and people from the Indian sub-continent to a similar degree.

Doctors say this suggests that the recent entry of refugees from high-risk countries and the presence of other ethnic minority communities in the population which had been linked with the rise in TB, was a 'minor factor' and that deteriorating socio-economic factors were responsible . . .

They recommend better health education programmes in high-risk areas, and improved contact tracing.

(The Independent, 13 April 1995)

Diet and health

In June 1991 the National Children's Home charity commissioned a survey on the eating habits of low-income families in the UK. The results suggested that 1 in 5 parents regularly denied themselves food through lack of money, and 1 in 10 children under the age of five went without enough to eat at least once a month. The report claimed to have found a direct relationship between those on the lowest income and those with the poorest diet.

ACTIVITY 53

1 Politicians often claim that it is possible to eat healthily on Income Support level. How far do you agree with this claim?

In a group in your school or college, design a diet to feed yourselves for three or four weeks on the amount of money you would have if you were on Income Support. Is this diet healthy, or are there deficiencies?

2 Read the article below:

COULD LOTTERY FEVER DAMAGE OUR HEALTH?

The National Lottery could be gambling with the nation's health, say researchers.

Medical experts fear the millions of pounds spent each week may be at the expense of more important items – even food . . .

In an editorial in the latest issue of the British Medical Journal, public health specialist Martin McKee calls for research into the social and medical implications of the lottery.

His observations are certain to become a lively talking point over the possible impact of the game. 'Anything that makes poor people in Britain even poorer, especially if they do not derive benefits in kind, becomes an important public health issue,' he says.

However, Lottery organiser Camelot said yesterday that it believes people are merely spending 'loose change in their pocket'.

Mr McKee wants research into 'the extent to which changes in disposable income affect consumption of other goods relevant to health – such as fruit and vegetables on the one hand and tobacco and alcohol on the other'.

He adds: 'Many believe the lottery will widen inequalities. Lotteries tend to gather money from poor people to be spent on amusements for wealthy people . . .'

(The Daily Mail, 22 August 1995)

3 Read the 'Food, diet and health' article below to give you a worldwide perspective on the relationship between poverty and disease. Choose one aspect and investigate it further:

FOOD, DIET, AND HEALTH

The existence of hunger and malnutrition and the persistence of diseases for which medical science has found the cure reveal the inequalities in the modern world. While food supplies are sufficient to meet the world's aggregate minimum requirements, they are so inequitably distributed among the different countries and among the people of each country because of income disparities that the lives of hundreds of millions are affected.

Interactions between nutrition and infection to produce the 'malnutrition/infection complex' create the greatest public health problem in the world. Infection influences nutritional status through its effects on the intake, absorption, and utilization of nutrients and in some cases on the body's requirement for them. A child's rate of growth may be retarded by too little food and/or too many infections or parasites. Malnutrition may result in lowered immunity. Infection can lead to loss of appetite, decreased efficiency of food and nutrient utilization, increased energy requirements, and decreased growth. The relationship between diarrhoeal diseases and physical growth has been clearly shown. These interrelationships produce the malnutrition and infection cycle so prevalent in many developing countries. The vulnerability of malnourished people to environmental health risks has been widely documented. Hence the importance of improved water supplies, sanitation, and safe food to reduce water-related and foodborne diseases and of programmes to control disease vectors supported by education and health care.

It is now widely accepted that chronic hunger is due more to lack of purchasing power or of land on which to produce food than to the non-availability of food. Alleviation of poverty is at the forefront of the development agenda, but waiting for its decline to alleviate malnutrition may take decades. The results of poverty – hunger, sickness, debility, early death – are centred on nutrition. Malnutrition results, and preventing malnutrition is an aim that can be monitored.

Nutrient deficiency diseases

Iodine

Goitre and cretinism are clinically obvious and easily recognizable forms of this deficiency. But the more pervasive effects of milder deficiency on the survival and physical and mental development of children and the intellectual ability and work capacity of adults are now being recognized. About 1,000 million people are affected in more than 80 countries; the Andes, Alps, Great Lakes basin of North America, and Himalayas are particularly iodine-deficient areas, but coastal areas and plains may also be deficient. Excessive intake of goitrogens (for example through eating cassava) interferes with the normal intake and metabolism of iodine and may amplify the effects of iodine deficiency.

Vitamin A

Vitamin A deficiency, leading to xerophthalmia and sometimes blindness, continues to be a widespread problem among children. This deficiency also decreases resistance to infections and thus increases mortality. Analyses of food supplies from different regions show that the availability of vitamin A is limited and the problem exacerbated by any tendency to withhold vegetables from children for cultural or other reasons. The problem is most pronounced in Asia because the overall availability of vitamin A is less than that required and any maldistribution of foods high in vitamin A within a population worsens the problem. Xerophthalmia continues to be a major problem in about 40 countries.

Iron

Anaemia, whose dominant cause is iron deficiency, remains a major problem. Estimates made in 1980 suggest that it affects close to 200 million children between 0 and 4 years of age, 217 million between 5 and 12 years, 174 million men, and 288 million women (including 54 million pregnant women). Most are in Southern Asia, although the proportion of those affected is high in Africa; in both these regions half or more of all children in both age groups and close to half of all women are affected. More than three-fifths of all pregnant women are affected in these two regions. Anaemia also affects significant proportions in each of the above groups in other developing countries. In many areas of the tropics or subtropics, dietary iron deficiency due to low intake and/or poor absorption may be complicated by hookworm infection, which causes intestinal blood loss and may lead to profound iron deficiency anaemia.

Others

Fluoride deficiency increases the incidence of dental caries. (On the other hand, excess of fluoride leads to mottling of teeth and in severe cases to bone damage.) Rickets, which is still widespread in parts of Northern Africa and the Eastern Mediterranean and is reported to be increasing in Mexico, is attributable to insufficient exposure to sunlight and lack of vitamin D in the diet. Ascorbic acid deficiency is a problem in some drought-affected populations, especially in Africa. Vitamin B12 deficiency, which causes anaemia and, if severe, neurological disorders, may occur in those consuming exclusively vegetarian diets.

(WHO, 1992)

Education and health

Living in poverty magnifies the stresses and anxieties of daily living in health-damaging ways and reduces people's capacities for making healthy choices. For example, smoking is now predominantly a habit of the poor, which contributes to the health inequalities described above. Particularly high smoking rates are found among people who are unemployed and young adults with children, particularly lone parents. Health-education campaigns exhorting people to stop smoking may be considered to be 'blaming the victims' and may, therefore, do more harm than good. This means that a wide range of other policies should be considered, from those concerned with eradicating poverty to a ban on tobacco advertising and an increase in cigarette prices.

ACTIVITY 54

1 Can you think of health-education campaigns which are likely to be effective in changing the habits of poorer people?

2 How will the educational background of the target group affect the way health-promotional advice is presented to them? Can you find examples of health-promotional advice aimed at target groups from two different educational backgrounds?

Cultural expectations and health

Despite the multi-racial nature of British society, both now and in the past, many routinely collected statistics on health do not provide information on ethnic groups. Although there is a lack of meaningful routine statistics on the health status of different ethnic groups, there is sufficient evidence to demonstrate the poorer health suffered by certain minorities. However, these minorities do generally have lower rates of mortality than do people in their country of origin.

Figure 3.38 provides information on general-practitioner-consultation rates by sex and ethnicity. It shows that for all complaints listed together, the differences between the ethnic groups are fairly minor, although the consultation rate for Indian males is well above average. However, males and females of Indian and Caribbean origin and Irish males have much higher consultation rates for serious complaints. It is difficult to determine the reasons for these differences. Although there are some diseases, such as sickle-cell disease, which are specific to certain ethnic groups because of the higher frequency of a gene, these genetic diseases account for only a tiny minority of cases of ill-health within the group. Cultural differences such as diet are often suggested as explanations, but research indicates that the diets of many ethnic minorities are more healthy than the majority, with lower levels of saturated fats and cholesterol, and higher levels of fibre. Often, there are also lower levels of smoking and drinking in ethnic-minority groups.

Although it is likely that poverty may at least partly explain the poorer health of ethnic minorities, it is most likely that there is an interaction of social and cultural influences involved here. For example, it could be that minority ethnic groups are deterred by a

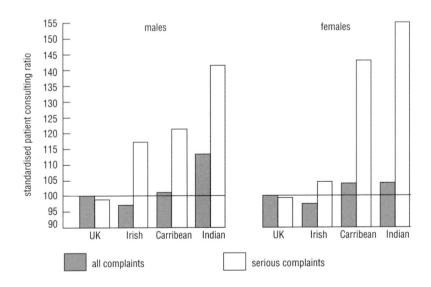

Figure 3.38 Standardised patient consulting ratios in general practice by sex and ethnicity, 1981–82 (all ethnic groups = 100)

Source: Morbidity statistics from general practice 1981–82 (series MB5 No. 2), HMSO, London, 1990

range of cultural barriers, institutionalised racism and socioeconomic disadvantages from seeking help from general practitioners in all but the most serious of cases.

ACTIVITY 55

An interesting class exercise or opportunity for research would be to investigate different cultural perceptions of health and illness among fellow students or within your community. Some questions you might ask could be:

- What value do different ethnic-minority groups attach to 'health'?
- What approaches do people have towards 'becoming healthy' or being in 'perfect health'?
- How is illness/disease viewed?
- What is ill-health attributed to?
- What contact have people had with health (and care) services in the UK? Have these been positive or negative in any respects?

Other questions may be asked about different perceptions of specific illnesses, diseases, medical conditions or childbirth/death practices and beliefs. Did any clear differences in health beliefs occur between members of various ethnic-minority, cultural or religious groups? Or were there more similarities than differences? How might you explain your findings?

ASSESSMENT OPPORTUNITY

1 Produce a report on two examples of infectious disease which includes the following:
- a description of the cause(s) of each disease
- an explanation of the modes of transmission of each disease

- a description of methods for the control and prevention of each disease
- an evaluation of the role of any socioeconomic factors affecting health and each disease

Your report could be written; in poster form; as a booklet or leaflet; oral; or any combination of these.

2 Write notes on four other non-infectious diseases or illnesses, including causes and the role of socioeconomic factors.

PROCESSES AND RESPONSES IN DISEASE AND ILLNESS

The stages of the disease process

1 *Transmission and infection*: the acquisition of the pathogen (see above for methods of transmission).
2 *The incubation period*: the time between infection and the appearance of signs and symptoms. During this time, the pathogen will be multiplying.
3 *Signs and symptoms*: signs are the objective abnormalities that can be seen by someone other than the patient, whereas symptoms are the subjective abnormalities felt only by the patient.

ACTIVITY 56

Which of the following are signs, and which are symptoms?
- a high body temperature
- headache
- rash
- shivering
- lethargy

4 Crisis: the turning point of a disease, after which the patient either improves or

deteriorates. Since the advent of antibiotics infections seldom reach the point of crisis.

5 *Convalescence and recovery*: the phase during which signs and symptoms disappear.

ACTIVITY 57

Can you think of examples of diseases for which this phase takes

(a) a few days
(b) a few weeks
(c) months or even years?

ACTIVITY 58

Consider the following diseases: chicken pox, the common cold; myalgic encephalomyelitis (ME); 'flu; measles; gonorrhoea. Find out about:

(a) the method of transmission
(b) the length of the incubation period
(c) the signs
(d) the symptoms
(e) the usual length of convalescence and recovery.

Stress

Stress represents an inadequate adaptation to change, or an unsuccessful attempt on the part of individuals to cope with, and adapt to, the changed circumstances of their lives.

ACTIVITY 59

Examples of factors causing stress (*stressors*) include the following:

• bereavement
• the birth of a child
• moving house

Can you think of other examples of stressors?

The stress response is affected by a number of factors which include:

• the characteristics of the individuals
• their physical environment
• the social support available to them
• their economic status
• their cultural background

Not all these factors present themselves as negative factors in relation to the stress response. The importance of each factor lies in each individual's ability to adapt and respond to the stressor.

STRESS AND PERSONALITY

Different people can tolerate different levels of arousal.

At one end of the scale are those who actively seek out maximum stress, who take life-threatening risks, for example stunt performers, racing drivers, mountaineers. Such people are characterised by, among other things, a very low level of anxiety and a high degree of emotional control.

At the other extreme are those who find too much arousal in everyday life and seek to minimise it. Some people who find ordinary life too stressful may develop panic attacks or phobias, and need psychological treatment. (See the section on mental illnesses above.)

Too high arousal – excessive stress – leads to poor performance. Too much stress affects a complex task more than a simple task, but very high arousal will affect even performance of the simplest task. This relationship between performance and arousal is known as the Yerkes–Dobson Law (see Figure 3.39).

ACTIVITY 60

Too high arousal may be controlled by advance planning and rehearsal of the stressful situation. Levels of arousal are cumulative, so a lot of minor 'hassles' will add to the overall level of arousal.

1 Think of a stressful situation coming up, e.g. an important interview, examination, driving test.

2 Think of all the stressful things that have happened in previous such situations, and list them.

3 Then make a list of stressful things that might happen, e.g. for an interview:
   • *stressful things that happened in previous interviews*: couldn't answer the questions; clothes felt wrong
   • *stressful things that could happen in this interview*: might get up late and miss the bus, might not be able to find the interview room

4 Go through your lists and work out a way of being absolutely sure that none of these things would actually happen at your important interview.

THE PHYSIOLOGICAL RESPONSE TO STRESS

Biologically, stress is any stimulus which creates an imbalance in the body. The stress may come from the external environment, for example heat, loud noise or a lack of oxygen, or it may originate within the body in the form of stimuli such as high blood pressure, pain or unpleasant thoughts. Fortunately, the body has many regulating devices that oppose the forces of stress and bring the internal environment back into balance, but if the stress is extreme or prolonged it triggers a wide range of bodily changes called the *general adaptation syndrome*. This syndrome does *not* maintain a constant internal environment. It does just the opposite. For example, blood pressure and the blood sugar level are raised above normal. The purpose of these changes is to gear the body up to meet an emergency.

The emotional centres of the cerebral cortex are connected to the hypothalamus. When the hypothalamus senses stress, it triggers a series of events leading to the 'alarm' or 'flight, fight or fright' reaction which is the body's initial response to a stressor. The hypothalamus stimulates the production of the hormone *adrenalin* which has the following effects:
• an increased heart rate
• the constriction of blood vessels in the skin and around the gut
• a dilation of the blood vessels of the heart and skeletal muscles
• the conversion of glycogen into glucose in the liver
• sweating
• the dilation of the bronchial tubes
• decreased urine production

These responses are rapid and short-lived.

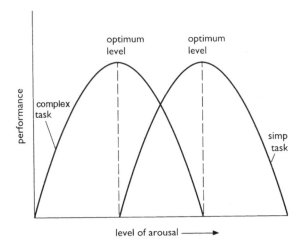

Figure 3.39 The Yerkes–Doson law of arousal
Source: Thomson et al., 1995.

ACTIVITY 61

1 Describe the appearance of a person who has just been frightened badly. Link these characteristics to the effects of adrenalin as listed above.

2 The function of adrenalin is to mobilise the body's resources for immediate physical activity. Large amounts of oxygen and glucose are brought to the organs which are most active in warding

off danger. These are the brain, the skeletal muscles and the heart. Non-essential activities decrease. How do the effects of adrenalin listed above help with these processes?

3 These physiological responses may no longer be appropriate to our modern lifestyle. What does this mean?

If the stressor is not removed, there is a *resistance reaction*. This is a long-term reaction which accelerates the body's metabolism to provide energy to counteract stress. If the stressor is still not removed, a stage of *exhaustion* results. In this stage, the body's resources become depleted; the adrenal gland cannot function properly; and blood glucose levels drop. It is at this stage that *psychosomatic disorders* develop (see below).

STRESS-RELATED ILLNESS

Stress and how we manage our own stress levels has a direct link to our general well-being. Various illnesses may be said to be either caused or triggered by stress, including:

- stomach ulcers, which may sometimes be caused by too much acid being produced in the stomach at a time of anxiety or worry
- heart attacks: it is thought that the fat released into the bloodstream when the body responds to demands gets trapped in the walls of the heart's own vessels. This gradually narrows these tubes, and when increased demand is placed on the heart, the narrowed tubes prevent the flow of oxygen, causing the heart muscle to die
- skin disorders such as eczema and psoriasis
- myalgic encephalomyelitis (ME): the role of stress has been well documented in this very distressing condition

Myalgic encephalomyelitis is sometimes called *post-viral fatigue syndrome*. In April 1990, it was estimated that 150,000 people in the UK were affected by ME, and studies affirmed that

people in the caring professions made up the largest group affected, with three times as many women as men suffering from ME. The label 'yuppie flu' was given to ME by the press, although it was rejected by ME victims as insulting. The media have given relatively little attention to ME compared with other illnesses affecting a similar proportion of the population.

No one definite cause is known, but various theories have suggested the following:

- a persistent viral infection
- damage to the immune system following a viral infection
- a neurotic disorder, e.g. hyperventilation

The main symptoms are:

- muscle fatigue
- exhaustion
- headaches
- dizziness

Other symptoms common to many people with ME are:

- muscular pains
- fever
- depression
- bowel and digestive problems

There is no diagnostic test, although enteroviruses can be traced in the colon of more than half of ME sufferers. Diagnosis is by a process of elimination of other illnesses and diseases.

The medical profession has little to offer in terms of scientific explanation or treatment of ME. The following treatments are among the more common:

- anti-depressants: these are often prescribed, but the long-term use of these drugs is not recommended
- a sugar- and yeast-free diet: many sufferers follow this, in common with sufferers from *candida albicans*, a yeast infection of the gut. It is thought that stress can lead to a weakening of the immune system, thus allowing this infection to flourish
- relaxation techniques such as meditation,

the Alexander technique and yoga are often practised
- homoeopathy
- acupuncture
- herbal treatments, e.g. with evening primrose oil
- counselling: this can enable a person to lead a less stressful lifestyle, thereby reducing their propensity to further bouts of ME

CASE STUDY: HOLLY

Before becoming ill with ME, Holly, aged 32, had led an active life both at work as a social worker and outside her job, having many interests which occupied most of her spare hours. She made little time for relaxation, and her diet was high in sugar and carbohydrates. Her emotional history had been stressful. When she became ill, she suffered from most of the common symptoms of ME and was bedridden for three months. After numerous setbacks and relapses, she is now in the fifth year of her illness and has used diet, homoeopathy, herbal treatments and counselling as her path to recovery. The most difficult experiences for Holly were the financial implications of being ill. She lost her job and has been living on state benefits; she has found her practical circumstances difficult to reconcile with her need for relaxation and a reduction in stress. After five years out of work it will be difficult for her to find a job, particularly with this history of ill-health. She says that counselling has empowered her to face the stresses and difficulties which the future might hold without becoming ill again.

ACTIVITY 62

Study Holly's story, then answer the following questions:
1 What advice and recommendations should be made to a person with ME pre-disposal factors to help that person avoid contracting ME?

2 What support should be made available to people with ME by
 (a) the NHS;
 (b) the DSS;
 (c) the workplace;
 (d) friends and family?

3 Many ME sufferers feel isolated as there is still a lot of ignorance about the illness. How could this be combated?

Coping with stress

PSYCHOLOGICAL METHODS

Lazarus and Folkman (1984) found two major forms of coping strategy:
- emotion-focused coping, using ego defence mechanisms
- problem-focused coping

Defence mechanisms

These are means of emotion-focused coping; while useful in the short term, they are unhealthy and undesirable in the long term. See Table 3.9 on p. 184.

CASE STUDY: A FAMILY UNDER STRESS

A woman describes her situation to a member of the social services department:

I've come with my little one who's having terrible nightmares and wetting the bed. We've got no money, my husband's been made redundant, it's completely changed him, he just sits around watching old films on TV. His temper is terrible too, he keeps shouting and slamming doors. My eldest boy is all right, but they keep ringing up to say he's not attending school, well why should he if there's no jobs to go to afterwards, they're even concerned he might be trying drugs – well, not my boy, I don't believe that – the school just pick on him, his teacher is always criticising, she's useless. Why don't they think of me? I can't take much more.

Table 3.9   Examples of ego defence mechanisms

Defence mechanism	Description	Example
Repression	Repression of painful or frightening memory out of consciousness. (But repressed memories can still affect behaviour)	A child who has been abused may push the memory out of consciousness but then be disturbed for years by bad dreams
Rationalisation	Making an excuse and believing it. Not giving the real reason	'I can't speak in public because I've got a cough'
Reaction formation	Concealing a motive from oneself by giving strong expression to the opposite motive	People who crusade with fanatical zeal against loose morals, alcohol etc. may themselves at one time have had difficulty with these problems
Projection	Protects us from recognising our own undesirable traits by assigning them in exaggerated amounts to other people	'I hate that group of people' becomes 'they hate me'. An element of paranoia and prejudice
Intellectualisation	Used to distance oneself from suffering	Used by e.g. doctors
Denial	When a reality is too unpleasant to face, an individual may deny it exists	Someone refusing to accept they have a serious illness, or that a relationship is over
Displacement	Choosing a substitute object for the expression of feelings	When angry with parents/partner, slam the door or kick the cat.
Regression	Returning to an old childhood habit	Eating or curling up in bed when upset
Sublimation	Finding a substitute activity to express an unacceptable impulse. This is a constructive defence mechanism and could be called problem-focused	Rechannelling aggression by playing sport

Source: Thomson et al. 1995.

ACTIVITY 63

1 Read the above case study of a family trying to deal with its problems using emotion-focused coping.

2 Identify the defence mechanisms being used by the family members.

3 What are the possible strengths in this family?

4 What might a counsellor suggest as more conscious and constructive ways of dealing with their problems?

Role-play is a possibility here (for example, one person could take the role of the mother and one person could take the role of the counsellor).

Problem-focused coping

These are *conscious* ways of trying to adapt to stress in a positive and constructive way. They include:

* searching for information
* problem solving
* seeking help from others
* recognising true feelings
* establishing goals and objectives

Grasha (1983) described the problem-focused mechanisms as in Table 3.10.

PRACTICAL METHODS

ACTIVITY 64

Before you read any further, imagine yourself to be in a stressful position. For example, you have an end-of-unit test in a fortnight on a topic you find particularly difficult. What might you do to cope with the stress this generates? Within the class you may find that some people choose methods which are beneficial to their health whereas others choose methods which are detrimental to their health.

1 Look at the list below of beneficial methods and discuss their effectiveness (or course, different people will favour different approaches):

(a) *Changes in work patterns.* For example, you plan a revision timetable (and stick to it!) which allows you to spend an hour each evening going through your work with a friend.

(b) *Exercise.* For example, you make time to go for an early morning swim.

(c) *The use of relaxation techniques.* For example, you start attending yoga classes.

(d) *A healthy diet.* You make time to enjoy a regular, well-balanced meal.

(e) *An increase in leisure pursuits.* For example, you make time in your

revision timetable for relaxing with friends.

2 *Detrimental practices* may include the increased use of tobacco, alcohol, tranquillisers or sleeping pills, or the illegal use of drugs. For each of these substances, list the harmful effects they may cause (see the above 'Self-inflicted' diseases section).

3 Design and use a questionnaire to find out the range and effectiveness of methods for coping with stress that people use.

ASSESSMENT OPPORTUNITY

1 Prepare and give a presentation on an investigation into processes and responses involved in disease and illness which includes:

- a description of the stages of the disease process, including signs of inflammation
- a description of methods of achieving immune status
- an explanation of the immune-system process

2 Produce a report which explains the effect of stress and describes the methods of coping with stress.

Table 3.10 Problem-focused mechanisms

Coping mechanism	Description
Objectivity	Separating feelings from thoughts
Logical analysis	Analysing problems; making plans
Concentration	Putting aside upsetting thoughts to concentratge on the matter in hand
Empathy	Seeing how others feel in a situation and taking account of this
Suppression	*Not* repression: this is holding feelings back consciously until the time is right to express them
Substitution of thoughts and emotions	*Consciously* to substitute thoughts for how we really think in order to deal with a difficult situation

SOURCES OF INFORMATION

Information may be found from a local community physician, health centres, health-promotion departments, WHO, UNICEF and any standard publications listing information on health statistics (see the section in this chapter 'Sources of information for determining patterns of disease').

When possible, invite local health professionals in to talk to your group or arrange interviews with them.

REFERENCES AND RESOURCES

Beaglehole, R., Bonita, R. and Kjellstrom, T. (1993), *Basic Epidemiology*, Geneva: WHO.

Benzeval, M., Judge, K. and Whitehead, M., (ed) (1995), *Tackling Health Inequalities: an Agenda for Action*, Poole: BEBC.

Blackburn, C. (1991), *Poverty and Health: Working with Families*, Oxford: OUP.

Black Report (1980), *Inequalities in Health*, London: Penguin.

Gray, A. (ed.) (1993), *World Health and Disease*, Buckingham: Open University Press.

Health Education Council (1987), *The Health Divide*, London: HEC.

Martinez, C. A., Barua, D. and Merson, M. H. (1988), 'Control of diarrhoeal diseases', *World Health Statistics Quarterly*, vol. 41, no. 2, pp. 74–81.

McConway, K. (ed) (1994), *Studying Health and Disease*, Buckingham: Open University Press.

Molla, A. M. et al. (1985), 'Rice-based oral rehydration solution decreases the stool volume in acute diarrhoea', *Bulletin of WHO*, vol. 63, no. 4, pp. 751–6.

Oppenheim, C. (1993), *Poverty: the Facts*, London: Child Poverty Action Group.

PHA (1995), *Poverty and Health – Tools for Change*, Birmingham: PHA.

Thomson et al. (1995), *Health and Social Care*, 2nd edn, London: Hodder and Stoughton.

Timmreck, T. C. (1994), 'An introduction to epidemiology', Boston: Jones and Bartlett.

Tolba, M. K. et al. (ed) (1992), *The World Environment 1972–1992: Two Decades of Challenge*, London: Chapman and Hall, on behalf of the United Nations Environment Programme (UNEP).

Tortora, G. and Anagnostakos, N. (1987), New York: Harper and Row.

Waddington, I. (1989), 'Inequalities in health', *Social Studies Review*, January.

West, R. (1994), *Obesity*, London: Office of Health Economics.

Which? Consumer Guides (1991), 'Understanding back trouble', Sevenoaks: Hodder and Stoughton.

World Health Organization (1987), *WHO Expert Committee on Onchoceriasis – 3rd Report*, Technical Report Series 752, Geneva: WHO.

World Health Organization (1992), *Our Planet, Our Health: Report of the WHO Commission on Health and Environment*, Geneva: WHO, HMSO.

UNEP (1989), *Environmental Data Report 1989/90*, Oxford: Blackwell.

UNEP (1992), *The World Environment 1972–1992*, London: Chapman and Hall.

UNICEF (1986), *The State of the World's Children 1986*, Oxford: OUP.

USEFUL ADDRESSES

OPCS publications, official reports and other government documents are available from:

HMSO
49 High Holborn
London WC1V 6HB
Tel.: 0171 873 0011 (enquiries); 0171 873 9090 (orders)

There are also HMSO shops in Manchester, Birmingham, Bristol, Edinburgh, Belfast and Cardiff.

WHO publications are available from:

World Health Organization
1211 Geneva 27
Switzerland

For epidemiological journals:

International Journal of Epidemiology
Journal Subscriptions Department
Oxford University Press
Walton Street
Oxford OX2 60P

Journal of Epidemiology and Community Health
British Medical Journal
BMA House
Tavistock Square
London WC1H 9JR

Bournemouth English Book Centre (BEBC)
PO Box 1496
Poole
Dorset BH12 3YD

Office of Health Economics
12 Whitehall
London SW1A 2DY

(PHA)
138 Disbeth
Birmingham B5 6DR
Tel.: 0121 643 7628

4

PHYSICAL SCIENCE FOR HEALTH CARE

This chapter develops an understanding of the laws of physics covering forces and machines, sound, light and electricity. The applications of these laws to the care setting are described.

Wherever and whenever possible, practical work should be carried out and accurate records maintained. You should keep a notebook for this purpose, and these records will then form part of your Assessment Opportunity work.

MECHANICS IN CARE CONTEXTS

The application of the laws of force and motion to the human body and to care contexts

UNITS

For ease of communication, it is important that scientists use the same system of *units of measurement*. The one most frequently used is the Système International (SI). Table 4.1 gives some of the more commonly used base units, and Table 4.2 gives some of the commonly used *prefixes*.

ACTIVITY I

1 The most fundamental quantities in any physical science are *mass*, *length* and *time*. Check which units are used to record these quantities (see Table 4.1).

2 Refer to Table 4.2, and decide which units you would use to record the following:
  - a person's height
  - a person's weight
  - the width of a cell
  - the distance between two hospitals

MASS, WEIGHT AND GRAVITY

Mass is a quantity of matter. It is measured in kilogrammes (kg), and is constant wherever

Table 4.1 Commonly used base units of the SI system

Physical quantity	Abbreviation	Name of unit	Symbol for unit
Length	l	metre	m
Mass	m	kilogramme	kg
Time	t	second	s
Temperature	T	kelvin	K
Current	I	ampere	A
Charge	Q	coulomb	C
Resistance	R	ohm	Ω
Voltage (potential difference)	V	volt	V
Work	W	joule	J

Table 4.2 Commonly used prefixes of the SI system

Prefix	Sub-multiple	Symbol
centi-	10^{-2}	c
milli-	10^{-3}	m
micro-	10^{-6}	μ
nano-	10^{-9}	n
pico-	10^{-12}	p
	Multiple	
kilo-	10^{3}	k
mega-	10^{6}	M
giga-	10^{9}	G

the body is situated in the universe. A mass is pulled downwards towards the earth. This is because all bodies are attracted to each other. The force which pulls masses together is *gravity*. Usually, this force is too small to notice, but because the mass of the earth is so large, the force becomes noticeable. A large mass is pulled towards the earth with greater force than a small one. The strength of the force pulling an object towards the earth is called its *weight*. Like all forces, this is measured in *newtons* (N). A kilogramme of mass is pulled towards the earth by a force of 9.81 N. (To make calculations easier, we usually say the strength of gravity on earth is 10 N/kg.) The following equation is used to calculate weight:

weight = mass × strength of gravity (g)

ACTIVITY 2

What is the weight of a person with a mass of 60 kg

(a) on earth
(b) in space where there is no gravitational force?

NB: in a care setting (for example, a GP's surgery), if a person is asked their weight, they will give their mass in kilogrammes and not their weight in newtons!

CENTRES OF GRAVITY AND EQUILIBRIUM

The centre of gravity of a body is the point through which its whole weight may be considered to act. If the body is supported either exactly under or exactly above that point, it will balance. This is because the forces on each side are equal. The body is then said to be in *equilibrium*.

A body is said to be in *stable equilibrium* if, when given a small displacement and then released, it returns to its original position; for example, if someone in a lying position is

pulled up a little and then released, they will fall back into the lying position. A body is said to be in *unstable equilibrium* if, when given a small displacement and then released, it moves further from its original position – for example, if a standing person is pushed and falls over. A body is said to be in *neutral equilibrium* if, when given a small displacement and then released, it remains in its new position – for example, if a person on a stool is swivelled round to face a different direction.

For a body in stable equilibrium, the stability is increased by having a large base area or a low centre of gravity, or both. The correct stance adopted by a carer when lifting a person *manual handling* illustrates this. The legs should be positioned apart to give a large base area, and the knees should be bent to lower the centre of gravity (see Figure 4.1).

Lifting a person on a *stretcher* gives a large base area and a low centre of gravity.

ACTIVITY 3

1 A body is unstable when its centre of gravity lies outside its base: in other words, when a line drawn vertically downwards does not pass through the base (see Figure 4.2). Draw simple diagrams of people in different positions to illustrate stable and unstable postures. In each case, indicate the base and the approximate centre of gravity.

2 Read through the guidelines for lifting for people working in the health services. (Suggested sources are given at the end of this chapter.)

FRICTION

Friction is a force which acts when two surfaces are in contact. The particles of the two surfaces are attracted, so when one surface is dragged over the other, work has to be done to overcome this attraction.

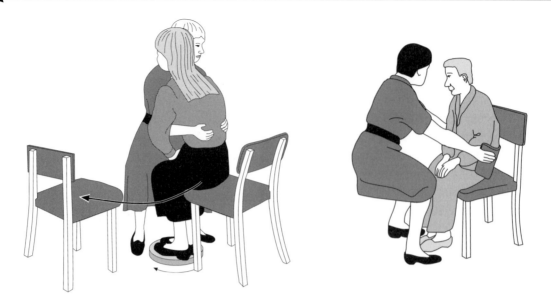

Figure 4.1 Correct lifting procedures – making a single-nurse transfer or lift safe and comfortable for nurse and patient
Source: Nursing Times, 18 January 1995, vol. 91, no. 3.

Catheter insertion

A catheter is any flexible tube which may be inserted into a narrow opening in the body so that fluids may be introduced or removed. For example, a urinary catheter is inserted into the bladder through the urethra to allow urine to drain away. Catheters can also be placed in the blood vessels. There is friction between the molecules of liquid moving along a catheter, but there is an even greater attraction between the molecules of liquid and the surface of the walls of the catheter. This means that liquid flows more slowly near the walls and faster in the middle. The narrower the diameter of the catheter, the more the friction will slow the flow of liquid. Thick liquids are subject to more friction between particles than thinner liquids. This friction inside a liquid is known as *viscosity*, and a less viscous liquid will flow more rapidly than a more viscous liquid.

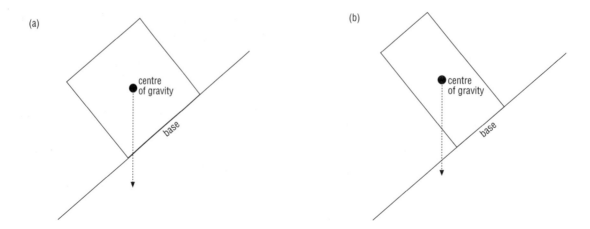

Figure 4.2 Stable and unstable objects compared: (a) stable object, (b) unstable object

ACTIVITY 4

1 What are the disadvantages in using a catheter tube with a wide diameter?

2 To reduce the friction between two moving surfaces, a *lubricant* can be used. Find out about the lubrication of the joints of the body.

3 Several lifting devices are now available to make it easier to move patients (see Figure 4.1 for an example of a swivelling low-friction board). Find out about the range available. Draw diagrams of these, and explain how they work.

SCALAR AND VECTOR QUANTITIES

A *scalar* quantity has magnitude only, but a *vector* quantity has magnitude and direction. Examples of scalar quantities are mass, distance, time and energy. Force and weight are examples of vector quantities.

SPEED, VELOCITY AND ACCELERATION

Speed is a scalar measurement. It is a measurement of length travelled per unit time, but it gives no information about the *direction* of travel.

Average speed can be calculated by using the following formula:

$$\text{average speed} = \frac{\text{distance moved}}{\text{time taken}}$$

ACTIVITY 5

Using this formula, calculate the approximate average speed of a red blood cell if it takes 60 seconds to travel around the body – i.e. from the right atrium, through the pulmonary circulation, back to the left ventricle, through the systemic circulation, down to the foot, and back again to the right atrium. You will have to make a rough estimate of this distance.

The *rate of flow* (the speed at which a fluid moves) has to be calculated when a nurse administers *intravenous fluid* (i.e. a 'drip' – see Figure 4.3). When an intravenous order is written, it usually specifies the amount of fluid to be absorbed per hour. The nurse must then calculate the number of drops per minute required to give the hourly volume prescribed. This differs according to the administration set used (the relevant information, such as the 'drop factor' is printed on the box containing the administration set).

The following equation can be used to calculate the flow rate:

$$\text{flow rate (drops per minute)} = \frac{\text{volume to be given/hour} \times \text{drop factor}}{\text{time of infusion in minutes}}$$

$$\text{i.e. flow rate} = \frac{\text{volume}}{\text{time}}$$

Velocity expresses speed in a specified direction (in a straight line). Because it specifies both magnitude and direction, velocity is a vector quantity.

Average velocity can be calculated by using the following formula:

$$\text{average velocity} = \frac{\text{displacement}}{\text{time}}$$

where *displacement* is the distance travelled in a specified direction (in a straight line).

NB: the difference between speed and velocity only becomes important when an object does not move in a single straight line.

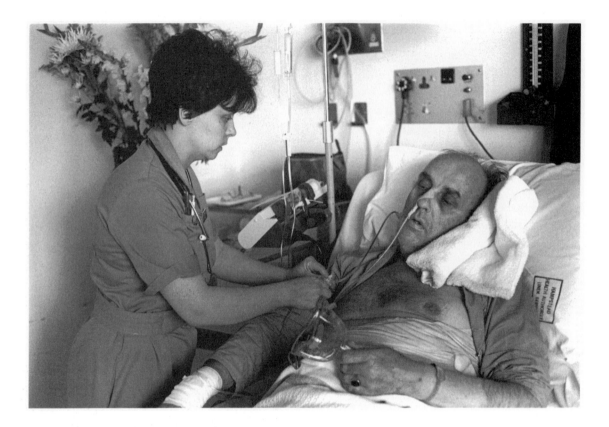

Figure 4.3   Intravenous fluid administration

ACTIVITY 6

A nurse walks around a ward from A to B to C, as shown in Figure 4.4. She travels at an average speed of 1 metre per second.

1 How far does she walk?

2 How long does this take her?

3 What is her displacement in the direction AC?

4 What is her average velocity in the direction AC? (Express your answer in metres per second (m/s).)

Acceleration tells you how fast velocity is changing. If velocity is decreasing, acceleration is negative. If velocity is increasing, acceleration is positive.

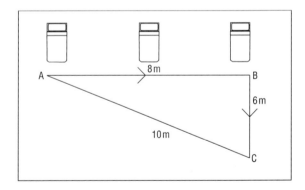

Figure 4.4   Calculating velocity

Acceleration can be calculated by using the following formula:

$$\text{acceleration} = \frac{\text{change in velocity (m/s)}}{\text{time taken (s)}}$$

The units in which acceleration can therefore be expressed are *metres per second per second*, but this can be shortened to m/s^2 or ms^{-2}.

NEWTON'S LAWS OF MOTION

1 If a body is at rest, it will remain at rest; and if it is in motion, it will continue to move in a straight line with constant velocity unless it is acted upon by a resultant external force. (See the 'Friction' section on pp. 189–191 above.)

2 The acceleration of a body is directly proportional to the resultant force acting on it and inversely proportional to the mass of the body:

force = mass × acceleration

In other words, the harder you push an object, the faster it accelerates, and ends up going faster. The heavier the object, the slower it accelerates; it does not end up going as fast. (Think, for example, of pushing a car!)

3 If a body A exerts a force on body B, then B exerts an equal and opposite force on A.

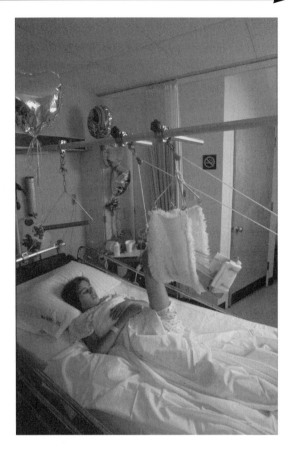

Figure 4.5 Traction

The relationships between work, energy and power

WORK

Work is energy transfer. It can be calculated using the following equation:

work = force applied × distance moved in direction of force

Work is measured in *joules* (J). 1 joule of work is done when a force of 1 N moves its point of application through a distance of 1 metre.

NB: work is done only if a force is actually moving an object.

ACTIVITY 7

Traction is the application of a pulling force, and is usually used as a means of counteracting the natural tension in the tissues surrounding a broken bone (see Figure 4.5). Considerable force may be exerted with weights, ropes and pulleys to ensure that a broken bone is kept correctly positioned during the early stages of healing. Draw a diagram of this process, using arrows to show the exertion of equal and opposite forces.

ACTIVITY 8

Calculate how much work is done when you climb up a vertical 10 metre ladder. (NB: you will need to work out your weight in newtons first.)

ENERGY

Energy is the capacity to do work. It is measured in joules. Energy cannot be created or destroyed (this is *the principle of the conservation of energy*), but it can be changed from one form into another.

Potential energy

Potential energy is energy due to position. This is accumulated in a system as a result of previous work being done on the system. For example, if a body is lifted vertically, then it gains gravitational potential energy. This can be calculated using the following equation:

gravitational potential energy gained
= weight × vertical height gained

(Remember: weight = mass × gravity.)

Other examples of potential energy include:

- the energy stored in a stretched elastic band
- the energy stored in a spring

Kinetic energy

Kinetic energy is the energy possessed by a moving body. For example, a swinging pendulum has kinetic energy. It has most kinetic energy at the bottom of its swing, since this is where it is going fastest. At the top of its swing, where it momentarily stops, its kinetic energy is zero. At this point, all its kinetic energy has been converted into potential energy.

Kinetic energy can be calculated using the following equation:

kinetic energy $= 1/2 \, mv^2$

(where: m = mass and v = velocity).

To stop a moving object, the force applied must equal the kinetic energy of the object. In other words, the work needed to stop a moving object depends on the square of its velocity. For example, if a bicycle and rider have a combined mass of 70 kg and are travelling at 5 m/s, their kinetic energy is:

$1/2 \times 70 \text{ kg} \times (5 \text{ m/s})^2 = 875 \text{ J}$

ACTIVITY 9

1 Calculate the kinetic energy if the cyclist travels at twice the above velocity, i.e. 10 m/s. Then, calculate the cyclist's kinetic energy at other velocities and draw a graph to show the relationship between velocity (on the x axis) and kinetic energy (on the y axis).

2 The fact that kinetic energy is determined by the *square* of the velocity means that injuries arising from road accidents become considerably worse when the velocity of a vehicle increases only slightly. Find out how the following absorb the car's driver's kinetic energy:
- crumple zone
- seat belt
- air bag

Energy transfer

Although energy cannot be destroyed (see the principle of the conversation of energy mentioned above), whenever energy is *transferred*, some is wasted. For example, if a block is dragged up a slope, kinetic energy will be converted into potential energy. However, friction will cause some energy to be 'lost' as *heat*. In the body, chemical energy from our food is converted into work by our muscle cells. There are actually many energy transfers between molecules (for example, from glucose to ATP, and between different molecules in the muscle). During each of these different energy transfers, some energy goes into the surroundings as heat. This is why vigorous exercise makes you hot.

ACTIVITY 10

Figure 4.6 shows the energy transfers which take place as a cyclist goes up a hill. Draw a similar diagram to show the energy changes which take place when a person climbs a ladder and comes down a slide.

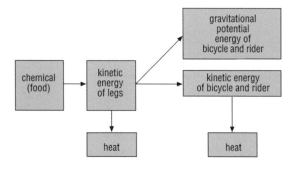

Figure 4.6 Energy transfers that occur when a cyclist climbs a hill
Source: Macmillan Work Out Series: Work Out physics GCSE, H. J. P. Keightey, Macmillan, 1987.

Energy in food

The energy contained in food can be worked out from the amount of heat given out when it is burnt. This can be tested in a *Heat of Combustion* apparatus. A known mass of food is burnt, and the heat given out heats a known quantity of water. This energy should be expressed in *kilojoules* (kJ). (4.2 kJ of energy are required to raise the temperature of 1 *kilogramme* of water by 1 °C.)

(NB: although you should use the SI unit, i.e. the joule, an alternative unit sometimes used is the *calorie* (*cal.*).

1 calorie = 4.2 J

i.e. a calorie is the amount of energy required to raise the temperature of 1 gramme of water by 1 °C.)

Approximately 7,000 kJ, the energy required to boil 100 cups of tea, are required to maintain our basal metabolic rate (i.e. just our 'ticking over' processes), but the exact amount varies from person to person.

ACTIVITY 11

1 During periods of complete rest, for example sleeping in bed, what are the processes taking place in the body which require energy?

2 Find out how much energy is required for half an hour of the following activities:
- tennis
- sleeping
- walking

3 Find out the approximate daily energy requirements of the following groups of people:
- a newborn baby
- a 10-year-old child
- an adult male in a sedentary occupation
- an adult female in a manual occupation

4 Find out how much energy a gramme of each of the following foods contains:
- butter
- bread
- apple
- chicken
- potato chips

5 If possible, use a computer diet programme to calculate your energy consumption on a typical day.

6 If a person's energy consumption is greater than their energy output, the excess energy will be stored as *fat*. What advice would you give to someone who wishes to reduce their fat reserves?

7 Write a list of instructions which would enable a Heat of Combustion apparatus to be used to calculate the energy content of food. What sources of error would there be?

8 To find out how much energy is stored in a peanut, start by putting 25 cm^3 of water in a boiling tube and measuring its temperature. Then, put a peanut on the end of a mounted needle. Heat it

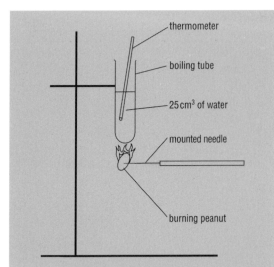

Figure 4.7   Measuring the energy in a peanut

with a Bunsen flame, and as soon as it starts to burn, hold it under the boiling tube (see Figure 4.7). Record the new temperature of the water. Calculate the rise in temperature by subtracting the first from the second temperature. Work out the quantity of energy transferred to the water from the burning peanut as follows:

(a) 4.2 joules raise 1 g of water by 1 °C;

(b) 25 cm^3 of water has a mass of 25 g;

(c) the rise in temperature = T °C; therefore,

(d) the energy from the peanut = (4.2 × 25) × T) joules.

Explain why this experiment is very inaccurate.

POWER

Power is the rate of doing work. It is measured in *watts* (W). 1 watt is a rate of working of 1 joule per second.

Work is calculated using the following formulae:

$$\text{power} = \frac{\text{work done}}{\text{time taken}}$$

$$\text{or} \quad = \frac{\text{energy transferred}}{\text{time taken}}$$

$$\text{or} \quad = \text{force} \times \text{velocity}$$

$$\text{or} \quad = \frac{\text{force} \times \text{distance}}{\text{time taken}}$$

ACTIVITY 12

You can measure your power output during a run upstairs. Find your weight in newtons (look back at the section on weight on pp. 188–189 above). Measure the vertical height of the stairs. Run up the stairs as fast as you can, timing yourself in seconds.

1 Calculate energy transferred (force used × distance moved): your weight in newtons × height of the stairs in metres.

2 Calculate the power output: (your weight × height of stairs)/time taken in seconds.

3 What weight of peanuts should you eat to give you the energy needed?

Lever systems and machines

A *machine* is something that makes work seem easier. It transfers energy from one point to another. The efficiency of a machine can be calculated by using the following formula:

$$\text{efficiency} = \frac{\text{useful output of energy}}{\text{input of energy}}$$

(NB: because efficiency is a ratio it has no units.)

In practice, no machine is 100% efficient – i.e. the input energy is always more than the useful output energy. This is because work must be done against friction, so some energy will always be 'lost' to the surroundings as heat.

LEVERS

A lever is a machine. It may be defined as a rigid rod that moves about on some fixed point called a fulcrum (a pivot). A lever is acted upon at two different points by two different forces: the *resistance* (the load) and the *effort*. The resistance may be thought of as the force which has to be overcome, whereas the effort may be thought of as the force which has to be exerted to overcome the resistance. In producing body movement, bones act as levers and joints function as the fulcrums of these levers.

There are three classes of lever. Examples of each class may be found within the body.

1 *First-class levers.* The pivot is between the effort and the load (see Figure 4.8). If the pivot is nearer to the load, the lever is a *force multiplier* (the effort is less than the load). If the pivot is nearer to the effort, the lever is a *distance multiplier* (the load moves more than the effort.) An example of a first-class lever is a *seesaw*.

There are not many first-class levers in the body, but one example is the head resting on the vertebral column. When the head is raised, the front part of the skull (the face) is the load, the joint between the

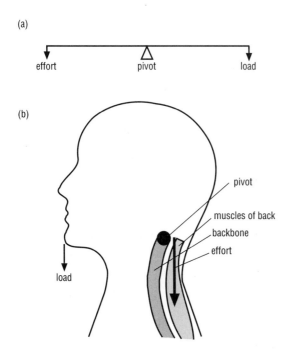

Figure 4.8 First-class levers: (a) the principle; (b) a human head

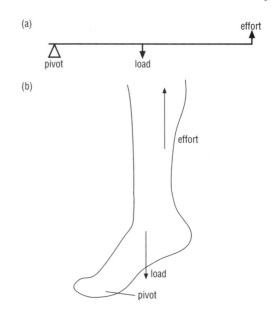

Figure 4.9 Second-class levers: (a) the principle; (b) a foot

atlas (the top vertebra) and the skull is the pivot, and the contraction of muscles at the back is the effort.

2 *Second-class levers.* The load is between the effort and the pivot (see Figure 4.9). Here, the effort always moves more than the load. This lever is a *force multiplier*: the effort is less than the load but moves through a larger distance. An example of a second-class lever is a *wheelbarrow*.

There are very few examples of second-class levers in the body, but one example is the raising of the body on the toes. The body is the load, the ball of the foot is the pivot, and the contraction of the calf muscles to pull up the heel is the effort.

3 *Third-class levers.* The effort is between the pivot and the load (see Figure 4.10). The load always moves more than the effort. The lever is a *distance multiplier*: the load force is *less* than the effort force.

Third-class levers are the most common levers in the body. An example is the flexing of the forearm at the elbow. The weight of the forearm is the load, the contraction of the biceps is the effort, and the elbow joint is the pivot.

(a)

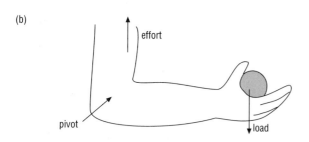

(b)

effort

pivot

load

Figure 4.10 Third-class levers: (a) the principle; (b) an arm

(a)

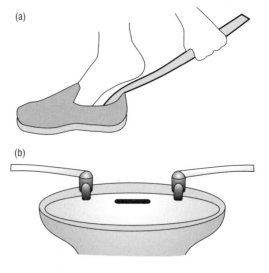

(b)

(c)

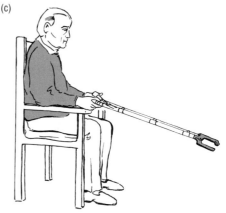

Figure 4.11 Aids for the physically disabled based on levers: (a) a long-handled shoe horn; (b) long-handled taps; (c) long 'pinchers' for picking up objects

The mechanical advantage of a lever can be calculated using the following formula:

$$\text{mechanical advantage} = \frac{\text{load (L)}}{\text{effort (E)}}$$

$$\text{or} = \frac{\text{distance of E from pivot}}{\text{distance of L from pivot}}$$

ACTIVITY 13

Draw a see-saw, wheelbarrow and drawbridge, showing the position of the pivot, the load and the effort.

Many common aids for the disabled are based on levers. Look at the pictures of some examples in Figure 4.11 and classify them as first-, second- or third-class levers.

AN INCLINED PLANE

A ramp, or inclined plane, is a simple machine. Energy is not saved by pushing a weight up a slope instead of lifting it straight up the vertical height, but it does make it easier to do the work (which is the definition of a machine).

ACTIVITY 14

Ramps are used to give wheelchair access to buildings (see Figure 4.12).

1 Do a survey of the wheelchair access in your school or college building. Produce maps to show clearly any parts of the building(s) which are *not* easily accessible, and make suggestions as to how this situation could be improved.

2 You can work out the *mechanical advantage* of using a ramp. If no energy is lost, this is equal to:

$$\frac{\text{distance moved by effort}}{\text{distance moved by load}}$$

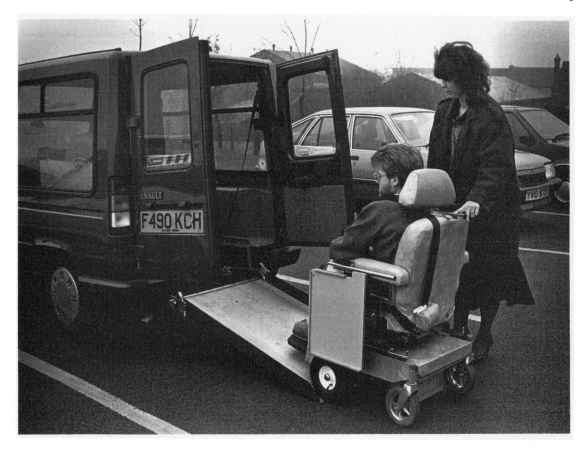

Figure 4.12 An inclined plane used for wheelchair access

So, by measuring the two distances involved (see Figure 4.13), you can work out how much easier the ramp makes the work. Do these measurements and calculations for ramps in your building.

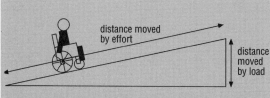

Figure 4.13 Estimating the mechanical advantage of a ramp

NB: in practice, because of friction, some energy will be lost, so working out the mechanical advantage in this way only gives you a rough estimate. To calculate the *real* mechanical advantage, you would have to measure the *effort force* you need to use against the *load force*.

THE HYDRAULIC PRESS

Hydraulic machines are *force multipliers*: they can convert a relatively small pressure into a considerable force.

force = pressure × area

In other words, if you exert a particular pressure on a large area, you will produce a larger force than if you were to exert the same pressure on a small area. By changing the area that a liquid acts against, large forces can thus be produced (see Figure 4.14).

Hydraulic machines use *oil* to transfer energy from a pump to a piston. Pneumatic systems use *compressed air* to transfer energy from a pump to a piston. Examples of hydraulic presses in health care are lifts for raising patients, dentists' chairs and operating tables.

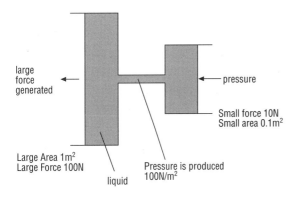

Figure 4.14   The principle of hydraulic machines

ACTIVITY 16

With reference to the above information, and using diagrams if necessary, explain why:
*   if a solid is stretched or squashed, it will only change its shape slightly
*   liquid will flow and take up the shape of any container it is put in
*   a gas fills and takes up the shape of any container that it is put in
*   heating changes a solid into a liquid and a liquid into a gas
*   if a gas in a closed container is heated, the pressure on the walls of the container will increase

ACTIVITY 15

What other examples of hydraulic machines can you find?

Fluid mechanics

KINETIC THEORY

All matter consists of very small, moving particles.

In *solids*, the particles are not moving around, but they do vibrate slightly. Here, the particles are close together, with strong forces between them. If a solid is heated, the particle vibrations increase.

In *liquids*, the particles vibrate, and they can also move around one another. The particles are joined together in small groups and are not as close together as the particles in a solid. The forces between the particles are not as strong as the forces between the particles of a solid. If a liquid is heated, the particles move faster.

In a *gas*, the particles are free to move around. There are hardly any forces between the particles, and they are a long way apart. The particles move around very quickly, and if the gas is heated they will move even faster (see p. 12).

PRESSURE

Liquids are virtually incompressible when subjected to pressure, but gases *may* be compressed. This is because, in a gas, the particles are far apart and can easily be pushed closer together, but in a liquid, the particles are already close, so a large force must be exerted to get them any closer.

ACTIVITY 17

To try compressing a gas, put your finger over the end of a bicycle pump and squeeze the pump. You will feel some movement. Now fill the pump with water and try the same thing. This time, there will hardly be any change.

When any part of a confined liquid is subjected to pressure (for example, the water in the pump in the above example), the pressure is transmitted equally to all parts of the vessel containing the liquid. This explains why *water mattresses* may be used in preference to *air mattresses* for bedridden patients. If the former type of mattress is used, the pressure from the weight of the patient will be distributed equally to all parts of the bed, whereas if an air mattress is used, most of the pressure will be concentrated at those points at which the patient is in contact with the mattress.

Because fluid cannot be compressed, and because any pressure on a liquid contained in a vessel is transmitted equally to all parts of the vessel, fluid in a confined volume can be used to 'cushion' against external forces. A biological example of this type of 'shock-absorber' is that of *amniotic fluid* (see Figure 4.15). This is found within the *amniotic sac*, and it entirely surrounds the foetus. By the time the baby is ready to be born, there is about 1 dm^3 of fluid.

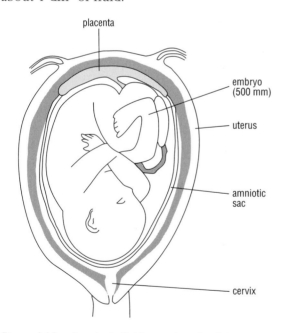

Figure 4.15   Amniotic fluid protects the foetus

A second biological example of this type of shock absorber is that of the *cerebrospinal fluid* (CSF) which protects the brain and spinal cord (i.e. the central nervous system). There are between about 80 and 150 cm^3 of cerebrospinal fluid, which is a clear liquid of watery consistency. This fluid protects the brain and spinal cord from jolts which would otherwise cause them to hit against the bony walls of the skull and vertebrae. Normally, cerebrospinal fluid is absorbed into the blood system as fast as it is formed so that the pressure remains constant. If, however, there is a build-up of cerebrospinal fluid, a *lumbar puncture* can be used to drain off fluid so as to release the pressure.

The eye disorder *glaucoma*, which is the second most common form of blindness (after cataracts), results from the fact that the fluid within the eye cannot be compressed. In the eyes of people with this disorder, there is a build-up of the aqueous humour (see Figure 5.34, which occurs in Chapter 5 on p. 274) because this liquid does not return to the bloodstream as quickly as it is formed – as should happen. As the fluid accumulates, because it cannot be compressed, it puts pressure on the neurones of the retina. If the pressure continues over a long period of time, glaucoma can progress from mild visual impairment to a point where neurones of the retina are destroyed and the person becomes blind. Glaucoma can be treated through drugs or laser surgery.

THE MEASUREMENT OF PRESSURE

Gas pressure can be measured using a *manometer*. This is a tube with a U-bend which contains a liquid, usually coloured water or mercury. The gas whose pressure is to be measured is fed into one end. The pressure of the gas pushes against the liquid in the tube. The height of the liquid it can support is a measure of its pressure (see Figure 4.16).

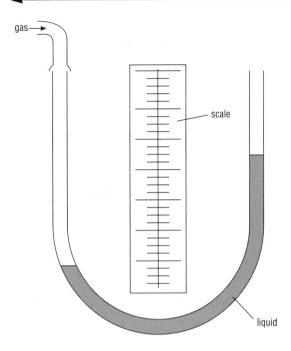

Figure 4.16   A manometer

2 With reference to Figure 4.16, construct your own water manometer to compare the maximum pressure produced by different people exhaling. (Make sure you use a long enough tube!)

GAS LAWS

The gas laws are used to explain the behaviour of gases when temperature, volume or pressure change. When the temperature, T, of a gas is raised, either the pressure, p, or the volume, V, or both, increase. These variables are related by the equation:

$$\frac{p_1 V_1}{T_1} = \frac{p_2 V_2}{T_2}$$

where 1 represents the initial state of the gas and 2 represents the final state. NB: the temperature (T) must be in Kelvin (i.e. temp in Kelvin = temp in centigrade + 273 e.g. 27 °C + 273 = 300 K).

Boyle's law

For a fixed mass of gas at constant temperature,

ACTIVITY 20

1 Figure 4.17 shows a mercury column sphygmomanometer which incorporates a mercury manometer. Find out how this works (see Thomson et al. (1995), Chapter 3, p. 174), and, if possible, use one to measure your blood pressure.

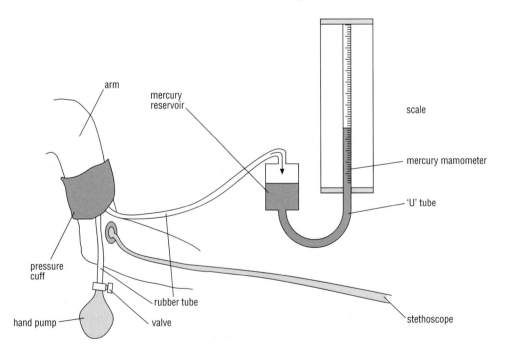

Figure 4.17   A mercury column sphygmomanometer

$$p_1 V_1 = p_2 V_2$$

or $\quad p \propto \dfrac{1}{V}$

(i.e. p is proportional to 1/V).

The pressure law
For a fixed mass of gas at constant volume,

$$p \propto T$$

Charles's law
For a fixed mass of gas at constant pressure,

$$V \propto T$$

ACTIVITY 21

Draw graphs to show the relationships described by the three laws above.

BREATHING

From Boyle's law above, it can be seen that an increase in volume will result in a decrease in pressure for a fixed mass of gas. This can be shown to happen during the process of *inhalation* (breathing in). The volume of the thorax is increased by two movements:

1 The muscles around the edge of the diaphragm contract and pull downwards so that if flattens.
2 The lower ribs are raised upwards and outwards by contraction of the external intercostal muscles which run obliquely from one rib to the next. The internal intercostal muscles are relaxed at this time.

The volume of the lungs increases as the volume of the thorax increases. This is because the lungs are thin and elastic. This increase in volume causes a decrease in pressure (Boyle's law). Because the pressure of the external air is higher, air rushes into the lungs (see Figure 4.18).

Breathing out is largely a passive process. The muscles of the diaphragm relax so that it resumes its domed shape. The external intercostal muscles relax, and the internal intercostal muscles contract. The volume of the thorax and lungs, therefore, decreases. This causes an increase in pressure, and so air leaves the lungs.

ACTIVITY 22

Set up and use the bell-jar model of breathing illustrated in Figure 4.19. Write an account of how it functions, mentioning any changes in volume and pressure.

Pleural effusion
Between the pleural membranes is the *pleural cavity* (see Figure 4.18). This contains a lubricating fluid that allows the membranes to move freely on one another during breathing. In certain conditions, the pleural cavity may fill with air, blood or pus, or excess pleural fluid may be formed (*pleural effusion*). Air in the pleural cavity, most commonly introduced in a surgical opening of the chest, may cause the lung to collapse. This occurs because it is not possible to produce the drop in pressure necessary to draw air *into* the lungs. There are various methods for draining away air or liquid, but the basic principle is always the same: to allow air and excess fluid to escape from the pleural cavity while preventing any reflux.

RESPIRATORS AND VENTILATORS

If a patient is unable to breathe, a device may be used to maintain breathing movements for them – for example, in the case of paralysis. There are different types of devices, some of which are described below.

1 *A drinker respirator (iron lung)*. The patient is enclosed, except for the head, in an airtight container in which the air pressure is increased and decreased by changing the volume of the container (see Figure 4.24 again). This draws air in and out through the normal air passages.

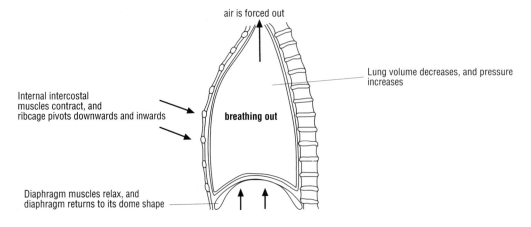

air is forced out

Lung volume decreases, and pressure increases

Internal intercostal muscles contract, and ribcage pivots downwards and inwards

breathing out

Diaphragm muscles relax, and diaphragm returns to its dome shape

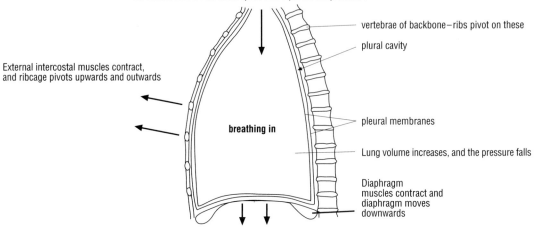

Air rushes in to fill the extra space and equalise the pressures

vertebrae of backbone – ribs pivot on these

plural cavity

External intercostal muscles contract, and ribcage pivots upwards and outwards

breathing in

pleural membranes

Lung volume increases, and the pressure falls

Diaphragm muscles contract and diaphragm moves downwards

Figure 4.18 Breathing (a) in, (b) out

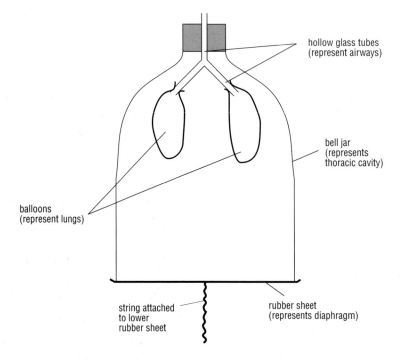

hollow glass tubes (represent airways)

bell jar (represents thoracic cavity)

balloons (represent lungs)

string attached to lower rubber sheet

rubber sheet (represents diaphragm)

Figure 4.19 The bell-jar model of breathing

2 *A cuirass respirator.* This is a respirator which works on the same principle as an iron lung but leaves the limbs free.

3 *A positive pressure respirator.* This is a respirator which blows air into a patient's lungs via a tube passed either through the mouth into the trachea, or through a tracheostomy.

ACTIVITY 23

Which of the respirators described above has a mechanism *least* like natural breathing?

If the airways are blocked with mucus, they may be cleared with a *suction tube*. Figure 4.20 shows how this works. In the past, a nurse

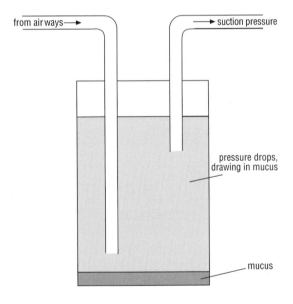

Figure 4.20 A suction tube

would place the tube in her mouth and suck, but now, because of the risk of infection, a suction pump is used instead.

BUOYANCY

Buoyancy describes the ability of an object to float in a liquid or gas. An object will only float if it is less *dense* than the liquid or gas. Density is the mass per unit volume, and can be measured in g/cm^3 or kg/m^3. The density of water is 1 g/cm^3.

ACTIVITY 24

How would you write the density of water in kg/m^3?

The formula

mass = volume × density

can be rearranged to find either volume or density, i.e.:

$$\text{volume} = \frac{\text{mass}}{\text{density}}$$

$$\text{density} = \frac{\text{mass}}{\text{volume}}$$

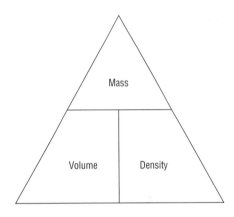

Figure 4.21 The formula triangle for volume, mass and density

When working out which formula to use, you may find it helpful to use the formula triangle shown in Figure 4.21. Cover up the quantity you wish to find, and the arrangement of the other two is shown.

ACTIVITY 25

1 If you can obtain regular shapes of different types of wood, work out their different densities.

2 A steel ship will float even though steel is denser than water. Can you explain this?

3 A *urinometer* is a type of hydrometer that measures the *specific gravity* of urine, i.e. the ratio of the density of urine to that of water). This indicates the *concentration* of urine present. Use a hydrometer of the type sold for wine-making to investigate the density of different concentrations of sucrose solution. Write an account of how it functions. (NB: because a urinometer requires at least 20 cm^3 of urine to function, it has generally been replaced by a *refractometer* which only requires one drop and is more accurate.)

Archimedes' principle

Archimedes (287–212 BC) was a Greek mathematician and physicist who was responsible for the law of physics which states that the apparent loss in weight of a body immersed in a fluid is equal to the weight of the displaced fluid.

ACTIVITY 26

You can prove Archimedes' principle by carrying out the following investigation.

Tie a thread around an object. Weigh it and calculate its mass:

$$mass = \frac{weight}{g}$$

(where g = 10 N/kg).

Fill a beaker, large enough to take your object, with water from a measuring cylinder, right to the top, noting the exact amount of water you put in. Immerse your object in the beaker, letting the water that it displaces overflow. Measure how much water is left in the beaker, and work out how much water has been displaced.

• What is the volume of your object?
• What is the density of your object?

Suspend your object from the thread again and measure its weight when it is

immersed in water. Is the weight that the object has lost in the water compared with its weight in the air equal to the weight of water it displaced?

What possible sources of error are there in this experiment, and how could you improve its accuracy?

(NB: the object weighs less in the water because of the *upthrust* or lifting force the water provides. Any liquid or gas produces upthrust.)

FLOW

A characteristic of liquids is that they can *flow* (i.e. move in a stream). This allows them to be used to transport energy (such as heat) and chemical reagents. The rate at which a fluid flows through a system can be controlled in two ways: obstructions can be used, or the pressure pushing the liquid can be adjusted.

ACTIVITY 27

1 What is transported in the blood flow?

2 What is responsible for (i) pushing and (ii) obstructing blood flow?

Measuring blood flow
Non-invasive techniques

1 *Pulse.* The pumping action of the heart causes a regular pulsation in the blood flow. Because the arteries have muscular walls, they alternately expand and recoil as the blood flow varies, and this can be felt in arteries both near the surface and lying over a bone or other firm tissue. The pulse is strongest in arteries closest to the heart. Figure 4.23 shows the places at which the pulse may be determined. A trace can be made (see Figure 4.22) which shows not only the pulse rate but rhythm and volume.

Taking the pulse by hand: the pulse is usually

checked during the course of a physical examination because it can give clues to the patient's state of health. Two fingertips are pressed against the wrist just below the base of the thumb to feel the pulse in the radial artery. The features that should be noted are:

- *the rate* – between 60 and 80 beats per minute in fit individuals. The pulse rate usually corresponds with the heart rate, which varies according to the person's state of relaxation or physical activity
- *the rhythm* – an abnormal rhythm may indicate a heart disorder; when the heart is beating very fast, some of its beats may be too weak to be detectable at the pulse
- *the character* – if the pulse feels 'thready' or weak, it may be a sign of shock; if the pulse feels very full or 'bounding', it may be a sign of respiratory disease
- *the vessel wall* 'this should feel soft when the pulse is felt; a wall that feels hard may be a sign of *arteriosclerosis*

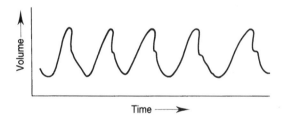

Figure 4.22 The trace of a carotid pulse
Source: Thomson et al., 1995.

ACTIVITY 28

1 Usually, the pulse is counted for 15 seconds and then converted into beats per minute. What is the formula for making this conversion?

2 Compare the following in a person who takes regular exercise (e.g. competes at a high level in a sport) and a person who does not take exercise.

- the resting pulse rate
- the pulse rate after a set exercise (e.g. one minute of 'step ups')
- the time taken for the pulse rate to return to the resting rate (plot the pulse rate against time on a graph)

NB: for safety reasons, make sure that the exercise you suggest is easily within the capabilities of your subjects.

2 *Doppler ultrasound.* This technique depends on the fact that sound waves reflected from moving objects change in frequency, and that therefore there is a change of tone. You may have noticed this when a siren on a vehicle moves past you and you hear a sudden fall in pitch, i.e. the frequency of the siren note is higher when it approaches you than it is when it recedes from you (see Figure 4.24). To measure the speed and direction of movement of the blood, ultrasound waves (high-frequency sound waves) are directed from a transmitter on to blood vessels (see Figure 4.25). These waves are reflected from the moving red blood cells and detected by a receiver. The faster the blood is moving, the greater the change in the frequency of the waves. Abnormal changes in frequency can indicate a blockage due to a clot (thrombosis) or a narrowing of the blood vessels.

Invasive techniques

A catheter can be inserted into the blood vessels to measure blood flow. The catheter can be manipulated through the chambers of the heart. Sometimes, a small balloon is inflated at the end of the catheter so that it will be moved along by the bloodstream. Dye can be injected along the catheter and X-rays taken to investigate blood flow.

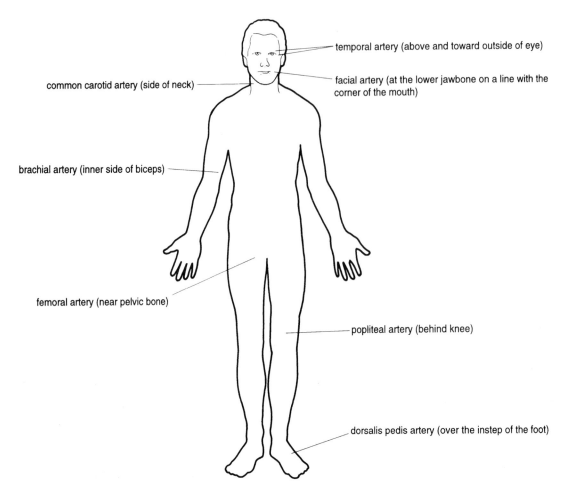

temporal artery (above and toward outside of eye)

facial artery (at the lower jawbone on a line with the corner of the mouth)

common carotid artery (side of neck)

brachial artery (inner side of biceps)

femoral artery (near pelvic bone)

popliteal artery (behind knee)

dorsalis pedis artery (over the instep of the foot)

Figure 4.23 Locations for pulse measurement
Source: Thomson et al., 1995.

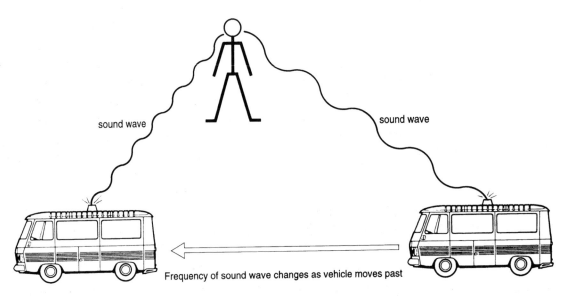

sound wave

sound wave

Frequency of sound wave changes as vehicle moves past

Figure 4.24 An example of the Doppler effect
Source: Thomson et al., 1995.

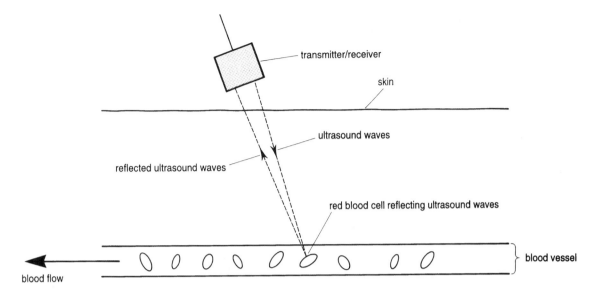

Figure 4.25 Doppler ultrasound measuring blood flow
Source: Thomson et al., 1995.

ASSESSMENT OPPORTUNITY

1 Produce a record of an investigation into mechanics in care contexts, including:
   - a description of the application of force and motion to the human body
   - an explanation, using calculations, of the relationships between work, energy and power
   - an explanation of examples of lever systems and machines
   - an explanation of the applications of fluid mechanics

2 Write a report describing the principles of fluid mechanics relevant to two applications from care contexts, one of which involves mobility and access for clients with disabilities.

ELECTRICITY, MAGNETISM AND THEIR INTERACTION

This topic should involve a considerable amount of carefully supervised practical work which should give you a sound working knowledge. The practical work you do will obviously be dependent in part on the facilities available in your centre.

The study of electricity is concerned with the behaviour of charged particles, electric fields and magnetic fields.

Electrostatic forces

In Chapter 1 (on chemical science) you will have seen that an atom has negatively charged particles known as *electrons* and positively charged particles known as *protons*. If the number of protons equals the number of electrons, then the atom is uncharged.

If two materials are rubbed together, it is possible that electrons may be rubbed off one and onto the other, giving the former a positive charge and the latter a negative charge. The charge these materials have is known as *static electricity*. If the charges on two materials are alike (i.e. both positive or both negative), they will repel one another. If the charges are different (i.e. one positive and the other negative), they will attract each other. Coulomb's law states that the force between two charged bodies is dependent on the amount of charge on each body and their distance from each other. The following equation shows the relationship between these parameters:

force between charged bodies

$$(F) = \frac{k \times q_1 \times q_2}{r^2}$$

where:
F = force between charged bodies
k = a constant
q_1 = the charge at point 1
q_2 = the charge at point 2
r = the distance between point 1 and point 2

ACTIVITY 29

Draw a sketch graph to show force (F) against distance apart (r). Assume that the two charges (q_1 and q_2) remain constant, so that you can calculate F from the equation:

$$F = \frac{1}{r^2}$$

(i.e. there is an inverse square relationship).

Walking on a nylon carpet can result in electrons rubbing off the carpet and onto you. Because the charge is static (i.e. stays on you), you will not notice it. However, if you touch a *conductor*, such as a metal post connected to the ground, this will allow electrons to flow from you into the ground (*discharge*). You will feel this as a small electric shock.

Care is taken in operating theatres to prevent the build-up of static charges, because they could produce a spark which could ignite the explosive vapours released by some anaesthetics.

ACTIVITY 30

1 Rub a perspex rod with a piece of wool and observe what happens. Try to explain your observations in terms of the loss or gain of electrons.

2 Find out about a Van de Graaff generator, and if possible, see one in action.

3 The space around a charged object in which it can affect other objects is called its *electric field*. *Field lines* can be drawn around a charged object to show the direction of the force involved. Arrows are then drawn on the field lines to show the direction in which the force would act on a positively charged object. Figure 4.26 shows the electric field around a

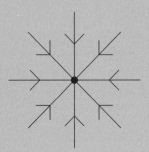

Figure 4.26 Electric field lines around a negatively charged object

negatively charged object. Draw the electric field you would find around a *positively* charged object. (NB: the closeness of the lines drawn will indicate the strength of the field: the closer the lines, the stronger the field.)

4 A metal post was mentioned above as an example of a *conductor*. Materials that do not allow a flow of electrons through them are called *insulators*. Compile a table giving a number of examples of materials which are conductors, and a number of examples of materials which are insulators.

ELECTRIC CURRENTS

An electric current is a flow of electrons. The amount of charge involved is measured in *coulombs* (C).

The *current* is the measure of how quickly the charge is moving. It is worked out as the amount of charge that flows past a particular point in a particular period of time (i.e.

current = charge passing per second). The unit it is measured in is the *ampere* (A):

current in amperes =

$$\frac{\text{charge passing (in coulombs)}}{\text{time interval (in seconds)}}$$

For example, if a total charge of 3 coulombs passes a point in a wire in 6 seconds:

$$\text{current} = \frac{\text{charge}}{\text{time}} = \frac{3 \text{ C}}{6 \text{ s}}$$

$$= 0.5 \text{ C per second}$$

$$= 0.5 \text{ A}.$$

An *ammeter* can be used to measure electric currents. The charge passing through per second is displayed either digitally or on a dial.

ELECTRIC CIRCUITS

Figure 4.27a shows a simple electric circuit. Figure 4.27b shows a parallel circuit; in this, the electrons split up, half going one way and half the other, and that means that, for the split part of the circuit, the current is halved. Figure 4.27c shows a circuit connected in series; all parts of this circuit would have the same current.

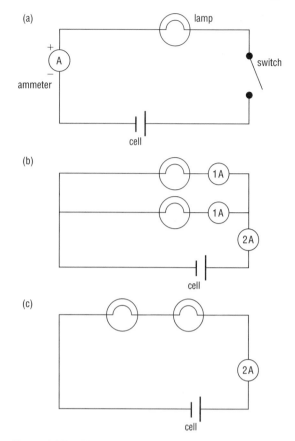

Figure 4.27   Electric circuits: (a) a typical example; (b) a circuit connected in parallel; (c) a circuit connected in series

---

ACTIVITY 31

1 Make the circuits shown in Figure 4.27. Note the readings on the ammeters and the brightness of the lamps, and record your observations. Explain your results in terms of the flow of electrons.

   Make up other circuits, predicting in advance what current will go to each light in your circuits.

2 If a current of 2 A is passing through a circuit, how much charge flows past any point in 10 seconds?

VOLTAGE

In electrical circuits, the energy to move the electrons around the circuit comes from the cell. The energy that the cell gives to the electrons is measured as *voltage* or *potential difference*. This is calculated by measuring the difference in the electrical potential energy on either side of the cell. The units used are *volts* (V), and measurement is carried out using a *voltmeter* which is connected across a cell. The potential difference (in volts) between two points is the work done in joules moving 1 coulomb (C) of charge between them:

$$\text{Potential difference (V)} = \frac{\text{work done (W)}}{\text{charge moved (Q)}}$$

$$1 \text{ V} = \frac{1 \text{ J}}{\text{C}}$$

As electrons flow through a lamp, their electrical energy is converted into heat and light energy. This energy loss can be measured by connecting a voltmeter across a lamp. The total energy lost around a circuit is equal to the energy *provided* by the cell.

ACTIVITY 32

1 Set up the circuits shown in Figure 4.28 using cells with a potential difference of 1.5 V. Record the voltages using voltmeters as shown. Does the total potential difference provided by the cell(s) equal the totals of the potential differences across each lamp? What can you conclude about the potential difference across a lamp connected in series compared with that of an identical lamp connected in parallel?

2 120 J of work (W) are done when 10 C of charge (Q) passes through a bulb. What is the potential difference (V) across the bulb?

OHM'S LAW

If the potential difference across the source of electrical energy is increased, for example by adding more cells or by increasing the voltage of the power pack, then the *current* will increase: if, for example, the potential difference is doubled, then the current is doubled. In other words, the current flowing through a metallic conductor is *proportional to* the potential difference, provided the temperature and other physical factors remain constant. This is known as Ohm's law. Ohm's law does not hold if a non-metallic conductor is used.

ACTIVITY 33

1 Draw a sketch of a graph to show the relationship between current (amperes) (on the y axis) and potential difference (volts) (on the x axis).

2 Set up a circuit as shown in Figure 4.29. Use a number of conductors, for example graphite, lead and different types of wire. For each one, adjust the voltage from the power pack, or increase the number of cells, and then record voltages and currents. Plot a graph of current (I) against voltage (V) for each material used.

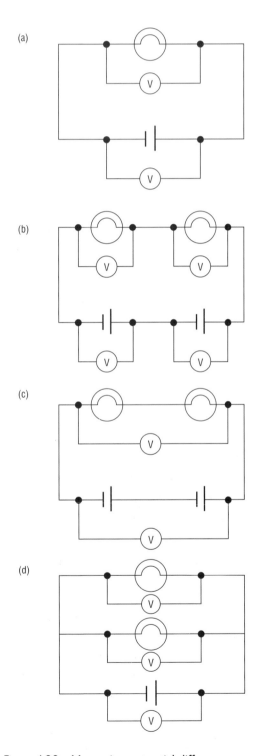

Figure 4.28 Measuring potential differences

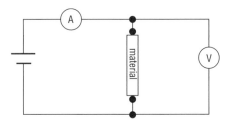

Figure 4.29   A circuit to test Ohm's law

RESISTANCE

Electrons will flow along a conductor if there is a potential difference, or voltage, across the ends of the conductor. However, different conductors allow different amounts of current to flow, even when the voltage is kept constant. The movement of electrons through a circuit is resisted by the atoms of the materials through which they pass. This is known as *resistance*. If a material has a high resistance, only a small current will flow. If a material has a low resistance, a larger current can flow at the same voltage.

Resistance is measured in units called *ohms* (Ω), and can be calculated by using the following equation:

$$\text{resistance} \atop (R) = \frac{\text{potential difference(voltage)(V)}}{\text{current (I)}}$$

ACTIVITY 34

Look back at the formula triangle in Figure 4.21 and work out how to manipulate this formula so as to make it involve *resistance*, *voltage* and *current* instead.

A conductor with resistance is known as a *resistor*. In a series circuit, the total resistance is the sum of the resistance of each of the individual resistors. In a parallel circuit, because there are alternative routes for the electrons, the total resistance will always be less than that of any individual resistor, and can be worked out using the following equation:

$$\frac{1}{\text{total resistance}} = \frac{1}{R_1} + \frac{1}{R_2} + \frac{1}{R_3}$$

ACTIVITY 35

1 Set up resistors in series and in parallel to test the rules given above.

2 How could you arrange three resistors, each with a resistance of 4 Ω, to make a 6 Ω combination in a circuit?

3 What is the value of the resistance (R) in the circuit shown in Figure 4.30?

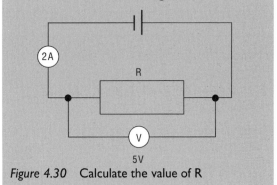

Figure 4.30   Calculate the value of R

ELECTRICAL POWER

As electrons flow through a wire, some of their energy is transferred to the atoms in the metal, and this causes heating. The rate of this energy transfer, i.e. the *power* output, can be calculated using the following equation:

$$\begin{array}{cccc} \text{power} & = & \text{potential difference} & \times & \text{current} \\ (P) & & (V) & & (I) \\ (\text{watts}) & & (\text{volts}) & & (\text{amperes}) \end{array}$$

To enable you to make other calculations, the following equations may also be useful:

$$\text{power} = I^2 R$$

$$\text{power} = \frac{V^2}{R}$$

ACTIVITY 36

1 Which household electrical appliances can you think of which use the heating effect of an electric current?

2 A 60 W, 240 V lamp is connected to a 240 V mains. What current does it take? What is its resistance?

FUSES

A *fuse* is a safety device. If a current exceeds a certain amount, the heat generated causes the thin tin-plated copper wire in the fuse to melt. This breaks the electrical circuit and disconnects the appliance from the supply. Fuses fitted to household appliances are usually 5 A, 10 A or 13 A.

ACTIVITY 37

1 Obtain material from your electricity-supply company on electrical safety information, including information on the use of fuses and earth-leakage circuit breakers, and how to wire a plug. Produce posters to inform the public of the hazards of electricity, and how to avoid these.

2 What fuse would you put in a plug if the plug was connected to an appliance labelled 750 W 250 V? (Clue: you need to find the current.)

CAPACITORS

Capacitors store charge. They form an important part of virtually every electrical circuit. The charge on a capacitor is proportional to the potential difference (voltage) across it. *Capacitance* (C) can be defined as the amount of charge stored by a capacitor per unit potential difference across it; i.e.:

$$C = \frac{\text{charge (Q)}}{\text{voltage (V)}}$$

(remember: Q = current (I) × time).

The unit of capacitance is the *farad* (F). 1 farad is equal to 1 coulomb per volt.

Capacitors have a wide range of uses which depend on their ability to store charge. For example, they are used in electronic circuits in which voltages vary with time.

DEFIBRILLATION

In Chapter 5 (the physiology chapter) you will see that the heart is controlled by electrical signals (see Chapter 5, p. 239). It is therefore not surprising that an electric current travelling through the body close to the heart can disrupt this control. A small shock may lead to the heart stopping for a short time before the natural rhythm is restored by impulses from the sinoatrial node. A greater shock, however, may lead to *ventricular fibrillation*, which is when the muscles of the ventricles contract rapidly in a completely disorganised and uncoordinated way. In this state, the heart cannot pump blood around the body, so death results. Fibrillation also occurs in heart-attack victims. It can only be stopped by giving the heart a controlled electric shock of exactly the right current, frequency and duration. This is brought about by the discharge of a capacitor and is known as *defibrillation* (see Figure 4.31). This brings the heart to rest so that the sinoatrial node can once again produce coordinated contractions, provided fibrillation has not caused any permanent damage to the cardiac muscle.

ACTIVITY 38

Defibrillation can only be administered by qualified medical staff. Interview a professional who is familiar with this process to find out more about this aspect of their work.

ALTERNATING AND DIRECT CURRENTS (AC, DC)

In the circuits described above, the current was flowing in one direction only, i.e. it was a *direct* current. However, the electricity from a mains supply reverses direction at a set frequency, and this is an *alternating* current. Although the mains supply in the UK is referred to as a 240 V supply, the voltage actually varies from +240 V to −240 V, with the current alternating at 0.02 s intervals. An

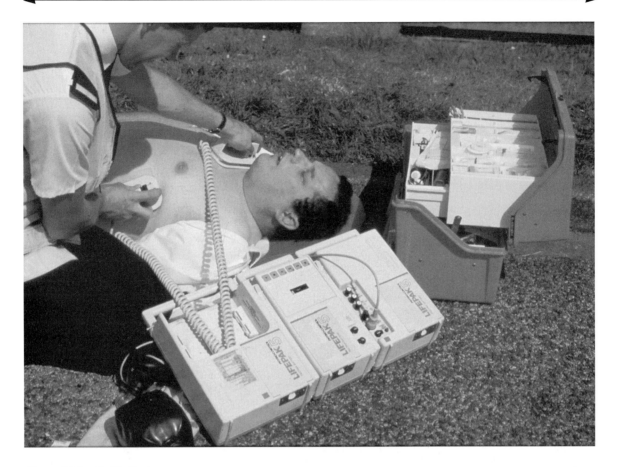

Figure 4.31   Defibrillation

alternating current helps to overcome the problems of energy loss associated with transmitting large currents at low voltages. See Figure 4.32.

The application and functioning of an oscilloscope in care contexts

An *oscilloscope* is a cathode ray tube (see Figure 4.33) designed to display electronically a wave form correlating with the electrical data fed into it. When a filament (cathode) is heated, electrons are emitted from the surface of the metal. This is known as *thermionic emission* and is a process similar to the evaporation of molecules from the surface of a liquid. These electrons can be directed into a beam by positioning two positively charged anodes, *focusing* and *accelerating* respectively, close to the filament. The whole of the interior of the tube is under a vacuum,

because air molecules would deflect the electrons. (The cathode–anode assembly is called an *electron gun*.) The beam is then passed through X-plates which produce an electric field that deflects the beam horizontally, and through Y-plates which produce an electric field that deflects it vertically. When the beam strikes the fluorescent screen at the end of the tube, a spot of light is produced. When an alternating current is connected across the Y-plates, a vertical line appears on the screen; and a waveform is displayed if the timebase, which moves the spot horizontally across the screen, is then switched on. The control grid regulates the number of electrons that reach the anode, and hence the brightness of the spot on the screen.

An oscilloscope can be linked to *monitoring devices*, such as an *electrocardiograph* (monitors heart beat) and an *electroencephalograph* (monitors electrical activity from different parts of the brain), and to *measuring devices*, for example

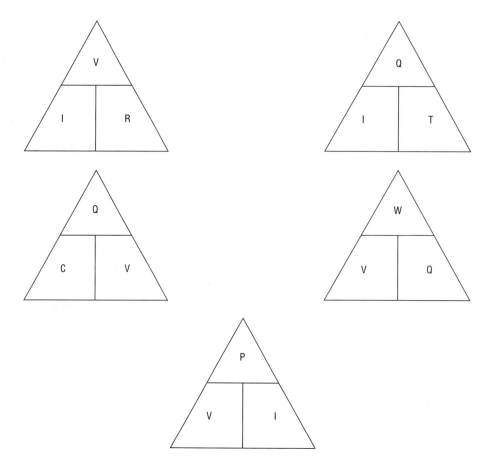

Figure 4.32   Formula triangles to help you with electrical calculations

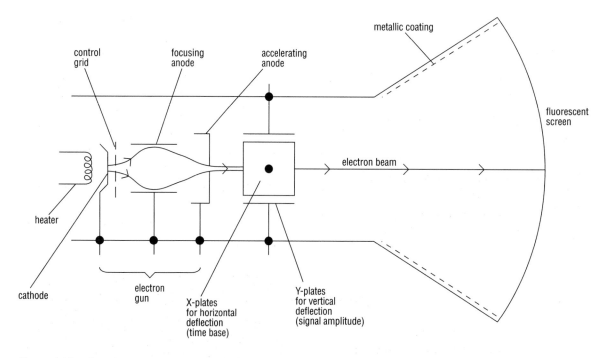

Figure 4.33   A cathode ray tube

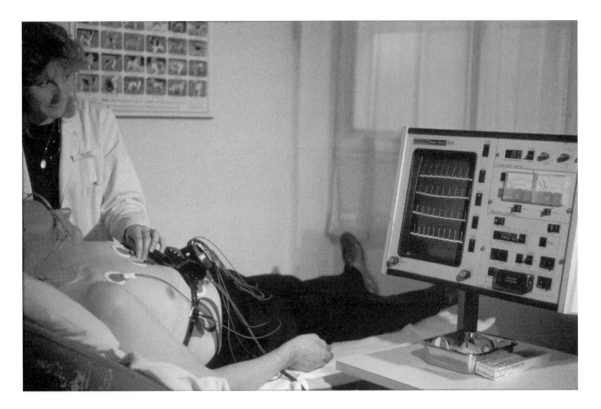

Figure 4.34   An oscilloscope linked to an electrocardiograph

devices for measuring blood pressure or respiration during surgery (see Figure 4.34).

ACTIVITY 39

If possible:

1 use an oscilloscope in the laboratory. For example, you could use it to display the changing voltage caused by sound waves.

2 observe the use of an oscilloscope for a medical purpose. Produce a report explaining exactly what it is measuring or monitoring.

Magnets and magnetic fields

Everyone is familiar with magnets. Think briefly of the times that you have seen the effect of magnetic force, and you may think of

a compass, or of a simple bar or horseshoe magnet attracting pins.

A magnet always has two *poles*. These are the points where the magnetism is the strongest. If a magnet is suspended so that it is free to turn, the *north-seeking pole* or *north pole* of the magnet will swing to point to the north pole of the earth. The other end is the *south pole*, which points towards the south pole of the earth. Unlike poles attract (i.e. a north pole of a magnet attracts south poles, and the south pole of a magnet attracts north poles), and like poles repel (i.e. a north pole will repel a north pole, and a south pole will repel a south pole).

The *magnetic field* around a magnet appears to come from the poles.

ACTIVITY 40

1 You can investigate the magnetic field around a bar magnet using either a compass or iron filings. If using iron

FURTHER STUDIES FOR HEALTH

filings, sprinkle them on the surface of a thin card held just above your bar magnet. Draw the pattern they form. The same pattern will be produced if you use a plotting compass and trace out the path of the needle as it moves around the compass. The lines traced are known as flux lines. Arrows can be used to show the direction of the force on a magnetic north pole, and the closeness of the lines (as already mentioned) indicates the strength of the field: the closer the lines, the stronger the field. Don't forget that the field lines you have drawn only give a 2-dimensional representation: in reality, the magnetic field around a magnet is, of course, 3-dimensional.

2 Test a number of different metals to find out which can be attracted by a magnet.

Permanent magnets are made from *ferromagnetic* materials. A ferromagnetic material effectively consists of many tiny individual bar magnets, or *domains*. These regions are about 20 millionths of a metre in size. An electron spinning around the nucleus of an atom produces a tiny magnetic field. In each domain the spinning electrons are arranged in a way that lines up their magnetic fields. When a material is unmagnetised, these domains are aligned at random, so that their magnetic fields cancel one another out. When the material is then subjected to a strong magnetic field, the domains line up. And when the material is then removed from the external magnetic field, the domains remain lined up, so that the material is permanently magnetised.

Materials which retain their magnetism after they have been removed from the external magnetic field are said to be magnetically *hard* (e.g. steel), whereas materials which lose their magnetism when removed from the external magnetic field are said to be magnetically *soft* (e.g. iron).

ACTIVITY 41

Compare the strength and permanence of iron and steel magnets by attaching a piece of steel wire and a piece of iron wire to a strong bar magnet. Which picks up the most iron filings? Then use unmagnetised pieces of iron and steel. To magnetise them, stroke them in one direction only with the strong magnet. Which piece keeps its magnetism longest?

The interaction between magnetism and electricity

When a current is flowing along a wire, the movement of electrons produces a circular magnetic field around the wire. The strength of the magnetic field is directly proportional to the amount of current flowing.

ACTIVITY 42

Set up an apparatus as shown in Figure 4.35 to find the pattern and direction of the field lines surrounding a current.

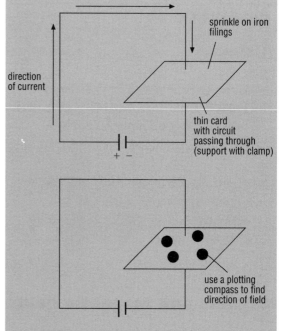

Figure 4.35 Examining the field lines around a current

Electromagnets may be made by coiling a wire (*solenoid*) around a bar of magnetic material and passing an electric current through the wire. The type of metal used as the magnetic core will depend on the function of the electromagnet. For example, a magnetically soft material such as iron is used in 'relays' in microelectronics, whereas a magnetically hard material, such as steel, is used in loudspeakers.

ACTIVITY 43

Make your own solenoid by coiling a wire around a pencil. Put a 12 V lamp in the circuit to restrict the current, and then pass a few amperes through the wire. Use a plotting compass to plot the magnetic field around the solenoid.

Try changing the following factors, and test how the strength of the magnetic field is affected:

• the number of turns in the coil
• the strength of the current

Replace the pencil with an iron nail, and again note the change in the strength of the magnetic field.

MOTORS

If a current is flowing through a wire, there is a magnetic field around the wire. If the wire passes through another magnetic field, there will be an interaction between the two magnetic fields. In this way, a force is produced.

Electric motors basically consist of a coil which can rotate in a magnetic field. A current passes through the coil, and the resulting forces on the coil cause it to rotate. The direction of the current is reversed after every half-revolution. This ensures continuous rotation.

The speed of the rotation can be increased by increasing the current, by increasing the number of turns in the coil, or by increasing the strength of the magnetic field.

ACTIVITY 44

Find out how a simple electric motor can be made. If you have the necessary equipment you could try this.

THE MASS SPECTROMETER

A *mass spectrometer* uses the interaction of charged particles with magnetic and electric fields to measure the masses of atoms and to find their relative abundance. Figure 4.36 shows how it works. Molecules are vaporised by heating and then bombarded with a stream of high-energy electrons. This splits the molecules into ionised fragments. The ions are then accelerated by being passed through an electric field, and are then sorted according to their relative masses by being passed through a *magnetic* field. The relative abundance of each type of ion is measured. The *mass spectrum* of a particular compound is unique, so the trace obtained can be used to identify the compound. In pathology laboratories, a mass spectrometer may be used to identify traces of toxins such as lead or arsenic.

ACTIVITY 45

1 If possible, visit an analytical laboratory to see a mass spectrometer working. If you can keep a trace of a mass spectrum, label it to explain what it shows and write an account to explain how it was produced.

2 A *cyclotron* is a type of particle accelerator in which the particles spin under the effect of a strong vertical magnetic field. Some hospitals have their own small cyclotron to produce isotopes for medical use (see the next section). Find out more about how they work, and about their other uses.

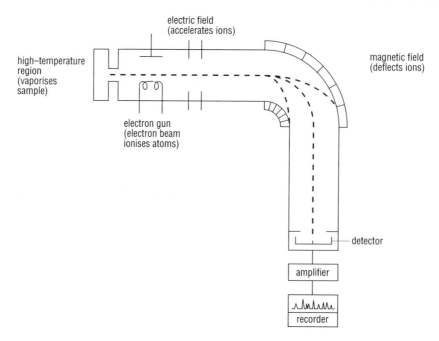

Figure 4.36 A diagram of a mass spectrometer

THE PROPERTIES OF WAVES AND PARTICLES

(NB: wherever possible, try to organise visits and invite in visiting speakers on this topic, depending on your local facilities. There are also many excellent videotapes available.)

Electromagnetic waves

Electromagnetic waves are characterised by oscillating electric and magnetic fields. They are produced by energy changes in atoms or electrons, and in a vacuum they all travel at the speed of light (300,000,000 m/s). They travel as *transverse waves*: in other words, the oscillations occur at right angles to the direction in which the wave is travelling – like the wave passing along a rope when it is shaken up and down.

Electromagnetic waves are grouped according to their *wavelength* or *frequency*: the shorter the wavelength, the higher the frequency and the more energy the electromagnetic radiation carries. Figure 4.37 shows the *electromagnetic spectrum*. Below is a description of the various types of electromagnetic wave, starting with those with the longest wavelength.

RADIO WAVES

These are electromagnetic waves with wavelengths over 1 mm. They are produced by electrons vibrated by electronic circuits, radio and TV transmitters, and stars and

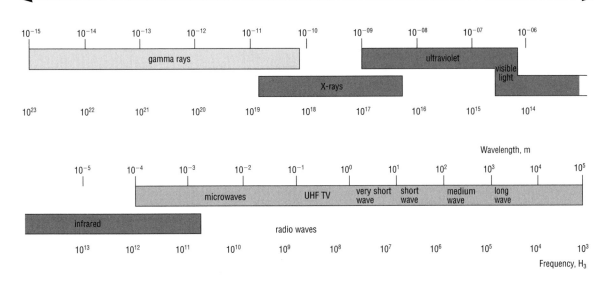

Figure 4.37 The electromagnetic spectrum

galaxies. They can be detected with a radio aerial.

MICROWAVES

These are short-wavelength radio waves. Telephone links between cities use microwaves, as does communication to satellites. They are also used in cooking. Microwaves pass through air, glass and plastic without causing any heating, but are reflected by metals.

INFRARED WAVES

Infrared radiation is given off by hot objects. This cannot be detected by the human eye, but it can be detected as warmth.

VISIBLE LIGHT RAYS

Human eyes are sensitive to visible light. There are three types of cell in the eye (*cones* – see Chapter 5, pp. 275–277) that react to colour: one type is sensitive to red light, one to blue light and one to green light.

ULTRAVIOLET WAVES

Ultraviolet light is contained in sunlight, but it cannot be detected by the human eye. Fluorescent material can convert ultraviolet radiation into visible light. For example, some washing powders contain chemicals which

fluoresce, and when ultraviolet light shines on white clothing which has been washed with these powders, it glows in the dark.

X-RAYS

These are produced when electrons slow down very quickly. Some of their kinetic energy is then converted into electromagnetic energy. X-rays are high-energy waves which can penetrate solids and can be detected by photographic film.

GAMMA WAVES

Gamma rays have the shortest wavelength (and the highest frequency). They are produced by changes in the nuclei of radioactive atoms, and they carry large amounts of energy.

Medical applications associated with electromagnetic waves

Many branches of medicine utilise electromagnetic waves. They are used particularly in *diagnostic radiography* and other medical imaging techniques, in *therapeutic radiography*, and in *physiotherapy*.

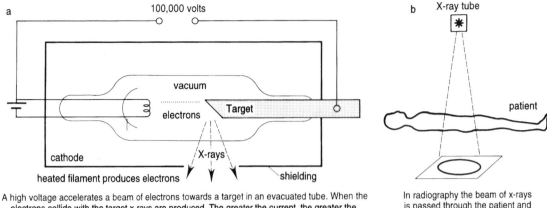

A high voltage accelerates a beam of electrons towards a target in an evacuated tube. When the electrons collide with the target x-rays are produced. The greater the current, the greater the number of electrons hitting the target and the more intense the x-rays. The higher the voltage the greater the penetrating power (or energy) of the x-rays.

In radiography the beam of x-rays is passed through the patient and on to the photographic film which is developed to produce an image.

Figure 4.38 The production of X-rays
Source: Thomson et al., 1995.

MEDICAL IMAGING TECHNIQUES

Diagnostic radiography

X-radiography is probably the best-known imaging technique. It is likely that you have had at least one X-ray examination. Figure 4.38 shows how X-rays are produced. A high voltage accelerates a beam of electrons (negative particles that are found in atoms) towards a target, in a tube from which all the air has been removed. (Because electrons are so small it is important that there are no comparatively large air molecules around which could deflect them from their pathway.) The electrons collide with a tungsten target and cause the production of X-rays. The greater the current, the greater the number of electrons hitting the target and the more intense the X-rays. The higher the voltage, the greater the energy and penetrating power of the X-rays. X-rays are directed onto the area of the body under investigation, and pass through it to record an image on photographic film. The more dense tissues, such as bone, absorb more X-rays than less dense body tissues. This means the strength of X-rays reaching the photographic film varies, which leads to the production of images of varying densities known as *radiographs* (see Figure 4.39). *Radiographers* are responsible for producing the radiographs,

and specialist doctors known as *radiologists* interpret these radiographs.

X-rays are used in determining the nature of a disorder (diagnosis). For example, bone fractures show up clearly, as do problems affecting joints and cartilage, such as the damage caused by osteoarthritis and

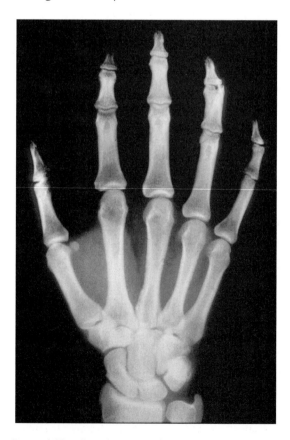

Figure 4.39 A radiograph of a normal right hand

osteoporosis. *Chest X-rays* are commonly taken because the size of the heart and lungs can be seen, as can areas of inflammation or fluid.

QUESTION

What diseases do you think could be diagnosed and investigated with a chest X-ray?

As well as having an important diagnostic role, X-rays are also used in *screening tests*. These are any simple tests carried out on a large number of apparently healthy people to separate those who possibly have a specified disease from those who do not.

QUESTION

Can you think of examples of screening tests which do *not* involve the use of X-rays?

An example of a screening test which involves X-rays is that of *X-ray mammography*. This is a technique in which low-dosage X-rays can be used to detect the presence of cysts and tumours in the breasts. It was first used in 1967.

Radio-opaque dyes (contrast media) can be used to show more detailed information than a simple X-ray. These dyes, which absorb X-rays, are injected into the tissue under investigation to highlight empty spaces and outline soft tissues. They are, therefore particularly valuable for examining hollow organs such as the bowel. The exact techniques used depend on the area of the body to be examined (see Table 4.3).

With *body scanning*, a detailed picture of the soft tissues of the body can be obtained by producing a *CAT scan* (see Figure 4.40). CAT stands for *computer axial tomography*. A series of X-rays, taken at fractionally different depths of tissue, is analysed by computer. This method produces images of a slice of the body. The most common use of the CAT scan is for examining the brain. Unlike conventional X-rays, the CAT scan can differentiate between normal tissues, abscesses and blood clots. The procedure is safe and quick, but unfortunately, the expensive equipment necessary is not widely available.

Thermography

Thermography is a technique for displaying images of infrared radiation (heat loss) from the skin (see Figure 4.41). This allows abnormalities in the skin temperature, and therefore in the underlying tissue, to be detected. Because tumours produce a change in the circulatory system around them, their location can be detected by using thermography.

THERAPEUTIC RADIOGRAPHY

See the 'Radiotherapy' section on p. 231 below.

PHYSIOTHERAPY

Diathermy

This involves the local heating of tissues using microwaves (frequency around 2,450 MHz (megahertz)). The radiation is absorbed directly into the tissue, and the frequency can be chosen to interact with particular molecules. Care must obviously be taken not to overheat the tissues. Diathermy is used in the treatment of joints, for example in arthritis, and of muscles and tendons, for example in strains. Many sports physiotherapists have a portable diathermy kit which can be used when applying emergency treatment on the field.

Infrared lamps

Infrared radiation may also be used by physiotherapists to heat tissue so as to reduce pain and improve circulation.

OTHER USES

Vitamin D production (UV lamps)

Ultraviolet light is required for the skin to produce vitamin D. If a person is not exposed

Table 4.3 Examples of techniques using contrast media

Technique	Body part examined	Method of administration	Examples of diseases diagnosed	Side effects
Angio-graphy/ Arterio-graphy	Blood vessels	Thin tube placed in the blood vessel (local anaesthetic and light sedation used). Dye injected. X-ray taken.	Blood clots, Artheriosclerosis, Arteriosclerosis, tumours	
Barium studies	Digestive tract	For the oesophagus, stomach and duodenum a barium meal is given. The patient fasts overnight then swallows a porridge-like drink containing barium. S/he lies on a table which can be tilted to coat the entire area under investigation and the stomach may be distended with air. Several X-rays are then taken over a period of about an hour. For small and large intestine a barium enema may be given.	Hernias, ulcers, colitis, tumours	Barium meal may cause constipation Barium enema may cause uncomfortable muscle spasms
Cystogram	Bladder and urethra	Dye is introduced to the bladder via a thin tube through the urethra. The patient is asked to urinate and a series of X-rays are taken.	Prostatic enlargement, urinary tract infection	Some discomfort
Hystero-salpingogram	Uterus and fallopian tubes	Dye enters uterus via a thin tube through vagina and cervix.	Blocked fallopian tubes	
Lymph-angiogram	Lymph system	Dye injected into a lymph vessel (usually at the top of the foot). This spreads throughout the lymph system.	Hodgkin's disease, Lymphoma	
Myelogram	Space surrounding spinal cord with vertebral column	Dye injected into the space (lumbar puncture). Table tipped to allow the dye to travel the length of spinal chord.	Spinal tumours	
Pyelogram	Kidneys	Patient dehydrated for four hours before dye is injected into a vein. This then travels through the blood to the kidney.	Kidney stone. Tumour	
Venogram	Vein	Dye is injected into vein in hand or foot.	Blood cot (e.g. deep vein thrombosis)	

Source: Thomson et al., 1995.

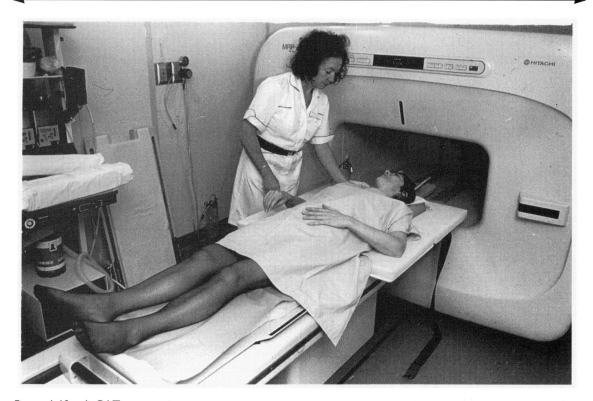

Figure 4.40   A CAT scanner in use

to sunlight, and the level of vitamin D in their diet is insufficient, they may develop a weakness of the bones known as *rickets*. For this reason, *UV lamps* are used in some parts of the world to enable people to synthesise vitamin D.

Sterilisation
Both UV light and gamma rays may be used for sterilising medical materials and instruments.

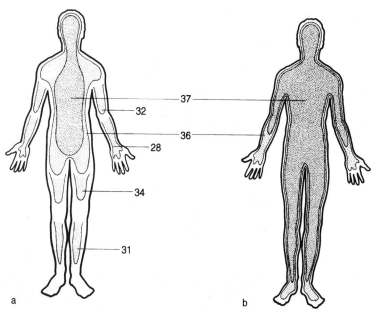

Figure 4.41   A thermogram showing heat loss from the skin (a) in a cold environment and (b) in a warm environment
Source: Thomson et al., 1995.

Safety procedures associated with electromagnetic waves

Electromagnetic waves can be potentially harmful if exposure is prolonged or the intensity is high. Even visible light, for example, can damage the retina at high intensities. Precautions associated with the heating effects of microwaves and infrared light should be taken, to prevent these actually cooking the tissues. Exposure to UV light can damage the eyes and cause sunburn or even cancer. Because of this, sunglasses and sun creams which filter out UV light should be used.

These are very strict safety procedures for people giving and receiving X-rays and gamma rays. For example, when an X-ray is being taken, the radiographer stands behind a screen, and over a certain part of the body, depending on which part is being examined, the patient wears a lead apron. These help prevent the scattered X-rays from entering the body. To check their radiation dose over a set period of time, each person working with X-rays and gamma rays wears a film badge (see Figure 4.42). This consists of a piece of photographic film in a special holder. It is pinned to the outside of the clothing for a period of 1 to 4 weeks before being developed. The degree of blackening indicates the extent of exposure to radiation.

Lasers and their medical applications

The word 'laser' is an acronym which stands for 'light amplification by the stimulated emission of radiation'. Ordinary light is used to stimulate the electrons of the atoms of the lasing medium. These then give out light of a particular wavelength when they return to their normal energy state.

Unlike ordinary light, a laser can produce a narrow beam of light which is very powerful, concentrating a large amount of energy over a small area. Laser light contains light of only

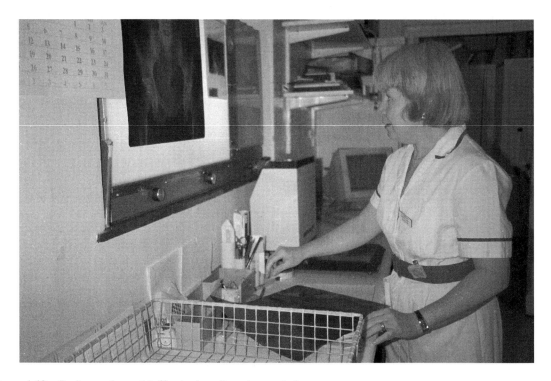

Figure 4.42   Radiographer with film badge clipped onto belt

one wavelength, and in lasers the light waves produced are all *in phase*, so the waves reinforce one another, making the light very bright.

Lasers are very useful in a wide range of applications. The energy of a laser can be used to cut, coagulate or destroy tissue. Because they are so accurate, lasers are often effective when a scalpel would not be suitable – for example, for delicate surgery on the fallopian tubes or brain. Lasers can be used to seal bleeding ulcers – by cauterising them – and to remove fatty deposits from arteries. They are also used in the removal of birthmarks.

Eye surgery is also often carried out with the use of lasers. For example, they have been useful in treating the eye disease which results from diabetes. The laser can stop bleeding in the eye which would lead to blindness. Lasers can also be used to repair small tears in the retina by a process known as *photocoagulation*. Only a few cells are targeted, and the operation is virtually painless. Eye defects, particularly short-sightedness, are increasingly being treated with lasers, which are used to remove microscopic portions of tissue from the front of the cornea, altering its shape and yielding a very precise change in its focusing power. (Further information on this

technique can be obtained from the Royal College of Opthalmologists – their address is given at the end of the chapter.)

ACTIVITY 46

1 What atoms may be used as 'lasing' material?

2 Produce a report on the use of lasers in cosmetic surgery.

3 Find out how lasers are used:
   (a) in a compact disc player
   (b) in the production of holograms.

Microscopy

The microscope is an invaluable tool for modern scientists. The most widely used microscopes are *light microscopes*, but the greatest magnification is obtained with an *electron microscope*.

THE LIGHT MICROSCOPE

Figure 4.43 shows how a light microscope functions. The mirror reflects light through

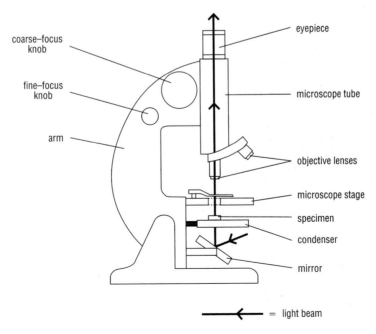

Figure 4.43   A light microscope

the specimen, the objective lens, the tube and the eyepiece lens, and into the eye. In this type of microscope, a *compound microscope*, magnification occurs twice: at the objective lens and at the eyepiece. (You can find the total amount by which the specimen has been magnified by multiplying together the magnifications of the objective lens and the eyepiece lens.)

The magnifying power of a microscope is not its most important feature, however. The degree of detail it allows to be seen, or its *resolving power*, is more relevant when viewing a specimen. If a microscope has high resolution, it allows two points which are close together to be seen as two separate points, whereas a microscope with lower resolution may be unable to distinguish the two points so that they would appear as a single point. The resolving power is inversely proportional to the wavelength of light used. Because the wavelength of light is limited, there is a limit to the resolving power of a light microscope. It cannot distinguish between points which are closer together than 0.2 μm.

ACTIVITY 47

1 Using Figure 4.43 to help you, trace the path of light waves through your microscope.

2 Write a list of instructions for:
   (a) setting up your microscope to view a specimen
   (b) making a temporary mount of a specimen

3 Find out about the history of the development of the light microscope.

4 If possible, use a *graticule* (a transparent scale) to allow you to measure with the microscope.

5 A light microscope can be modified to improve its performance. Find out how the following work:
   (a) oil immersion, and
   (b) the *phase contrast microscope*.

THE ELECTRON MICROSCOPE

An electron microscope (see Figure 4.44a)

(a)

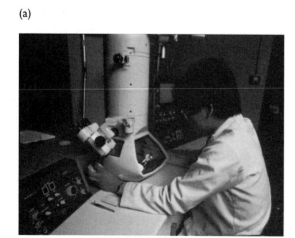

(b)

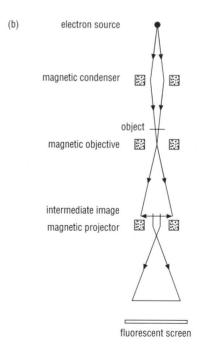

Figure 4.44   An electron microscope: (a) photograph, (b) diagram

uses beams of electrons instead of beams of light. Because electrons have a much shorter wavelength than light (0.05 nm (nanometre) compared with 500 nm), and electron microscope has a much higher resolving power than a light microscope. However, to prevent the electron beam from being deflected by air molecules, the microscope has to be kept under vacuum; and this, of course, means that only dead specimens can be observed with this type of microscope.

Figure 4.44b shows how an electron microscope functions. Whereas a light microscope uses glass lenses to focus the light beams, an electron microscope uses *electro magnets*. The electrons cannot be detected with the eye, so they are projected onto a fluorescent screen. In a *transmission electron microscope*, the prepared section is very thin, and some electrons can pass through it. If areas of the specimen then absorb electrons, these appear as dark areas on the image, and if, in other areas, the electrons are allowed to pass through, these areas appear bright on the image.

ACTIVITY 48

1 If possible, contact your local university or research laboratory and arrange to see an electron microscope being used.

2 The preparation of specimens for an electron microscope is much more time-consuming than the preparation of material for viewing with a light microscope. Find out about the former process, and write an account of the steps involved.

3 Although the transmission electron microscope is the type of electron microscope known as a *scanning electron microscope*. Figure 5.36b in Chapter 5 (photomicrograph of rods and cones in the eye) shows an example of a photoelectronmicrograph produced with

this latter type of microscope. Find out how the scanning electron microscope differs from the transmission electron microscope, and how the specimens are prepared.

4 Write out a table which makes a comparison between the light and electron microscopes in terms of: their advantages and disadvantages; the types of beam; the types of lenses; the pathway of the beam; and the preparation of specimens. (This will form part of the next Assessment opportunity below.)

Types of radioactivity and their medical uses

THE ATOMIC STRUCTURE

The nucleus of an atom consists of *protons* which have a positive charge and *neutrons* which have no charge. The number of protons is known as the *atomic number*, and this is the same for all atoms of a particular element. The number of protons and neutrons is known as the *mass number*. As you know, around the nucleus are *electrons*. These are negatively charged. Since the overall charge on an atom is neutral, the number of protons and electrons are equal (pp. 6–7).

ACTIVITY 49

1 The following example shows how the atomic number and atomic mass of an element may be written (56 is the atomic mass and 26 is the atomic number):

$^{56}_{26}$Fe (iron)

How many neutrons, protons and electrons does this element have?

2 For each of the following, give the atomic number, atomic mass, number of protons, number of electrons and number of neutrons:

$^{63}_{29}$Cu (copper)

$^{235}_{92}$U (uranium)

$^{226}_{88}$Ra (radium)

TYPES OF RADIOACTIVITY

If the number of neutrons is very different from the number of protons, the nucleus is very unstable. In this case it will rearrange to form a more stable atom, and in the process, give out radiation. These atoms are *radioactive* and are called *radioisotopes*.

There are four types of ionising radiation absorbed by human beings: *alpha particles, beta particles, gamma rays* and *X-rays*. Table 4.4 compares the four.

Isotopes are atoms of the same element but with a different mass number:

e.g. $^{238}_{92}$U, $^{235}_{92}$U.

ACTIVITY 50

1 Write a list of precautions to be taken when using radioactivity in the laboratory.

2 A Geiger–Müller tube may be used to measure levels of radiation. Find out how this works, and if possible use one yourself.

Table 4.4 A comparison of types of radiation

Type of radiation	What it consists of	Penetrating power	Effects on the body
Alpha (α)	2 protons and 2 neutrons (i.e. the nucleus of the gas helium); e.g.: $^{238}_{92}U \rightarrow ^{234}_{90}Th + ^{4}_{2}He + energy$ (Thorium)	Low. Can only penetrate a few sheets of paper	Causes large amounts of ionisation over short distances in body tissue. External sources will not pass through the skin, but internal sources (swallowed, breathed, through open wound) very dangerous
Beta (β)	Fast-moving electrons, formed when a neutron splits into a proton and an electron	Moderate. Stopped by a sheet of aluminium	Absorbed by approximately 10 mm of body tissue, therefore any damage is to the outside of the body. The organs such as the kidney, heart and lungs are protected unless the radioactive source is internal
Gamma (γ)	Part of electromagnetic spectrum (see above). Waves from the atomic nuclei	Very high. Stopped by thick blocks of lead or concrete and other dense materials	Can pass through the body and, therefore, can cause damage, whether from an internal or external source. Can kill living cells and cause cancers
X-rays	Part of electromagnetic spectrum (see above). Produced by electrons. (NB: this type of radiation does not come from radioactive elements but from a special X-ray tube)		

3 Find out what is meant by *radioactive decay* and *half-life*. Depending on your available facilities, you may be able to carry out an experiment to measure the half-life of radon or protactinium.

4 Use SATIS Unit No. 807, 'Radiation – how much do you get?', to find out about sources of radiation and to estimate your own radiation dose.

MEDICAL USES

Radioisotopes may be used for therapy or diagnosis.

Radiotherapy

Radiation can be used to treat cancers. However, doses of X-rays or gamma rays thousands of times higher than those received in diagnosis are needed. It is, therefore, important that the affected tissue only be irradiated and not the surrounding normal tissue. One way in which this is done is by aiming the beams at the tumour from several different directions, for example by rotating the radiation source around the patient. The dose received is critical: 10% lower than the optimum can have no effect, and 10% higher can cause severe problems.

Radioactive sources can also be *inserted* into the patient to destroy tumours. Other cancers can be treated with radioactive material given to the patients (*radiopharmaceuticals*).

ACTIVITY 51

1 It is important that this radioactive material accumulate in the organ or system it is required to treat. Find out about *monoclonal antibodies* or 'magic bullets' which have been used in recent years to carry radioactive chemicals to tumours.

2 What are the harmful side effects of using radiotherapy, and what can be done to overcome these?

Diagnosis

Radioisotope tracers may be used to diagnose disorders in the body. These are radioactive compounds which are introduced into the body. Their movements within the body can then be monitored by measuring the level of radioactivity in parts of the body, or by taking a radiograph. For example, the blood flow in the capillaries of the lungs can be imaged in this way: there is no radioactivity in any region where a clot is blocking the blood flow.

Magnetic resonance imaging (MRI) is the latest imaging technique used in hospitals (see Figure 4.45). This technique can produce

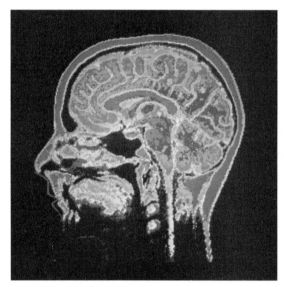

Figure 4.45 A lateral MRI scan of the head

images which are similar to, and in certain parts of the body (including the brain, spinal cord and heart) superior to, those of the CAT scanner, but without the radiation hazard. MRI offers an early diagnosis of many conditions, including cancer.

ASSESSMENT OPPORTUNITY

Produce a report exploring the properties of waves and particles, which includes:
* an explanation of the differences between electromagnetic waves, including laser light

- a summary of the medical applications and safety procedures associated with electromagnetic waves
- a description of lasers and their medical applications
- a comparison of light and electron microscopy
- an explanation of types of radioactivity and their medical uses

(b) the melting point of water, in degrees Kelvin?

2 If possible, use each of the following types of thermometer and write an illustrated account of how it works; when it might be used; and its advantages and disadvantages:
  - a thermocouple
  - a maximum–minimum thermometer
  - an electronic digital thermometer
  - a clinical thermometer
  - an alcohol-containing thermometer
  - a mercury-containing thermometer

THERMODYNAMICS

Thermal properties of matter

When heat energy is transferred to an object, its temperature may rise or it may change its state. In addition, it usually increases its size (expands) very slightly. As energy (in the form of heat) flows into the material, its *internal energy* increases. The internal energy is the total amount of energy, both kinetic and potential, possessed by all the individual particles in the matter (see the 'Kinetic theory' section on pp. 12 and 200 above).

It is very difficult to define *temperature*. Like mass and time, it is a fundamental quantity which cannot be defined in terms of any other quantity. A statement of the temperature of an object is a statement about whether it is in thermal equilibrium with other objects (i.e. whether there will be a flow of thermal energy from, or to, other objects).

The *specific heat capacity* of a material tells you how much its temperature will rise when you transfer heat to it.

Heat energy transferred (J) = mass (kg) × specific heat capacity ($J kg^{-1}K^{-1}$) × temperature rise (K)

Table 4.5 shows that water has an abnormally high specific heat capacity when compared with other substances ('$J kG^{-1} deg^{-2}$' in the table means 'joules per kilogramme per degree'). This means a lot of heat is needed to raise the temperature of a given mass of water. In other words, water is heated and cooled more slowly than expected and, in effect, buffers sharp temperature changes. This is of considerable biological importance to living cells and organisms, of which the major

Table 4.5 Examples of specific heat capacities

Substance	Specific heat ($J kg^{-1} deg^{-1}$)
Copper	390
Ice	2,110
Water	4,200
Biological tissue	c. 3,700
Air	950 (standard temperature and pressure)

Source: Physics for Biologists, G. Duncan, Blackwell Scientific Publications, 1975.

ACTIVITY 52

Measuring temperature (thermometry)
1 You will see from Table 4.1 that temperature should be measured in degrees Kelvin, which are the same size as degrees Celsius. However, 0 K is equal to −273 °C. What is
  (a) the boiling point, and

component is water. Fluctuations in the temperature of the environment will cause relatively slow changes in the internal temperature both of cells and organisms, and of the water in which aquatic species live (see p. 28).

The first law of thermodynamics states that: the change in the internal energy of a system is equal to the sum of: energy entering the system through heating, and energy entering the system through work being done to it. It was the work of Joule in the last century which first demonstrated the two ways of increasing the temperature of a body in a quantitative manner. Joule showed that the final temperature of a can of water depended on both the heat energy from the Bunsen flame applied and the mechanical energy dissipated during vigorous stirring.

As mentioned above, when a substance is heated it *expands*. This is because heating makes its molecules vibrate more, so they take up more room. For a given temperature rise, gases expand more than liquids, and liquids expand more than solids. Water has the unusual property of *contracting* as it is heated from 0 °C to 4 °C: it has its maximum density at 4 °C. Above this temperature the additional heat breaks some hydrogen bonds, and so the water molecules are less densely compacted.

ACTIVITY 53

Design an experiment which allows you to measure and compare the expansion, when heated, of a solid, water and a liquid other than water. NB: if you are actually going to carry out the experiment, you must check through all the *safety precautions* with your teacher before you start.

Changes in the state of matter

It was mentioned above that when heat energy is transferred to an object, the object may change its state. The heat energy put in increases the internal energy of the material. In other words, it increases the movement of the particles of the substance until the particles have sufficient energy to overcome the forces between them (completely in the case of liquid to gas, and only partly in the case of solid to liquid). When a substance is being heated and is changing state, its temperature, however, remains constant. The heat energy which has to be supplied to cause this change in state is called *latent* (hidden) *heat*. A substance's *specific latent heat* is the heat energy required to change the state of a certain mass of that substance without any corresponding temperature change. The SI unit is J kg^{-1}.

The latent heat required to convert a solid into a liquid is the *latent heat of fusion* or *melting*, and the latent heat required to convert a liquid into a gas is the *latent heat of vaporisation*. In most cases, the latent heat of vaporisation is greater than the latent heat of fusion. This is because of the large volume change that takes place when a liquid becomes a gas (see pp. 13–14).

ACTIVITY 54

1 Start with a bowl of crushed ice straight from the freezer and leave it at room temperature. Take the temperature at regular intervals, and plot a graph of temperature against time.

2 When a person sweats, the energy required to convert the liquid sweat into water vapour, i.e. the latent heat of vaporisation, comes from the body, which is therefore cooled. The evaporation of each gramme of water requires 2.5 kJ of energy. A person may produce up to 1,000 cm^3 per hour of sweat. If they are producing this maximum amount and it is all evaporating, how much energy will the person be losing?

3 Design an experiment to investigate the rate of evaporation on temperature loss. You could use boiling tubes containing water surrounded by cotton wool soaked ethanol, or water at different temperatures. You could use a hair dryer to vary wind speed.

Refrigerators use evaporation to produce cooling. In the coils around the icebox or cold plate in the fridge is a volatile liquid, i.e. one that evaporates very easily. This liquid evaporates, causing cooling, and the gas formed is pumped into the pipes at the back of the fridge where it is under pressure. It condenses back into a liquid, giving off heat. The liquid returns to the pipes in the icebox, and the process is continually repeated.

ACTIVITY 55

1 Find out what types of gas may be used to cool fridges. What precautions should be taken when disposing of these gases?

2 An increase in pressure raises the boiling point of a liquid and lowers its freezing point. *Autoclaving* involves heating things in steam under pressure to sterilise them. Because of the elevated pressure, temperatures of well over 100 °C can be obtained. If possible, arrange to see an autoclave being used, and produce an annotated sketch to explain how it works. (If you cannot see a large autoclave, you can examine a pressure cooker instead.)

3 The same principle of elevated pressure is used in the *canning process*. Produce a flow diagram to show the stages involved in this process.

Table 4.6 **Typical values for heat loss from the human body by different methods**

	Studying at 22 °C	Sunbathing at 32 °C	Walking at −18 °C
% of body clothed	85	15	95
Heat loss rate/W	170	400	400
% loss by:			
1 radiation	21	8	8
2 conduction and convection	67	10	50
3 evaporation	10	80	2
4 respiration and excretion	2	2	40

Source: University of Bath. Macmillan Science 16–19 Project: Medical Physics, M. Hollins, Macmillan, 1990.

Heat transfer

Heat energy may be transferred from one place to another by *conduction*, *convection* and *radiation*. Table 4.6 gives some typical values for these for energy loss from the human body.

CONDUCTION

Heat is transferred by physical contact between two bodies. For example, if a person is lying on the ground, heat will be lost from the body to the ground by conduction. Generally, the loss of heat by conduction is very low because of the *insulating* effect of the skin and clothing.

ACTIVITY 56

1 Look at a transverse section of skin under the microscope, and at Figure 3.25 from Chapter 3 (p. 161). The subcutaneous fat is a good insulator, and the hairs can be held erect by the contraction of the erector pili muscles which serves to trap a layer of air – also a good insulating material.

2 Clothing keeps us warm by trapping a layer of air. Design and carry out an experiment to investigate the

effectiveness of different types of
material as insulators.

3 The surface-area:volume ratio influences
the rate of heat loss by conduction. The
larger a person's surface area in relation
to their volume, the faster their heat loss.
Calculate the surface areas and volumes
of cubes with sides of (i) 1 cm and (ii)
2 cm. Which has the largest surface-
area:volume ratio?

   Who out of the following has the
largest surface-area:volume ratio:
(a) a newborn baby
(b) an adult?

4 Completely fill a 50 cm^3 beaker and a
1,000 cm^3 beaker with boiling water.
Take the temperature immediately, and
then at regular intervals. Plot a cooling
curve (i.e. temperature in °C against
time in minutes). Work out the
approximate surface-area:volume ratio
for each beaker. What conclusions can
you draw?

Table 4.7 The chilling effect of wind at various speeds

Air temperature (°C)	Apparent temperature (°C)		
+10	+9	−0	−3
+4	+3	−8	−12
−12	−14	−32	−38
Wind speed (m/sec)	2.0	9.0	18.0

Source: Climate and Environment Systems,
D.C. Money, Unwin Hyman, 1988

be. Air movement reduces the insulating
effect of ordinary clothes. This is because it
disturbs the warmed air trapped within the
fabric.

ACTIVITY 57

Find advertisements for clothing suitable
for use in exposed areas. What are the
features of these garments which protect
the wearer against the 'elements'?

CONVECTION

Convection is the transfer of heat energy by
the circulation of a fluid (a liquid or gas).
Because air temperature is usually lower than
the temperature of the human body, the air in
contact with the body becomes warm, rises
and is replaced with cooler air. The rate of
heat transfer by this method is linked to the
rate of air movement which continually
brings cooler air into contact with the body.
This means that the materials mentioned
above – i.e. hair and fabrics – which trap a
still layer of warm air reduce heat loss, not
only through decreasing conduction but also
through decreasing convection.

   This also explains the chilling effect of a
cold wind. Table 4.7 shows the chilling effect
of wind at various speeds, given as an *apparent*
temperature – which is how people feel it to

RADIATION

Radiation is the transfer of heat energy from
one place to another by means of
electromagnetic waves which lie in the long-
wave, infrared region of the electromagnetic
spectrum, beyond the visible spectrum (see
the 'Electromagnetic waves' section on
pp. 220–227 above). Heat energy from the
sun reaches us by radiation.

ACTIVITY 58

Black surfaces are good absorbers and good
radiators. Shiny surfaces are poor radiators
and poor absorbers. Use this information
to explain why dark-coloured skin is well
suited to a tropical environment, and how
a 'space blanket' functions.

ASSESSMENT OPPORTUNITY

1 Produce a record of an investigation into thermodynamics, including:
- an explanation of the thermal properties of matter
- an explanation of the relationship between energy and change in the state of matter

2 Write a report on heat transfer, providing physiological examples involved in the maintenance of body temperature.

REFERENCES AND RESOURCES

Whenever possible, visits should be made to appropriate local facilities, visiting speakers should be invited in, and relevant video tapes should be viewed.

A wide range of physics textbooks should be referred to when researching topics. These should include basic GCSE texts as well as standard A-level texts and specialised medical-physics texts. Some good examples of these are listed below, and it is likely that your school, college or local library will have others.

Fullick, P. (1994), *Physics*, Oxford: Heinemann.

Hollins, M. (1990), *University of Bath. Macmillan Science 16–19 Project: Medical Physics*, London: Macmillan.

Jones, G., Jones, M. and Marchington, P. 'Cambridge Coordinated Science: Physics' (1993) Publ. Cambridge University Press.

For further reading on manual handling:

Barker, A., Cassar, S., Garbett, J. et al. (1994), *Handling People: Equipment, Advice and Information*, London: Disabled Living Foundation.

Confederation of Health Service Employees (1992), *Lifting and Back Pain in Health Service Work*, Banstead: COHSE.

Corlett, E. N., Lloyd, P., Tarling, C. et al. (1992), *Guide to the Handling of Patients*, 3rd edn, London: National Back Pain Association/RCN.

'Lifting and handling', *Nursing Times*, vol. 91, no. 3.

RCN Advisory Panel for Back Pain in Nurses (1993), *Code of Practice for the Handling of Patients*, London: RCN.

USEFUL ADDRESSES

College of Radiographers
2 Carriage Row
183 Eversholt Street
London NW1 1BU
Tel.: 0171 391 4500

Institute of Physical Sciences in Medicine
Hospital Physicist's Association
2 Low Ousegate
York YO1 1QU
Tel.: 01904 610821

National Radiological Protection Board (NRPB)
Chilton
Didcot
Oxon OX1 0RQ
Tel.: 01235 831600
Fax.: 01235 833811

Royal College of Ophthalmologists
17 Cornwall Terrace
London NW1 4QW

Royal College of Radiology
38 Portland Place
London W1N 4JQ
Tel.: 0171 636 4432/3

5

PHYSIOLOGY FOR HEALTH CARE

BODY SYSTEMS INVOLVED IN THE TRANSPORT AND ELIMINATION OF METABOLIC PRODUCTS

You will remember from your work on the 'Health and social well-being' mandatory unit (see Thomson et al. 1995, Chapters 3, 4 and 7) that the cardiovascular system consists of the following tissues and organs:

* the heart
* the circulatory system: arteries, veins, capillaries
* the blood
* the lymph

The structure and action of the heart

STRUCTURE

ACTIVITY 1

Obtain a complete sheep's heart. Draw the external structure showing the coronary vessels which supply the cardiac muscle with blood.

Figure 5.1 shows the internal structures of the heart. Using a guide, dissect the heart. Relate the above diagram to the actual structure.

Cardiac muscle

Cardiac muscle is found only in the heart. It is capable of rapid, rhythmic contraction and relaxation. To allow the waves of contraction to spread over the heart, the muscle cells, or fibres, are branched and connected to one another (see Figure 5.2).

ACTIVITY 2

If possible, observe cardiac muscle under a microscope, and compare it with *voluntary* and *smooth* muscle.

ACTION

The cardiac cycle

The following is the sequence of stages of a heartbeat:

1 *Diastole.* The atria and ventricles are relaxed. Deoxygenated blood under low pressure enters the right atrium, and oxygenated blood enters the left atrium. The atria become distended as they become filled with blood. At first, the bicuspid and tricuspid valves are closed, but as the pressure in the atria increases, the valves are pushed open and some blood flows into the relaxed ventricles.

2 *Atrial systole.* When the diastole ends, the two atria contract simultaneously. This is called the atrial systole, and it results in more blood being pushed into the ventricles.

3 *Ventricular systole.* As blood is pushed into the ventricles, they contract almost immediately. This is called the ventricular systole. At this time, the bicuspid and tricuspid valves are closed. The ventricular pressure exceeds that of the aorta and the

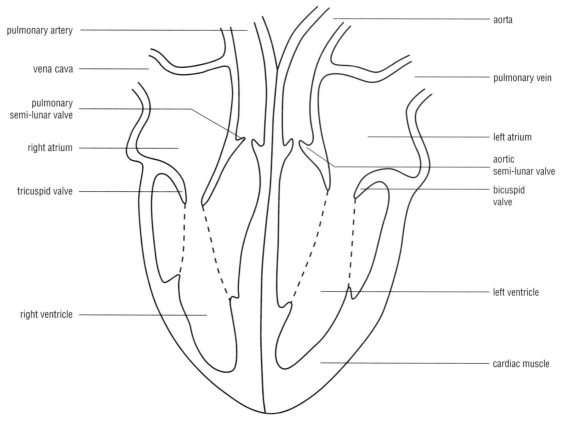

Figure 5.1   The structure of the heart: an internal view
Source: Thomson et al., 1995.

pulmonary artery, and the aortic and pulmonary valves are pushed open. Thus, blood is expelled into these vessels. During the ventricular systole the blood is forced against the closed atrioventricular valves, and this produces the first sound of the heartbeat ('lub').

4 *Diastole again.* The ventricular systole ends, and the ventricles and atria relax again. The high pressure developed in the aorta and

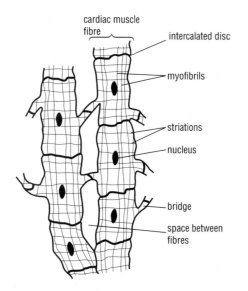

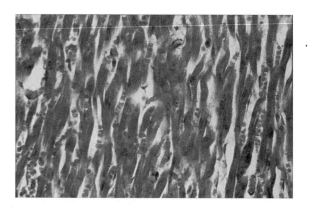

Figure 5.2   Cardiac muscle: (a) a diagram of the microscopic structure and (b) a photomicrograph
Source: (a) Stanley Thornes (Publishers) Ltd, *Understanding Biology for Advanced Level,* 2nd edition.

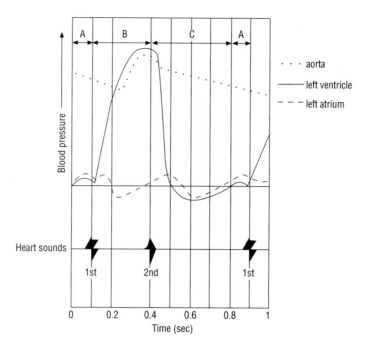

Figure 5.3 The cardiac cycle

the pulmonary artery tends to force some blood back towards the ventricles, and the aortic and pulmonary pocket valves close rapidly. This causes the second heart sound ('dub').

One heartbeat consists of one systole and one diastole, and lasts for about 0.8 seconds.

Figure 5.3 shows some of the changes that take place during one cardiac cycle.

ACTIVITY 3

1 From Figure 5.3:
   - calculate the heart rate (beats/minute)
   - explain what is happening in phases A, B and C
   - say what causes the first and second sounds of the heart beat

2 Copy Figure 5.1. Using the account above, draw arrows to show the direction of blood flow, and include short notes (annotations) on each label to describe points of interest.

Cardiac rhythm

The heart is *myogenic* i.e. it has an 'in-built' mechanism for initiating the contraction of the cardiac muscle fibres. This allows it to continue beating for quite some time when removed from the body and placed in an appropriate solution at 37 °C.

The stimulus for contraction originates at the *sino-atrial node* (S-A node), which is also known as the *pacemaker* (see Figure 5.4). A wave of electrical excitation passes from the S-A node across the muscle fibres of the atria, and this causes them to contract. The wave spreads at approximately 1 m/s. The fibres of the atria are completely separated from those of the ventricles, except for the region in the right atrium called the *atrioventricular node* (A-V node). The A-V node is connected to the *bundle of His*, a strand of modified cardiac fibres which gives rise to finer branches known as *Purkinje tissue*. Impulses are conducted rapidly along the bundle (5 m/s) and spread to all parts of the ventricles. Both ventricles contract simultaneously, and this starts approximately 0.15 s after the atria have completed their contraction.

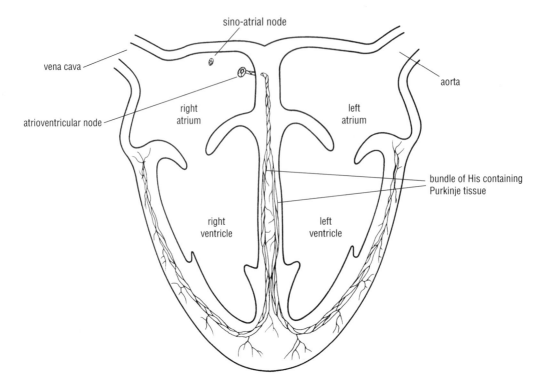

Figure 5.4 The structure of the heart, showing conduction tissue
Source: Thomson et al., 1995.

ACTIVITY 4

Redraw a simple diagram of the heart from Figure 5.4 showing the position of the S-A and A-V nodes and bundle of His. Put arrows on to show the direction of the spread of the wave of excitation described above.

Factors affecting cardiac output

Cardiac output is determined by the *heart rate* (beats per minute) and the *stroke volume* (the volume of blood expelled by the heart per beat).

Although the heart is myogenic (see above), it is connected to nerves which can cause the heart rate to speed up or slow down. Impulses from the *cardio-acceleratory centre* in the medulla of the brain pass along a sympathetic nerve and activate the sinu-atrial node, *increasing* the heart rate. Branches of the sympathetic nerve also stimulate the walls of the ventricles, and this increases their power of contraction, and hence stroke volume.

Impulses from the *cardio-inhibitory centre* in the medulla of the brain pass along the *vagus nerve* and activate the sinu-atrial node, *slowing down* heart rate.

With these two nerves supplying the heart, the rate can be altered depending on circumstances.

ACTIVITY 5

Exercise brings about an increase in the heart rate, and rest causes it to decrease. What other factors can you think of which will influence heart rate?

The microscopic structure of blood

Blood is found circulating within the cardiovascular system, i.e. within the heart and blood vessels.

Component	Appearance	Function	Nos. of cells mm^{-3}
Plasma	Straw-coloured liquid	Matrix in which a variety of substances are carried, e.g. vitamins, products of digestion, excretory products, hormones	
Red blood cells or *erythocytes*	Bioconcave discs full of the red pigment haemoglobin. No nucleus 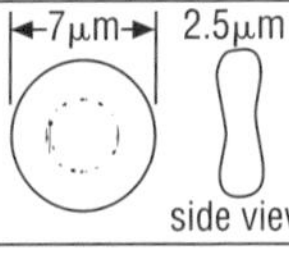 ←7μm→ 2.5μm side view	Carriage of O_2 and some CO_2	500,000
White blood cells or leucocytes (a) *Granulocytes*	Granlular cytoplasm. Lobed nuclei		
Neutrophils	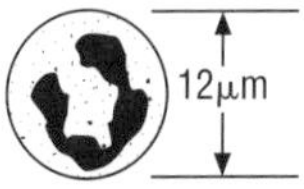 12μm	Engulf bacteria	4,900
Eosinophils	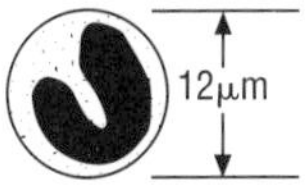 12μm	Anti-histamine properties	105
Basophils	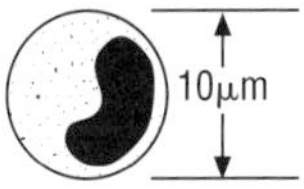 10μm	Produces histamine	35
(b) *Agranulocytes*	No granules seen under light microscope		
Monocytes	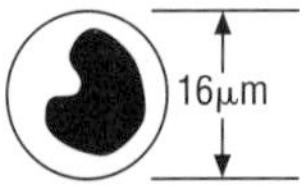 16μm	Engulf bacteria	280
Lymphocytes	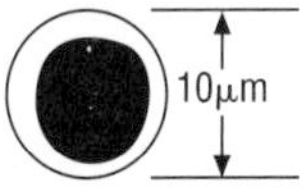 10μm	Antibody production	1,680
Platelets (thrombocytes)	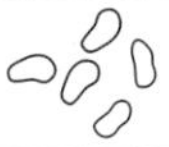 3μm	Clotting	250,000

Figure 5.5   The components of blood

ACTIVITY 6

1 Figure 5.5 shows the components of blood. Which of these can you identify in Figure 5.6? If possible, examine a prepared slide of blood under a microscope, and identify as many of the components as possible.

2 List three ways in which the structure of the red blood cells makes blood efficient at carrying out its main function.

3 Red blood cells have a lifespan of about three months. How are the waste products from their breakdown excreted?

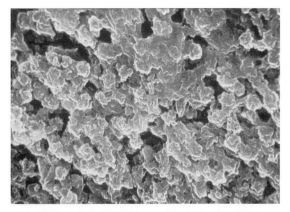

Figure 5.6   A photomicrograph of blood cells and platelets

The circulation of blood

THE CIRCULATORY SYSTEM

The role of the heart and circulatory system is to carry blood between various parts of the body. Each organ has a major artery supplying it with blood from the heart and a major vein which returns it.

ACTIVITY 7

Copy Figure 5.7 and add the names of the vessels numbered 1–19. Use arrows to show the direction of blood flow. Shade the vessels containing oxygenated blood red, and those containing deoxygenated blood blue.

Humans, in common with other mammals, have what is known as a *double circulation*. In other words, on a complete journey around the body, a blood cell passes through the heart twice: once when it is sent to the lungs (*pulmonary circulation*), and once when it is sent off to the rest of the body (*systemic circulation*).

ACTIVITY 8

1 Look at Figure 5.7 again and answer the following questions:
 • Which side of the heart pumps blood to the lungs, and which side pumps blood around the remainder of the body?
 • Which ventricle has to pump blood the furthest?

2 Look back at Figure 5.1. With reference to the last question, why is the wall of the left ventricle much thicker than the wall of the right ventricle?

3 Why are the walls of the atria much thinner than the walls of the ventricles? (Think again of the relative distances they have to pump blood.)

The flow of blood is maintained in three ways:

1 *The pumping action of the heart.*
2 *The contraction of skeletal muscle.* The contraction of muscles during movement squeezes the veins and increases the pressure of blood within them. Pocket valves in the veins prevent the backflow of blood and ensure that it flows to the heart.
3 *Inspiratory movements.* The pressure in the thorax is reduced when breathing in, and this helps to draw blood back to the heart.

ARTERIES, VEINS AND CAPILLARIES

Arteries carry blood away from the heart. *Veins* carry blood to the heart. *Capillaries* connect arteries and veins and form a network in the tissues.

ACTIVITY 9

1 Compare Figures 5.8 and 5.10. Can you see the structures labelled on the diagram in the photomicrographs?

2 Copy out the following table and complete it to compare the structures and functions of the three types of blood vessel.

ARTERY	VEIN	CAPILLARY
1 Thick muscular wall	Thin muscular wall	No muscle
2		
3		
4		

BLOOD PRESSURE

The pressure at which blood flows in the circulatory system is generated mainly by the pumping action of the ventricles. The arteries, having thick elastic walls, help to maintain this pressure by stretching during systole and recoiling during diastole. As the blood flows into the capillaries, the pressure drops. This is

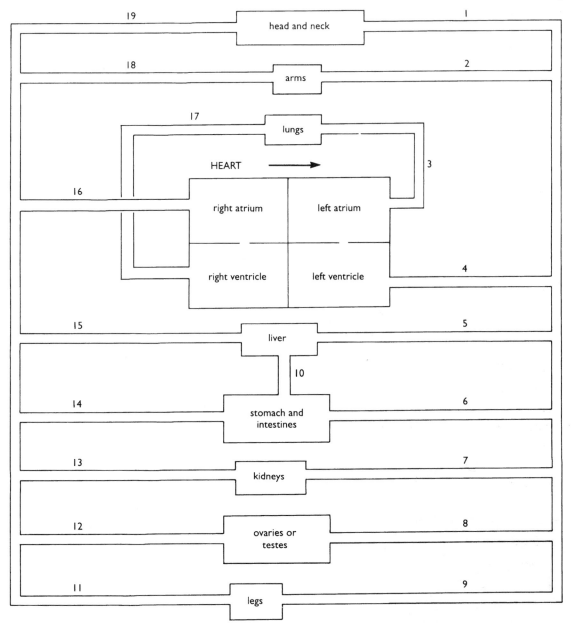

Figure 5.7 A general plan of the circulatory system
Source: Thomson et al., 1995.

because the narrower vessels offer a greater degree of resistance.

Blood pressure within the body can be controlled by messages from the brain causing *vasodilation* or *vasoconstriction* (the dilation or constriction of the arterioles which link arteries to capillaries). Blood pressure is also affected by changes in cardiac output (see 'Factors affecting cardiac output' on p. 240 above). The measurement of blood pressure is covered in Thomson et al. 1995, Chapter 3, pp. 174–5.

Functions of blood

The functions of each type of cell in the blood are shown in Figure 5.5.

A major role of blood is *transport*.

THE TRANSPORT OF OXYGEN

Complete the table in Activity 10 on p. 245 below. You should have written that oxygen is transported from the lungs to the respiring tissues by the haemoglobin in the erythrocytes. You should also have noted in

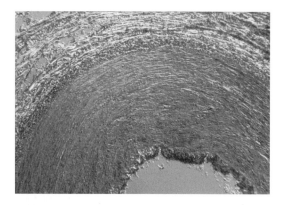

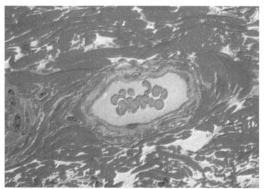

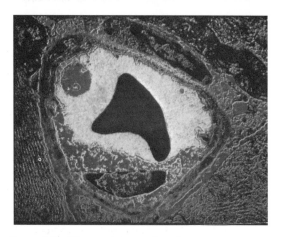

Figure 5.8 Photomicrographs of transverse sections of (a) artery, × 50, (b) vein, × 160 and (c) capillary, × 3,500

Oxygen combines with haemoglobin to form *oxyhaemoglobin*. This can easily break down again, or dissociate, to release the oxygen when needed. The amount of oxygen that can combine with haemoglobin is determined by the *oxygen tension*. This is expressed as *partial pressure*, and is the fraction of oxygen found in the air (see p. 24). Normal atmospheric pressure is approximately 100 kilopascals. As oxygen makes up around 21% of the atmosphere, the oxygen tension (partial pressure) of the atmosphere is around 21 kPa.

When haemoglobin is exposed to a gradual increase in oxygen tension, it absorbs oxygen rapidly at first, but more slowly as the tension continues to rise. This is shown by the sigmoid, or 'S'-shaped, *oxygen dissociation curve* (see Figure 5.9).

The fact that the oxygen dissociation curve is this shape, and that the relationship between oxygen tension and the saturation of haemoglobin is not linear (i.e. not a straight line) means that haemoglobin is very efficient at picking up oxygen when there is an increase in oxygen tension (i.e. at the lungs –

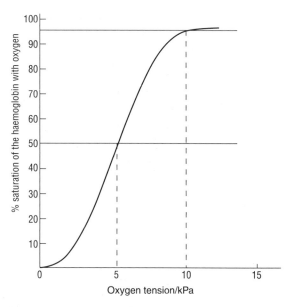

Figure 5.9 An oxygen dissociation curve for adult human haemoglobin
Source: Stanley Thornes (Publishers) Ltd, *Understanding Biology for Advanced Level*, 2nd edition.

your answer to the question above on how the erythrocyte is adapted to this function, that it has a large surface area relative to volume, which allows for a rapid uptake of oxygen; that it has no nucleus, which means that it can be packed with haemoglobin; and that it is small, which means that it can travel along the narrow capillaries.

ACTIVITY 10

Copy out the following table and complete it.

Materials transported	Examples	Transported to:	Transported from:	Transported in:
Respiratory gases	Oxygen			Haemoglobin in red cells
	Carbon dioxide			
Organic nutrients	Glucose			
	Amino acids			
	Vitamins			
Mineral salts	Calcium			
	Iodine			
	Iron			
Excretory products	Urea			
Hormones	Insulin			
	Anti-diuretic hormone			
Heat	Metabolic heat			

see Figure 5.11a), and very efficient at releasing oxygen when there is a decrease in oxygen tension (i.e. at the respiring tissues – see Figure 5.11b).

ACTIVITY 11

1 Draw graphs similar to Figures 5.11a and b to show that if the relationship between oxygen tension and the percentage saturation of haemoglobin were linear (i.e. a straight line instead of an S-shaped curve), there would be a less efficient uptake of oxygen at the lungs and a less efficient release of oxygen at the respiring tissues.

2 Study Table 5.1.

(a) Plot the data in the table as a suitable graph.

(b) The partial pressure of oxygen in the lungs is 12.5 kPa, and in the tissues it is 5.5 kPa. What is the percentage saturation
   (i) in the lungs,
   (ii) in the tissues?

(c) When the percentage saturation with oxygen reaches 100%, the oxygen content of the blood is $200 \text{ cm}^3 \text{ dm}^{-3}$. For each 1% fall in oxygen saturation, the blood's oxygen content also decreases by 1%. Calculate the volume of oxygen released as blood passes from the lungs to the tissues.

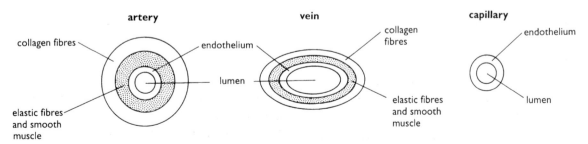

Figure 5.10 A diagram showing transverse sections of artery, vein and capillary

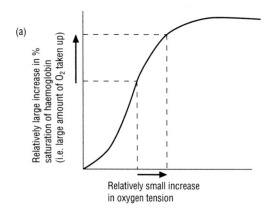

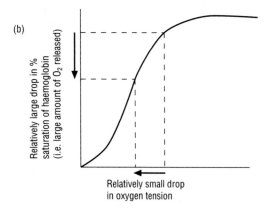

Figure 5.11 The oxygen dissociation curve means that haemoglobin is efficient at (a) picking up O_2 at the lungs, and (b) releasing O_2 at the tissues

Table 5.1 The percentage saturation of haemoglobin from adult humans, at different partial pressures of oxygen

Partial pressure of oxygen, pO_2, (kPa)	Percentage saturation with oxygen
0.0	0
1.0	8
2.0	18
3.0	31
4.0	44
5.0	58
6.0	70
7.0	80
8.0	86
9.0	91
10.0	93
11.0	95
12.0	97
13.0	97

ACTIVITY 12

Extension work

Find out

- the effect an increase in the partial pressure of carbon dioxide has on the oxygen dissociation curve.

    How does this help with:

    (a) the efficient uptake of oxygen at the lungs, and

    (b) the efficient release of oxygen at the respiring tissues?

- how the foetal oxygen dissociation curve differs from the adult curve, and how this difference enables the foetus to obtain oxygen

- the effect an increase in temperature has on the oxygen dissociation curve, and how this helps with the release of oxygen at the respiring tissues

- about the oxygen dissociation curve for the intramuscular oxygen carrier *myoglobin*

THE TRANSPORT OF CARBON DIOXIDE

There are three ways in which carbon dioxide is transported from the respiring tissues to the lungs.

1 *In solution.* About 5% of the carbon dioxide is transported in solution in the blood plasma.

2 *Combined with protein.* About 10% of the carbon dioxide combines with haemoglobin to form a compound known as *carbaminohaemoglobin*.

3 *As hydrogen carbonate.* The remainder of the carbon dioxide, about 85%, is carried in the plasma in the form of hydrogen carbonate. The formation of this compound involves a number of steps:

- First, carbon dioxide diffuses from the respiring tissues into the red blood cells where it combines with water to form carbonic acid. This step is catalysed by the enzyme *carbonic anhydrase*.

$$H_2O + CO_2 \xrightarrow{\text{carbonic anhydrase}} H_2CO_3$$

- The carbonic acid dissociates into hydrogen and hydrogen carbonate ions:

$$H_2CO_3 \rightarrow H^+ + HCO_3^-$$

- The hydrogen ions combine with haemoglobin (Hb) which releases its oxygen. (This oxygen can then be used by the respiring tissues)
- The hydrogen carbonate ions diffuse out of the red blood cells into the plasma where they combine with sodium ions (formed from the dissociation of sodium chloride) to form *sodium hydrogen carbonate*:

$$HCO_3^- + Na^+ \rightarrow NaHCO_3$$

- The loss of the negatively charged hydrogen carbonate ions from the red blood cell is balanced by the inward diffusion of negatively charged chloride ions (formed from the dissociation of sodium chloride). This is known as the *chloride shift*

The above events are summarised in Figure 1.26.

When the blood reaches the lungs, all these processes are reversed, which releases the carbon dioxide.

The structure of the kidney

THE MACROSCOPIC STRUCTURE

The kidneys are a pair of organs found in the abdominal cavity. They are embedded in fat and held firmly in place by the *peritoneum*, a thin layer of tissue lining the abdominal cavity. Each kidney is about 7–10 cm long and 2.5–4 cm wide in an adult. Inside, an outer dark *cortex* and an inner paler *medulla* can be seen (as in Figure 5.13).

ACTIVITY 13

Figure 5.12 shows the urinary system.

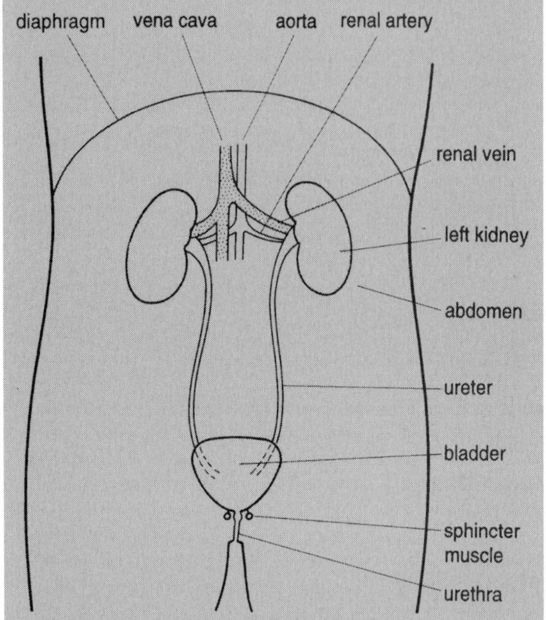

Figure 5.12   The urinary system
Source: Thomson et al., 1995.

1 Distinguish between the ureter and the urethra. What is the function of the bladder? What is the role of the renal vein?

2 The urea arrives at the kidney in the renal artery. Look back at Figure 5.7. How does the urea get to the kidneys from the liver? List the blood vessels it travels through. What other important chemical arrives in the renal artery?

3 Cut a kidney (e.g. from a lamb or pig) in half longitudinally with a sharp knife. Draw what you see, labelling as many structures shown in Figure 5.13 as you can see. (A nephron is too small to see.)

THE MICROSCOPIC STRUCTURE OF THE KIDNEY TUBULE

Each kidney has many blood vessels and approximately one million nephrons or

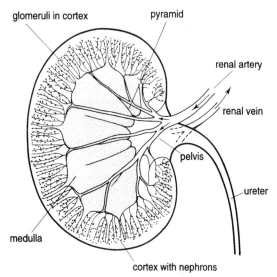

Figure 5.13 The macroscopic structure of the kidney
Source: Thomson et al., 1995.

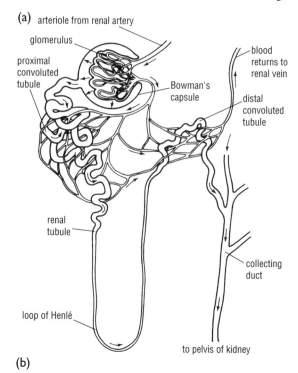

(b)

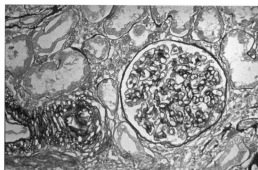

Figure 5.14 The microscopic structure of the kidney tubule: (a) a diagram, and (b) a photomicrograph
Source: (a) Thomson et al., 1995.

kidney tubules. It is these tubules that carry out all the regulatory functions listed above. The renal artery divides into many smaller arterioles, which eventually lead to the *glomeruli*, a small knot of capillaries in the Bowman's capsules.

ACTIVITY 14

Look at Figures 5.14a and b. Then examine a prepared slide of kidney cortex under a microscope. Can you find the Bowman's capsules, each containing a glomerulus, and transverse sections of the tubules of the nephron? There will also be blood vessels; you may be able to see some red blood cells.

The areas of the *nephron* (tubules of the kidney) differ in their appearance in transverse section (see Figure 5.15). These differences are related to the different functions of each section (see pp. 249–253 below).

THE ULTRASTRUCTURE OF THE BOWMAN'S CAPSULE

The *Bowman's capsule* can be envisaged as a hollow ball which has been pressed in at the

top to form a cup-shape. The *glomerulus* is found within this cup-shape. An electron microscope shows that there is a thin, porous *basement membrane* between the capillaries of the glomerulus and the capsule. The lining of the 'cup' (i.e. the inner layer of the Bowman's capsule) is composed of cells called *podocytes*. These are star-shaped, with each of the 'arms' (*primary processes*) having smaller branches (*secondary processes*) beneath them (see Figure 5.16). The secondary processes support the basement membrane and the capillary

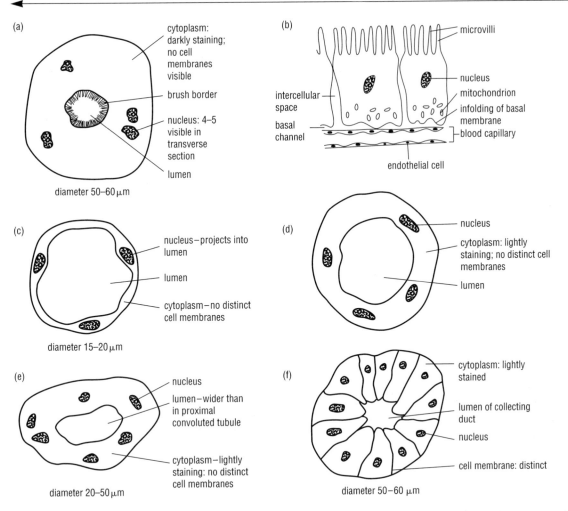

Figure 5.15 Diagrams of transverse sections of the kidney tubule: (a) a transverse section of the proximal convoluted tubule; (b) details of two cells from the proximal convoluted tubule; (c) the loop of Henle – a thin segment; (d) the loop of Henle – a thick segment; (e) the distal convoluted tubule; (f) the collecting duct
Source: Stanley Thornes (Publishers) Ltd, *Understanding Biology for Advanced Level*, 2nd edition.

beneath it. The gaps between the secondary processes form pores which facilitate the movement of materials (see p. 250 below).

The outer cells of the Bowman's capsule are unspecialised *squamous epithelial* cells.

The functions of the kidney

The kidney has several essential functions, the most obvious of which is *excretion* (see below). In addition to this, it is responsible for *osmoregulation* within the body (i.e. the regulation of the salt–water balance). This is also covered below. Another function which is

not covered here, however, is the regulation of the pH of the internal environment.

ACTIVITY 15

Distinguish between the following terms:
- excretion
- egestion
- secretion

EXCRETION

The kidneys produce urine and are the main organs of the urinary system. This system is

(a)

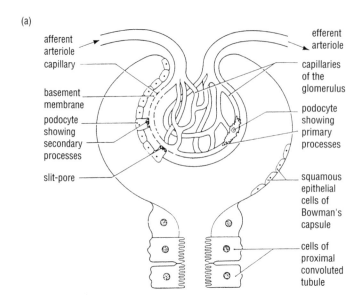

(b)

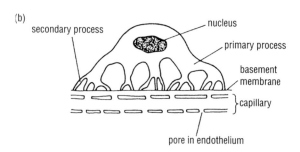

Figure 5.16 The ultrastructure of Bowman's capsule: (a) diagrams; (b) podocyte from visceral wall of Bowman's capsule
Source: (a) *Biological Science*, Stout, Green and Taylor (ed. Soper), Cambridge University Press, 1985; (b) Stanley Thornes (Publishers) Ltd, *Understanding Biology for Advanced Level*, 2nd edition.

often called the *excretory system* because an important function of the kidneys is the excretion of nitrogenous waste, mostly in the form of *urea*, dissolved in the urine. The body cannot store excess proteins, so amino acids that are not immediately required are broken down in the liver to make urea. This is carried in the bloodstream to the kidneys for elimination. All the blood in the body passes through the kidneys in five minutes.

Ultrafiltration

The blood pressure in the glomerulus is very high. This high pressure forces about one-fifth of the water of the plasma – and with it, small molecules – through the walls of the capillaries of the glomerulus and the walls of the Bowman's capsule into the capsule space (see the section 'The ultrastructure of the Bowman's capsule' above).

The liquid formed in the capsule space is called the *glomerular filtrate* or *fluid*, and the process by which it is formed is *ultrafiltration*.

ACTIVITY 16

1 Can you think of two reasons why the pressure of the blood in the glomeruli is so high?

2 How are the squamous cells that are found in the capillaries and Bowman's capsule adapted to their function?

3 Look at Table 5.2 and note the differences between the blood leaving the glomerulus and the glomerular filtrate. How do you account for these differences? (Think about the sizes.)

Table 5.2 The differences between the blood leaving the glomerulus and the glomerular filtrate

Blood leaving the glomerulus	Glomerular filtrate
Water	Water
Plasma proteins	–
Platelets	–
Red blood cells	–
White blood cells	–
–	Glucose
–	Amino acids
–	Urea
–	Minerals

Reabsorption

As the glomerular filtrate flows along the nephron, its composition changes. This is because there are many substances in it which are needed by the body and must therefore be *reabsorbed* back into the bloodstream. Much of the water and glucose, and most of the mineral salts and amino acids, are among the substances which must not be excreted. If there was not any reabsorption of the water, the body would be totally dehydrated in three minutes. Urea, other molecules and the water which is to be excreted are left in the nephron and eventually form urine. Most of the reabsorption occurs in the proximal convoluted tubule.

The role of active transport

Reabsorption takes place mainly by *active transport*: i.e. the movement of molecules is against a *concentration gradient*, and requires *energy*. If you look back at the description of the structure of the cells of the proximal convoluted tubule, you will see that they are ideally adapted for this purpose: they have a large surface area, intercellular spaces and numerous mitochondria to supply energy. Amino acids, glucose and ions from the filtrate in the *lumen* diffuse into these cells and then are actively transported into the intercellular spaces, from where they diffuse into the surrounding capillaries. Some sodium ions are also taken into the cells by active transport. This raises the osmotic pressure of the cells, so that water from the filtrate enters them by osmosis. About half the urea in the filtrate returns to the blood by diffusion.

ACTIVITY 17

Make a large copy of Figure 5.15b and draw in the pathways taken by the various compounds as described above. Use different coloured lines and a key to show whether movement is by diffusion, osmosis or active transport. Write a definition of each of these terms.

The loop of Henle

(As you read this account, continually refer back to Figures 5.13 and 5.14 to remind yourself of the positions of the structures mentioned.)

The loop of Henle plays an important role in the reabsorption of water. It causes a build-up of salt in the medulla by a method known as the *counter-current multiplier*. Because the collecting ducts pass through this area, water moves out of the filtrate by osmosis.

The counter-current multiplier hypothesis

The descending limb of the loop of Henle (see Figure 5.17) is narrow, and its walls are permeable to water. The walls of the ascending limb, on the other hand, are thick and not permeable to water. The mechanism is known as 'counter-current' because the fluids in the descending and ascending limbs are flowing in opposite directions.

Along the length of the ascending limb, sodium and chloride ions are removed from the filtrate by active transport. Some of these remain in the interstitial region (i.e. between the ascending and descending limbs), and some are pumped into the descending limb. This creates an area of high salt concentration in the medulla. The water leaving the permeable descending loop goes straight into a blood capillary, and so does not dilute this salt concentration.

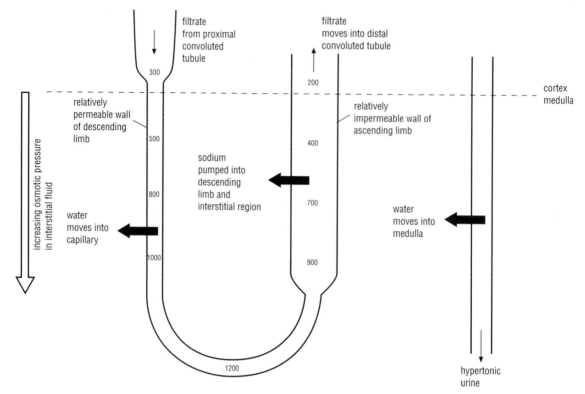

Figure 5.17 The counter-current multiplier of the loop of Henle
Source: Stanley Thornes (Publishers) Ltd, *Understanding Biology for Advanced Level,* 2nd edition.

ACTIVITY 18

If possible, study a computer simulation of the counter-current multiplier system.

OSMOREGULATION

This involves the control of the water–salt balance in the body.

Antidiuretic hormone (ADH)

The body controls changes in the amount of water in the body by regulating the permeability of the collecting ducts. The osmotic potential of the blood is detected by *osmoreceptors* in the hypothalamus of the brain. If the osmotic potential drops (i.e. less water, more salt), a message (in the form of a nervous impulse) is passed to the posterior pituitary gland, resulting in the release of *antidiuretic hormone* or ADH. This is carried in the blood to the kidneys where it causes the collecting ducts to become more permeable to water. More water can then leave the filtrate, resulting in more concentrated urine and an increase in the osmotic potential of the blood.

ACTIVITY 19

1 Find out the positions of the hypothalamus and posterior pituitary gland.

2 Draw a flow chart to illustrate the correction of a drop in the osmotic potential of the blood as described above.

3 Explain what would happen if the osmotic potential of the blood were to rise. Draw a flow chart to illustrate this.

4 A person who suffers from the uncommon disease of *diabetes insipidus* is

unable to produce sufficient ADH. What can you predict about the volume and concentration of the urine they produce?

5 To summarise your knowledge, complete Table 5.3, using + to show an increase and − to show a decrease.

Diuretics

Certain chemicals known as *diuretics* increase the urine volume by inhibiting the reabsorption of water. Some diuretics act directly on the nephron as they pass through the kidney. Others act by inhibiting the secretion of ADH as they circulate through the brain. Coffee, tea and alcohol are diuretics.

ACTIVITY 20

1 On one day, after urinating, drink 500 cm^3 of water. At 30-minute intervals over four hours, measure the volume of urine produced. On a second day, repeat the procedure but replace the water with strong tea or coffee. Plot the results on one graph (volume against time).

2 Find out why doctors may prescribe diuretics for a patient.

Aldosterone

Aldosterone is the hormone which acts in the kidney and is responsible for maintaining a more or less constant sodium level in the plasma. (It also has a secondary effect on

water absorption.) This control of aldosterone is very complex.

1 Any loss of sodium which causes a decrease in blood volume causes a group of secretory cells lying near the distal convoluted tubules in the kidney to release an enzyme called *renin*.

2 Renin enters the bloodstream and causes a plasma protein produced by the liver to form the hormone *angiotensin*.

3 Angiotensin stimulates the release of aldosterone from the adrenal cortex.

4 Aldosterone travels in the bloodstream to the kidney where it causes sodium ions to be actively taken up from the glomerular filtrate into the capillaries which surround the kidney tubules. This uptake will be accompanied by water, which enters by osmosis.

The sodium level of the blood and its volume is now restored.

ASSESSMENT OPPORTUNITY

Produce a report on an investigation into body systems concerned with the transport and elimination of metabolic products. The report should include:
- annotated diagrams describing the structure and action of the heart
- a description of the microscopic structure of blood
- an explanation of how blood is circulated

Table 5.3   A summary of ADH action

Osmotic potential of body fluids	ADH production	Permeability of collecting ducts	Reabsorption of water	Concentration of urine
High (more water; less salt)				
Low (less water; more salt)				

- an explanation of the role of blood in the transport of *two* different types of material
- annotated diagrams describing the structure of the kidney
- an explanation of the functions of the kidney

THE PROCESSING AND TRANSPORT OF NUTRIENTS

The components of a healthy diet

The following elements (*macronutrients*) are important in the diet:
- proteins
- carbohydrates
- fats

Water is also required, as well as fibre and *micronutrients*.

PROTEINS

Proteins contain carbon, hydrogen and oxygen, as well as nitrogen and sometimes sulphur. They are made up of *amino acids*, 10 of which cannot be made in the body and are therefore essential in the diet. There is a total of about 23 different amino acids. They are joined into peptide links which are broken down during digestion (see Figure 5.18). *Polypeptides* from proteins, which can contain hundreds of amino acids.

Table 5.4 shows the protein content of many common foods. Proteins have many important functions, and are major components in the structure of enzymes, haemoglobin and cell membranes.

CARBOHYDRATES

Carbohydrates are the simplest carbon compounds, with a formula of $C_nN_{2n}O_n$. Their basic building molecule is a simple sugar or *monosaccharide*. This can be built up into more complex compounds:

- disaccharides – comprising two monosaccharides, e.g. maltose and sucrose
- polysaccharides – comprising many monosaccharides, e.g. starch and glycogen

Plants manufacture *glucose*, a monosaccharide, in *photosynthesis*. The glucose is built up into more complex molecules. Storage materials like sucrose and starch are synthesised. These substances are present in large quantities in:
- cereal crops – wheat, oats, maize
- ground crops – potatoes, yams, carrots, turnips
- Leguminous crops – beans, peas

Carbohydrates are a primary source of energy.

FATS

Fats contain carbon, hydrogen and oxygen. The proportion of oxygen to the other elements is very low. *Lipids* is the correct term to use for this group of compounds, although in dietary terms they are often called fats.

Plants tend to have liquid fats (oils) which contain mainly unsaturated fatty acids. Animal fats are solid at room temperature and contain mainly saturated fatty acids. There is thought to be a link between the consumption of saturated fatty acids and cardiovascular disorder.

The terms *saturated* and *unsaturated* relate to the structure of the fatty acids which make up

(a)
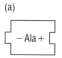

(b)
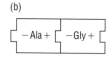

(c)
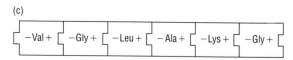

Figure 5.18 The formation of proteins: (a) a diagrammatic amino acid; (b) two amino acids forming a peptide link; (c) a polypeptide chain formed by amino acids

Table 5.4 The composition of food per 100 g (the percentage not accounted for is inedible waste, e.g. shell, bone, skin, water, etc.)

Type of food	kJ	Proteins (g)	Fats (g)	Carbo-hydrates (g)
Meat				
Bacon, grilled	1,722	24.9	35.1	0
Beef, sirloin, roast	1,182	23.6	21.1	0
Chicken, roast	621	24.8	5.4	0
Liver, lamb, fried	970	22.9	14.0	3.9
Luncheon meat	1,298	12.6	26.9	5.5
Pork chop, grilled	1,380	28.5	24.2	0
Sausage, beef	1,242	9.6	24.1	11.7
Dairy produce				
Butter	3,031	0.5	81.7	Tr
Cheese, cheddar	1,708	25.5	34.4	0.1
Eggs, raw, one	612	12.5	10.8	Tr
Ice-cream	814	3.6	9.8	24.4
Milk, whole	275	3.2	3.9	4.8
Yoghurt, fruit	441	5.1	2.8	15.7
Fish				
Cod, fried in batter	834	19.6	10.3	7.5
Kipper	855	25.5	11.4	0
Sardines, canned	906	23.7	13.6	0
Cereals				
Bread, white	1,002	8.4	1.9	49.3
Bread, wholemeal	914	9.2	2.5	41.6
Rice, boiled	597	2.6	1.1	32.1
Vegetables				
Beans, canned	355	5.2	0.6	15.3
Brussel sprouts, cooked	153	2.9	1.3	3.5
Cabbage, cooked	67	1.0	0.4	2.2
Carrots, cooked	100	0.6	0.4	4.9
Lettuce	59	0.8	0.5	1.7
Peas, boiled	291	6.0	0.9	9.7
Potatoes, boiled	306	1.8	0.1	17.0
Potato chips, fried	1,001	3.2	12.4	30.5
Tomatoes	73	0.7	0.3	3.1
Fruit				
Apples	199	0.4	0.1	11.8
Bananas	403	1.2	0.3	23.2
Oranges, peeled	158	1.1	0.1	8.5
Plums	155	0.6	0.1	8.8
Strawberries	113	0.8	0.1	6.0
Miscellaneous				
Apple pie	1,089	3.0	13.3	34.0
Buns, currant	1,250	7.6	7.5	52.7
Coffee, black, 900 ml	8	0.2	Tr	0.3
Fruit cake, rich	1,438	3.8	11.0	59.6
Rice pudding, canned	374	3.4	2.5	14.0
Sugar, white	1,680	Tr	0	105.0
Tea, black, 1000 ml	2	0.1	Tr	Tr

Data from The Composition of Foods, 5th edition (1991) are reproduced with the permission of The Royal Society of Chemistry and the Controller of Her Majesty's Stationery Office.

the fats. A typical unsaturated fatty acid is *oleic acid*. A typical saturated fatty acid is *palmitic acid* or *stearic acid*. Some fatty acids are essential in the diet since they cannot be synthesised in the body.

Fats are a secondary energy source in the diet. Sources of fat-containing foods will be found in Table 5.4.

FIBRE (ROUGHAGE)

The diet should contain fibre as well as the food materials discussed above. Fibre consists of the various types of cellulose that are found in plant foods. Cellulose cannot be broken down in the intestinal tract since humans do not possess the enzyme that can carry out the breakdown. Cellulose therefore remains undigested, and is eliminated in the faeces.

Research strongly indicates that a diet low in fibre is linked to diseases of the bowel. There are various theories put forward to account for this finding. Some researchers think that cancer of the bowel is caused by fewer eliminations of faeces associated with a low-fibre diet: the cells of the bowel would be in contact with carcinogens in the food for a longer period. Other researchers think that a diet high in fibre decreases the pressure on the bowel wall, and that it is this which helps to prevent bowel disease. A slow-moving bowel – because of lack of fibre – allows more water to be reabsorbed from the faeces, and this causes constipation.

ACTIVITY 21

Read the above section on 'Fibre' and answer the following questions:
- What is fibre?
- Why is it not digested?
- What can happen to people on low-fibre diets?
- What theories are there to explain the link between bowel disease and a low-fibre diet?
- Why is more water absorbed from faeces formed from a low-fibre diet?

VITAMINS

Vitamins are essential in small amounts in the diet. If they are missing from the diet, illnesses develop. These are called *vitamin deficiency diseases*.

- *Vitamin A.* Keeps skin and bones healthy, helps prevent infection of the nose and throat, and is necessary for vision in dim light. A lack of vitamin A causes poor night vision and increases the chances of infection of the nose and throat. Vitamin A is found in carrots, fish liver oils and green vegetables
- *Vitamin B1.* Helps the body obtain energy from food. A lack of it reduces growth and causes *beri-beri*, where the limbs become paralysed. Vitamin B1 is found in yeast, wholemeal bread, nuts, peas and beans
- *Vitamin B2.* Enables the body to obtain energy from food. A lack of it causes stunted growth, cracks in the skin around the mouth, an inflamed tongue and damage to the cornea of the eye. Vitamin B2 is found in green vegetables, cheese, yeast, eggs, milk and liver
- *Vitamin B12.* Enables the body to form protein and fat, and to store carbohydrate. A lack of it causes *pernicious anaemia*, a disease in which haemoglobin is not produced for red blood cells. This vitamin is found in liver, meat, eggs, milk and fish
- *Vitamin C.* Helps to heal wounds, and is needed for healthy gums and teeth. A lack of it causes scurvy, a disease where gums become soft and the teeth loose, and wounds fail to heal properly. Vitamin C is found in oranges, lemons, blackcurrants, green vegetables, tomatoes and potatoes. It is destroyed by cooking food
- *Vitamin D.* Enables the body to absorb calcium and phosphorus from food. These are needed to make bones and teeth. A lack of vitamin D causes rickets, leading to soft bones which bend under pressure. It is found in liver, butter, cheese, eggs and fish
- *Vitamin K.* Needed for the blood to clot in wounds. A lack of it causes a haemorrhage

when the skin is broken. It is found in cabbage and cereals, and is made by bacteria in the digestive system

INORGANIC SALTS

We need 15 minerals in our diets. Most of these are supplied by meat, eggs, milk, vegetables and fruit.

The following are some of these minerals:

	Daily requirement (mg)
Sodium chloride	5–10
Potassium	2
Magnesium	0.3
Phosphorus	1.5
Calcium	0.8
Iron	0.01
Iodine	0.00003

ACTIVITY 22

1 What other minerals are required in the diet in addition to those listed in the text?

2 Find out the functions of each of these minerals in the body.

3 Find out what deficiency diseases are caused by a lack of each mineral in the diet.

The morphology of the alimentary canal

The alimentary canal runs from the mouth to the anus (see Figure 5.19).

ACTIVITY 23

1 Before you read the information below on digestion, jot down briefly what you think is the function of each of the labelled parts in Figure 5.19.

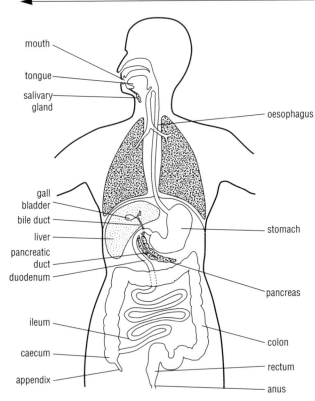

Figure 5.19   The alimentary canal
Source: Advanced Human Biology, Simpkins and Williams, Chapman and Hall, 1987.

2 • Which of your teeth pierce, grip and rip the food as it comes into the mouth?
• Which teeth cut and grind the food? Explain how the shape of each type of tooth is adapted to its special function.

3 The dental formula for humans is as follows:

$$\frac{2\ 1\ 2\ 3}{2\ 1\ 2\ 3}$$

Explain what this formula means.

4 How are the human set of teeth adapted to an omnivorous diet?

THE HISTOLOGY OF THE ALIMENTARY CANAL

The structure of the gut wall

A transverse section through the gut wall shows that the wall is made up of four layers: the *mucosa*, the *submucosa*, the *external muscle coat* (made up of circular and longitudinal muscle) and the *serosa* (Figure 5.20). Table 5.5 shows how these layers are modified in different regions of the alimentary canal.

The structure of a villus

Figure 5.21 details the structure of one villus. There are 20–49 villi to each square millimetre of the ileum wall.

ACTIVITY 24

1 Look at a prepared slide of the ileum – either a transverse section or a longitudinal section. Try to identify the tissue types and structures shown in Figures 5.20 and 5.21.

2 Label the parts A–G of the villus in Figure 5.21. Use the following labels: network of blood capillaries; lacteal vessel; Crypt of Lieberkühn; blood vessels supplying the villus; branch of lymphatic system; mucus-secreting goblet cell; epithelium.

The structure of the liver

(Strictly speaking, the liver and pancreas are not part of the alimentary canal but are important organs associated with it.)

The liver is a large, lobed structure which lies just beneath the diaphragm and partly overlaps the stomach. It receives oxygenated blood from the hepatic artery, and deoxygenated blood is removed in the hepatic vein. In addition it receives all the blood leaving the alimentary canal in the hepatic portal vein (refer back to Figure 5.7).

The liver consists of a large number of lobules. Each lobule contains many vertical series of liver cells. The blood supply to the lobules is from two sources, the hepatic artery and the hepatic portal vein. These vessels are at the periphery of the lobule. In the human liver the lobules are not clearly delimited

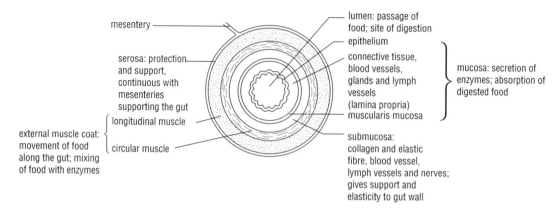

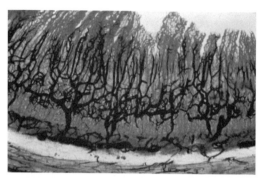

Figure 5.20 The main regions of the gut wall: (a) a diagram; (b) a micrograph

Table 5.5   A comparison of structures of the major regions of the alimentary canal

Layer	Oesophagus	Stomach	Small intestine	Large intestine
Mucosa (a) epithelium lining lumen	Stratified, squamous	Simple columnar	Simple columnar, absorptive and mucus cells	Simple columnar, absorptive and mucus cells
	Specialisation – a few mucus glands located in the lamina propria and submucosa	Specialisation – gastric glands located in lamina propria, four cell types: (i) mucus (ii) parietal (iii) peptic (iv) endocrine	Specialisation – (i) intestinal glands in crypts of Lieberkühn (ii) Paneth cells (iii) endocrine cells (iv) duodenal mucus glands	Specialisation – intestinal glands in lamina propria
(b) lamina propria	Some mucus glands	Many gastric glands	Intenstinal glands and prominent lacteals	Tubular glands
(c) muscularis mucosa	Present	Present	Present	Present
Submucosa	Some deep mucus glands	Present	Duodenal glands	Intestinal glands
External muscle coat (inner circular, outer longitudinal)	Transitional from striated muscle in upper region to smooth muscle in lower region	With additional innermost layer of oblique muscle. Circular muscle forms cardiac and pyloric sphincters	Present	Present
Serosa	Present	Present	Present	Incomplete serosa

Source: Biological Science, Stout, Green and Taylor (ed. Soper), Cambridge University Press, 1985.

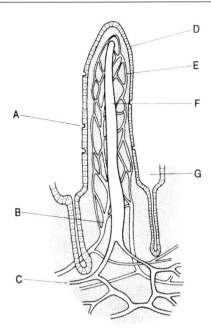

Figure 5.21 The longitudinal section of a villus
Source: Thomson et al., 1995.

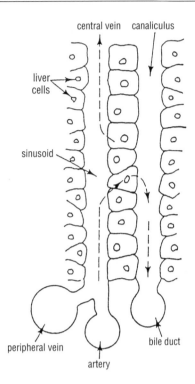

Figure 5.23 A diagram showing the flow of blood
in a sinusoid and canaliculus of a liver lobule
Source: Advanced Human Biology, Simpkins and
Williams, Chapman and Hall, 1987.

from each other. The liver cells are arranged
radiating out from a central blood vessel
which is a branch of the hepatic vein. The
hepatic vein drains the blood from the liver
cells in the lobules and releases it into the
general circulation. Between the liver cells are
other channels called *canaliculi* which receive
bile made by the liver cells and convey it to
the periphery of the lobule, to small bile
ducts. These lead to the gall bladder, and from
here the bile is taken to the duodenum in the
bile duct (see Figure 5.23).

ACTIVITY 25

Look at a microscope slide of a transverse
section of a liver.

The structure of the pancreas

The pancreas is situated just below the
stomach. It is connected to the small intestine
by the *pancreatic duct*. The cells which produce
the digestive enzymes (*exocrine cells*) are distinct
from the cells which produce hormones
(*endocrine cells*). These latter cells are grouped in
structures known as *islets of Langerhans* (see
Figure 5.24).

THE ACTION OF DIGESTIVE SECRETIONS IN THE STAGES OF DIGESTION

Digestion is the process by which insoluble
food consisting of large molecules is broken
down into soluble smaller molecules. These

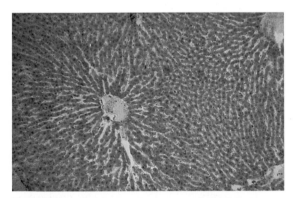

Figure 5.22 A transverse section of the liver to
show one lobule, × 90

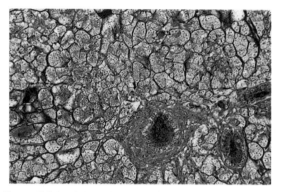

Figure 5.24   A histology of the pancreas

smaller molecules, in solution, pass through the walls of the intestine and eventually enter the blood stream. Digestion is brought about by *hydrolytic enzymes*. These are special proteins which are able to speed up the reactions causing the breakdown of proteins, carbohydrates and fats taken into the body in the diet. The elements of water, —H and —OH, are added to certain bonds in the large insoluble molecules. The bonds then break down, releasing the soluble small molecules.

1 *Proteins* are broken down into *amino acids*.
2 *Fats* are broken down into *fatty acids* and *glycerol*.
3 *Carbohydrates* are broken down into *glucose and other monosaccharides*.

In the alimentary canal, the mechanical breakdown of food into smaller pieces takes place first, and then chemical digestion and absorption follow. Each part of the alimentary canal is adapted to its own particular role in this sequence of events. The circular muscles, by contracting and relaxing alternately, push the food through the various regions of the alimentary canal, where it is first digested and then absorbed. The wave-like motion causing food to move along is called *peristalsis*.

The mouth

In the mouth, the *saliva* adds moisture to the food so that it is dealt with more easily, and it contains *amylase* which starts the enzymic breakdown of starch into disaccharide sugars. (If you chew a piece of bread for a couple of

minutes, you will taste it becoming sweet as sugars are formed from the starch.) The sight and smell of food, together with the arrival of food in the mouth, stimulates the salivary glands to produce saliva. The teeth have an important role both in ingestion and in starting the first stage of mechanical breakdown by thoroughly chewing the food. The food leaves the mouth as a *bolus*, a small ball of food which is then taken to the stomach via the *oesophagus* by peristalsis.

The stomach and small intestine

The lining of the stomach and small intestine is protected from the damaging effects of digestive juices by the secretion of mucus from goblet cells along the length of this part of the alimentary canal, and from Brunner's glands in the duodenum.

Further mechanical breakdown and digestion takes place in the stomach. Gastric juice containing protein-digesting enzymes is produced by gastric glands in the stomach wall. Hydrochloric acid is also produced here. This generates the acid environment required for the enzymes to work in the stomach, and kills bacteria which may contaminate ingested food. Food is kept in the stomach by the circular sphincter muscles, and is released into the duodenum in small amounts as a liquid chyme when the pyloric sphincter muscle relaxes.

The duodenum is about 30 cm long, and receives both pancreatic juice – containing enzymes – from the pancreas and bile from the gall bladder in the liver. Bile is a greenish fluid containing bile pigments which are the breakdown products of the haem part of haemoglobin. It also contains bile salts (sodium and potassium glycocholates) which help to emulsify lipids by causing them to break down into numerous very small droplets. This allows more surface area for the digestive enzymes to act upon. The bile also contains sodium hydrogencarbonate which neutralises the acid from the stomach and provides the slightly alkaline environment which is needed by the enzymes of the small intestine.

After the duodenum, there is the *ileum*, and these two parts make up the *small intestine* where almost all the digestion is carried out. Intestinal juice containing enzymes is produced by the cells in the *Crypts of Lieberkühn* between the villi in all the parts of the small intestine.

ACTIVITY 26

1 Redraw and complete Table 5.6. Then, draw three separate flow charts to show the different stages in the digestion of carbohydrates, proteins and lipids.

2 Look back at the section 'The components of a healthy diet' (see pp. 254–256 above). Choose a specific meal and then produce a poster which tracks its digestion.

THE ABSORPTION OF THE PRODUCTS OF DIGESTION

Some absorption takes place in the duodenum, but most takes place in the ileum. The latter is very well suited to its function. It has a large surface area created by the villi (see pp. 257 and 259 above), a thin epithelial layer and a good blood supply.

Some absorption takes place by *diffusion*, but most takes place by *active transport*. The latter requires energy, but allows movement to be in one direction only – i.e. from the gut to the circulatory system.

Glucose and amino acids

These compounds are transported through the epithelial lining of the villi and enter the blood capillaries. These capillaries merge to form the hepatic portal vein which takes blood to the liver.

Table 5.6   A summary of digestion

Region of alimentary canal	Digestive gland	Digestive juice	Enzymes	Substrate	Products
Mouth	Salivary gland				
Stomach			Pepsin		
				Milk protein	
Duodenum	Pancreas				Maltose
				Fats	
			Trypsinogen* ↓		
			Trypsin	Peptides	Amino acids
Duodenum Ileum		Intestinal juice	Enterokinase	Trypsinogen	Trypsin
					Amino acids
			Maltose		
			Sucrose		
			Lactase		
			Lipase		

* Trypsinogen is secreted in an inactive form from the pancreas. It is then activated by *enterokinase*, an enzyme produced in the intestinal juice

Fatty acids and glycerol

The fatty acids derived from digestion are insoluble in water. They form small, stable *micelles* of about 4–5 nm (nanometres) in diameter. These can be absorbed by the epithelial cells by diffusion. Inside the epithelial cells, they are converted into a form which can enter the *lacteals* (lymphatic capillaries). From here they are transported through lymphatic vessels to the *thoracic duct* where they enter the blood system. Some short-chain fatty acids follow the same route taken by glucose and amino acids.

Water

Most of the water you drink is absorbed in the stomach, but most of the water from digestive secretions, which can be up to 10 dm per day, is reabsorbed in the *large intestine* or *colon*.

Inorganic salts

Some inorganic salts are absorbed in the same way as glucose and amino acids, but others, such as sodium chloride, are absorbed in the form of *ions* in the colon.

Vitamins

Vitamins are absorbed in the small intestine. Fat soluble vitamins, such as A, D, E and K, are absorbed along with micelles of fat (see above). The water-soluble vitamins enter by diffusion.

ACTIVITY 27

In Activity 26 above, you were asked to produce a poster to show the digestion of a specific balanced meal. Now, taking the same meal, produce a poster to show how the end products of its digestion are absorbed.

ACTIVITY 28

Demonstrating a model gut
Introduction

In order that cells of the body can make use of the food that is eaten, the nutrients must pass out of the alimentary canal into the blood stream to be transported to where they are needed. The gut wall presents a barrier for the nutrients to cross. This exercise aims to reproduce what happens in the human gut, and to see whether both small and large molecules can pass through the gut wall. You will investigate starch (made up of large molecules) and glucose (made up of small molecules). You will be using visking tubing which has pores in its wall about the same size as those in the wall of the human gut.

Apparatus

You will need the following:
- Bunsen burner, tripod and gauze
- Water bath/beaker
- Thermometer
- Test tubes and rack
- Boiling tube
- 1% Starch–5% glucose mixture
- 1% starch solution
- Iodine solution
- Benedict's solution
- Teat pipettes
- Visking tubing
- Stop clock
- 0.1% amylase

Experiment 1

To investigate which molecules can pass through a porous membrane.

Method

Test 5 cm^3 portions of the starch–glucose solution with iodine and Benedict's solution separately. Carry out the same tests on some distilled water. Record your results. Heat the water in the beaker to 37 °C. You must maintain the temperature of the water at between 35 °C and 40 °C throughout the experiment. Tie a tight knot at one end of a length of visking tubing about 25 cm long. Using a teat pipette, fill the visking tubing three-quarters full with the starch–glucose mixture. Close the other end of the tubing with another knot. Rinse the outside of the tubing with water. Put the visking tubing and solution into the beaker of water. Make sure that the tubing is not totally immersed in the water bath. At the start of the experiment, test a sample of the water from the beaker with iodine and Benedict's solution, and record results. Take samples of the water from the beaker every 10 minutes, and test with iodine and Benedict's solution

Results
Record your results in a table (see below).
Conclusions
Record your conclusions from each of the tests.

1 Account for any changes you observe in the levels of glucose and starch in the water surrounding the visking tubing.

2 Why was the water kept at 37°C?

3 Why was the visking tubing rinsed before being placed in the boiling tube?

4 What do the results tell us about the properties of visking tubing?

5 Explain how your answer to (4) illustrates the importance of digestive enzymes?

6 Which part of the gut does the water in the boiling tube represent?

7 This exercise is only a simple demonstration of the way in which the human gut works. Note three ways in which the human gut *differs* from visking tubing.

Experiment 2
Demonstrating the digestion and absorption of a carbohydrate.

Method
Use the same apparatus as in the previous experiment. You will need two beakers of water. Set up two lengths of visking tubing. One is to contain a samples of the starch solution, and one will contain the starch–amylase solution. Test the water in the beakers as before over a period of 40 minutes.

Results
Record your results in a table.

Conclusions
What do you conclude from each of the tests you have carried out?

Answer the following:

1 Why is it important to have a test with visking tubing containing only starch solution?

2 What do you conclude about the action of amylase? Look up the structures of starch and glucose and explain your results.

3 What is the importance of your findings in relation to digestion and absorption in the human gut?

Sample	Colour: iodine test	Colour: Benedict's test
Starch–glucose mixture		
Water from beaker		
Solution after 10 minutes		
20 minutes		
30 minutes		
40 minutes		

THE FATE OF THE PRODUCTS OF DIGESTION

The products of digestion, once absorbed and carried to the liver, will be either *used*, *stored* or *excreted* depending on the body's current needs.

The use of the products of digestion
Respiration

All living systems require a constant supply of energy in order to maintain the processes of life, including the synthesis of large molecules, cell division, reproduction and movement. Respiration is the process by which cells release energy from food. *Carbohydrates*, mainly in the form of glucose, are the primary respiratory substrate, although when there is a shortage of these, fats will be used, and in conditions of starvation, proteins will be used. The energy which is released from these substrates is not used directly but is transferred to *adenosine triphosphate* (ATP) which is the short-term energy store in all cells.

Cell production (growth) and cell renewal (repair)

Cells in the body are constantly being produced or renewed. This requires the synthesis of large molecules from smaller molecules. For example, proteins will be formed from amino acids, large fatty acid molecules will be formed from smaller fatty acids, and monosaccharides, such as glucose, will combine to form disaccharides and polysaccharides. The synthesis of these molecules and the actual process of cell division (mitosis) require energy, and this comes from respiration.

(See p. 256 above for the uses of vitamins and minerals.)

ACTIVITY 29

List the uses of *water* within the body.

The storage of products

1 *As glycogen*. Within the liver, excess glucose will be converted into the storage polysaccharide *glycogen*. This is stored in the liver and muscles until it is needed, whereupon it can be converted back into glucose.
2 *As fat*. The body can only store a limited amount of glycogen. After this, any further excess glucose will be converted into fat. Any fat in the diet which is not required immediately for energy will remain as fat. Fat is well suited to its function as an energy store: it is light; a large amount of energy is stored in a compact space; and an unlimited amount can be stored. Fat is found in cells in *adipose* tissue which is found under the skin and around organs such as the kidneys and heart.
3 *As vitamins*. Unlike carbohydrates, fats and proteins, vitamins do not provide energy or serve as building materials. Most vitamins cannot be synthesised in the body, so they have to be obtained in the diet and then stored. Fat-soluble vitamins are generally stored in cells, particularly liver cells, so reserves can be built up. Water-soluble vitamins, by contrast, dissolve in the body fluids and are excreted in the urine. Thus, the body does not store these well.

The excretion and egestion of products

1 *As urea*. Proteins cannot be stored in the body. Excess proteins in the diet are, therefore, converted into urea in the liver. This passes, in the blood, to the kidneys where it is excreted in urine.

ACTIVITY 30

Look back to Figure 5.7 which shows a general plan of the human circulatory system. List the blood vessels that a molecule of urea passes through in its journey from the liver to the kidney.

2 *As roughage*. The cell walls of plants are made of the polysaccharide *cellulose*. Humans, in common with most other animals, do not have the necessary enzymes to digest this chemical. It is too large to be absorbed, so it therefore passes unchanged through the gut before being egested in the faeces.

Although of no nutritional value, cellulose does have a vital function within the diet as roughage. This is essential in creating enough bulk to allow the muscles of the gut to keep food moving along the gut by peristalsis. There is evidence to suggest that people with low-fibre diets are more likely to develop stomach cancer, because low-fibre food remains in the stomach for so long.

ACTIVITY 31

You have produced posters to show how a specific balanced meal is digested and absorbed. Now produce a third poster which shows the fate of the end products of digestion – i.e. assimilation.

ASSESSMENT OPPORTUNITY

Produce a summary of an exploration into the processing and transport of nutrients, which includes:
• annotated diagrams of the structure of the alimentary canal, including the liver and pancreas
• an explanation of the stages of physical (mechanical) and chemical digestion
• an explanation of the action of digestive secretions in the stages of digestion
• a description of the absorption of the products of digestion
• a description of the fate of the products of digestion

SENSORY AND COMMUNICATION SYSTEMS WITHIN THE HUMAN BODY

The role of the endocrine system in communication

THE PRINCIPLE OF HORMONAL COMMUNICATION

We possess two *coordinating* systems: the nervous system (described later in the chapter) and the endocrine system. The nervous system gives us rapid control, whilst the endocrine system regulates more long-term changes. The two systems interact so that the internal environment is kept constant and responses are made to changes in the external environment.

The endocrine system is made up of glands which are ductless and which secrete hormones directly into the blood stream. These hormones travel to particular organs, the target organs. Hormones are effective in small quantities. Most endocrine glands are influenced by the *pituitary gland*, which is linked to the hypothalamus. This can be considered as an important link between the endocrine and nervous systems.

ACTIVITY 32

1 In an outline diagram of the human body, indicate the positions of the major endocrine glands: pituitary, thyroid, parathyroid, pancreas, adrenal, ovary, testis.

2 Summarise the action of the anterior and posterior pituitary bodies in regulating the other glands. Explain the links with the hypothalamus.

3 Draw up a table with four columns:
   (a) Endocrine organ
   (b) Hormone produced
   (c) Target organ
   (d) Action
   Complete the table for all the glands listed above.

FEEDBACK MECHANISMS

Very little change can be tolerated within the human body. However, the external environment is almost constantly changing. This means efficient mechanisms are needed to prevent corresponding changes within the body. The maintenance of a constant internal environment is known as *homeostasis*.

Negative feedback

Although there is a huge variety of homeostatic functions within the body, they all work through the same basic mechanism:

- To control a factor, a *receptor* must detect any changes in the level of that factor
- The receptor must then communicate with an *effector* which will bring about the necessary corrections
- The changes back to the 'norm' or 'reference point' will then be detected by the receptor, and the system will be turned off

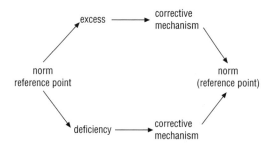

Figure 5.25   Negative feedback

This mechanism is known as *negative feedback* (see Figure 5.25). (NB: a *feedback system* is any circular situation in which information about the status of something is continually reported (fed back) to a central control region. The type of feedback system that *reverses* the direction of the initial condition is a *negative* feedback system.) A simple example of this control mechanism is a central-heating system controlled by a *thermostat*. The thermostat is the receptor, and the boiler and radiators are the effector. For example, when the temperature drops below the reference point which has been set, this is detected by the thermostat, which then causes the

effectors to be switched on. This causes the temperature to rise until the reference point is reached. This is detected by the thermostat, and the heating is switched off. The process is then repeated. In this way small changes are constantly occurring, but large, harmful changes are prevented.

ACTIVITY 33

1 Draw a flow diagram, like that shown in Figure 5.25, to illustrate the working of the heating system described above.

2 Draw a sketch graph to show how, on a cold day, room temperature would change with time if a thermostat-controlled heating system were in operation.

3 Refer back to the control of the amount of water in the blood by ADH (p. 252). Look at the flow chart you produced to illustrate the control of an increase in osmotic potential:
   - Identify the receptor and effector in this control system
   - Clearly mark the negative-feedback loop on your diagram
   - In the body, the communication between the receptor and effector/s may be nervous, hormonal or a combination of the two. Which of these forms does the communication take in this example?

An example of hormonal negative feedback: the control of the blood sugar level

The normal blood glucose level is 90 mg per 100 cm^3 of blood. The nervous system is especially sensitive to changes in this level. Carbohydrate taken in the diet is spasmodic, so there is a system which relies on the build-up and breakdown of glycogen in the liver to remove or add glucose to the blood (see Figure 5.26). This system is under hormonal control.

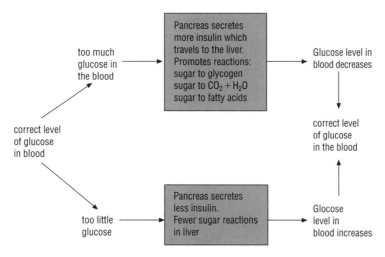

Figure 5.26   The control of the blood glucose level by insulin
Source: Advanced Human Biology, Simpkins and Williams, Chapman and Hall, 1987.

ACTIVITY 34

1   Look at the negative-feedback diagram (Figure 5.26) which shows the control of the blood sugar level by insulin. Summarise the information shown in the diagram.

2   Find out more about the role of the pancreas and the two hormones that are produced by the two different types of cell. What is the name of the second hormone secreted by the pancreas? How does it work with insulin to help regulate the blood sugar level?

3   Look at a microscope slide of a vertical section of the pancreas (Figure 5.24), and see if you can identify the two types of hormone-secreting cell. Can you see any blood vessels or capillaries? Why is it important for endocrine glands to have a blood supply?

Positive feedback

In homeostasis, fluctuations are corrected by negative feedback: i.e. the reactions of the body *counteract* any change. However, there are examples where the reaction of the body *intensifies* any change. This is known as *positive*

feedback. Most positive-feedback systems are destructive and result in various disorders. For example, if pure oxygen is breathed at pressures greater than atmospheric, as in diving, this can be very harmful and is exacerbated by positive feedback. In an effort to use up oxygen quickly, the metabolism rate in the tissues increases, which increases the amount of carbon dioxide produced. The increase in carbon dioxide then leads to an increase in breathing and heart rate, leading to even more oxygen being delivered to the tissues.

One of the few hormones which is an exception to the rule of negative-feedback control is *oxytocin* which causes contractions of the uterus during birth. As the output of this hormone increases, this brings about an even *greater* increase in its own output. Another hormone controlled by positive feedback is *luteinizing* hormone whose output rapidly increases to bring about ovulation.

HOW HORMONES CAUSE RESPONSES IN CELLS

Some aspects of hormone action are common to all hormone-mediated responses:

- The amount of hormone released depends on the need
- Information is received by hormone-secreting cells which determines the

amount and duration of the hormone release

- Target cells contain receptors that bind hormones
- The binding of hormones to receptors activates a specific chain of reactions
- The response feeds back to the hormone-secreting cells
- Hormones that have accomplished their tasks are degraded or excreted

Details of their methods of action and control vary from hormone to hormone. The examples below have been chosen to give you an idea of the range of these methods.

Thyroxine

Thyroxine regulates the growth and development of cells, and controls the metabolic rate. It is produced by the *thyroid gland*, and it is an example of a hormone whose production is controlled by a *releasing factor* produced by the hypothalamus (see Figure 5.27). Thyroxine functions by passing through the plasma membrane of its target cells (it can do this because it is a steroid, and therefore lipid soluble). It enters the nucleus where it combines with receptors. It can then activate specific genes to form proteins which are enzymes which bring about the hormone's characteristic actions.

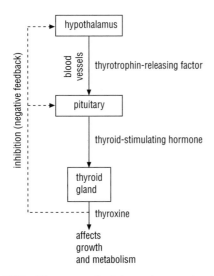

Figure 5.27 **The control of thyroxine production**

Insulin

The section on the control of the blood sugar level on pp. 266–267 above explains the function and control of *insulin*, which lowers the blood sugar level. The blood sugar level is detected directly by the insulin-secreting cells which can then make the necessary adjustments to the production of the hormone. There are specific insulin receptors on many cells, but when insulin combines with these receptors, the response depends on the type of cell. For example, in liver cells the transport of amino acids and the synthesis of glycogen is stimulated; in fat cells, glucose transport and lipid synthesis are stimulated; and in pancreatic cells, the secretion of *glucagon*, a hormone, is inhibited.

Adrenalin

The effects of adrenalin are described in Chapter 3. Adrenalin is the hormone which prepares the body to cope with emergencies. Under conditions of stress, the hypothalamus sends nervous impulses to the adrenal glands, bringing about an increase in the production of adrenalin. Like insulin, adrenalin has specific receptor sites on many types of cell, each of which responds differently to the stimulus. This leads to a number of physiological changes seen when the body responds to stress.

Antidiuretic hormone (ADH)

The control and action of ADH is described earlier in this chapter (see p. 253). ADH binds to receptor sites on the plasma membrane of the cells of the collecting ducts in the kidneys. This activates enzymes which bring about an increase in the permeability of the membranes.

Aldosterone

The control and action of aldosterone are also described earlier in this chapter (see p. 253). Because it is a steroid, and therefore lipid soluble, aldosterone passes through the plasma membranes of its target cells. It then binds to receptor sites in the cytoplasm. This hormone-receptor complex then moves into the nucleus where it interacts with specific genes. The proteins formed produce the hormone's characteristic effects.

ACTIVITY 35

Look back at Figure 5.27 which is a flow diagram to show the control of thyroxine production. Use the accounts above to produce similar diagrams to show how the production of insulin, adrenalin, ADH and aldosterone are controlled.

The nerve cell

Nervous tissue is composed of nerve cells, or *neurones*, which are capable of transmitting an electrical impulse. A neurone contains a *nucleus* which is found within a *cell body* (see Figure 5.28). Parts of the neurone known as *dendrons* transmit the impulse to the cell body, and parts known as *axons* transmit the impulse away from the cell body. Some neurones are covered with a fatty sheath and are known as *myelinated*; the remainder are unmyelinated.

Neurones are found throughout the body where they form the *nervous system*. This consists of the *central nervous system* (CNS) and the *nerves*. The central nervous system comprises the brain and the spinal cord.

• Neurones which conduct impulses from the internal and external environments towards the CNS are called *sensory neurones*

• Neurones which conduct impulses away from the CNS to effector organs like muscles and glands are called *motor neurones* (see Figure 5.28)

• Neurones which conduct impulses from sensory to motor neurones are called *intermediate neurones*

These three types of neurone can connect to form a *reflex arc* (see Figure 5.29) which is involved in an automatic response.

ACTIVITY 36

1 In Figure 5.29, identify the three types of neurone described. Compare the relative lengths of their axons and dendrons.

2 Describe the pathway of the impulse involved in the withdrawal of a finger from a pinprick.

3 Try one of the simplest reflexes, the knee jerk: sit with the right thigh crossed loosely over the left knee in such a way as slightly to stretch the extensor muscle of the leg. If someone now taps the right knee tendon (just below the knee cap), a sharp extension of the leg should result.

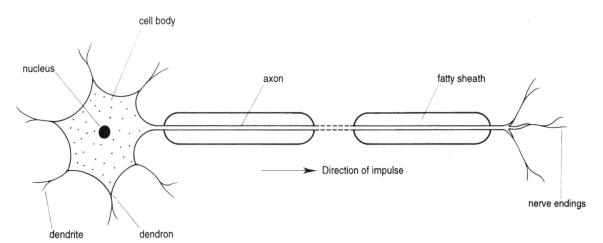

Figure 5.28   A motor neurone
Source: Thomson et al., 1995.

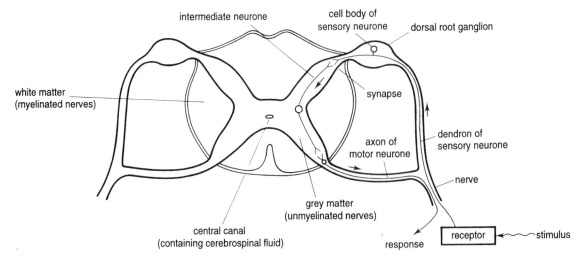

Figure 5.29 A transverse section through the spinal cord showing the reflex arc
Source: Thomson et al., 1995.

The nerve impulse

Messages are transmitted along the neurone by minute *electrical charges*. In the resting state, the neurone has a small positive charge on the inside and a small negative charge on the outside. This is known as the *resting potential*. The uneven distribution of charge is created by the cell membrane which pumps some ions out of the cell and other ions in. Energy, in the form of ATP, is required for this. The most important membrane pump is the *sodium–potassium exchange pump*. This pumps sodium ions (Na^+) out and potassium ions (K^+) in. Sodium ions then slowly diffuse back into the cytoplasm, and potassium ions slowly diffuse back out of the cell. However, the membrane is about 50 times more permeable to potassium ions than it is to sodium ions. Therefore, the potassium ions diffuse out of the cell more rapidly than the sodium ions diffuse in. As both ions have a positive charge, this results in the outer surface of the cell being positive relative to the inside. The membrane is said to be *polarised* because an electrical difference exists across it.

The cell membrane can be stimulated to become very briefly more permeable to sodium ions than to potassium ions. If enough sodium ions enter the cell, the charge will be reversed and the inside of the cell will become positive relative to the outside of the cell. The membrane is now *depolarised*. When the number of sodium ions entering the cell change, the potential across the membrane to a certain *threshold level*, an *action potential*, arises which generates an *impulse*. If there is only a very weak stimulus and the depolarisation does not reach the threshold level, then an action potential, and hence an impulse, is *not* produced. This is known as the 'all or nothing' law. Once the threshold level is reached: the stronger the stimulus, the more frequent the impulse production. However, once one impulse has been generated, before a second impulse can be generated the

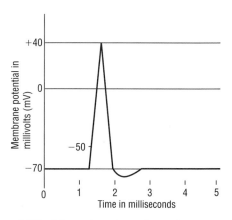

Figure 5.30 Nerve impulses: the action potential
Source: (a) *Advanced Human Biology*, Simpkins and Williams, Chapman and Hall, 1987.

membrane must first recover its resting potential. The time taken for this recovery is known as the *refractory period*.

Impulses travel faster through a myelinated nerve cell than an unmyelinated nerve cell, and the larger the diameter of the axon the faster they travel.

TRANSMISSION ACROSS A SYNAPSE

The small gaps between nerve cell endings are known as *synapses* (see Figure 5.29). These have a highly organised structure (see Figure 5.31). When the impulse arrives at the *synaptic knob*, it causes vesicles to move towards the *pre-synaptic membrane*. The vesicles become attached to this membrane and discharge a *transmitter substance*. At the majority of synapses, this is *acetylcholine*. Molecules of this diffuse across the *synaptic cleft* and become attached to specific sites on the *post-synaptic membrane*. This brings about the depolarisation of this membrane which, if the threshold level is reached, then generates an action potential.

ACTIVITY 37

Find out about the following:
* the effect of
  (a) amphetamines, and
  (b) beta-blockers
  on transmission across the synapse
* the transmission of the impulse at the nerve–muscle junction

---

The nervous system

Both the central and peripheral parts of the nervous system are made up of neurones. Neurones may be bundled together and wrapped in connective tissue to form *nerves*. The nervous system, as already mentioned, consists of the central nervous system (CNS) and the nerves (or *peripheral nervous system*). The

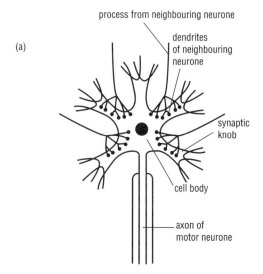

(a)

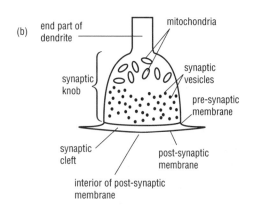

(b)

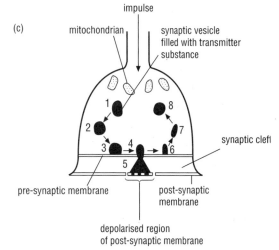

(c)

Figure 5.31   The structure of the synapse: (a) cell body of motor neurone (b) the synaptic knob (c) transmission across the synapse (one vesicle only shown)

central nervous system consists of the brain (see Figure 5.32) and the spinal cord (see Figure 5.29).

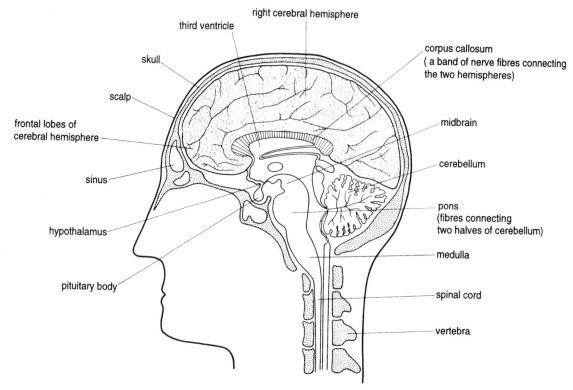

Figure 5.32   A section through the head to show the brain
Source: Thomson et al., 1995.

ACTIVITY 38

1   Find out the functions of each of the parts labelled in Figure 5.32.

2   Look at a prepared slide of the spinal cord (transverse section) under the microscope. How many of the features labelled in Figure 5.29 can you find? Under high power, look for the cell bodies in the grey matter.

The peripheral nervous system consists of not only the *somatic nervous system*, which activates voluntary responses, but also the *autonomic nervous system*, which controls activities of the internal environment which are normally involuntary. There are two different divisions to the automatic nervous system:

• the sympathetic nervous system
• the parasympathetic nervous system

Generally, these two have opposing effects on the organs they supply, and this enables the

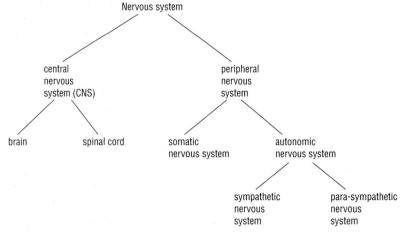

Figure 5.33   The organisation of the nervous system

Table 5.7   A summary of the effects of the sympathetic and parasympathetic nervous systems on the body

Region	Sympathetic	Parasympathetic
Head	Dilates pupils None Inhibits secretion of saliva	Constricts pupils Stimulates secretion of tears Stimulates secretion of saliva
Heart	Increases amplitude and rate of heart beat	Decreases amplitude and rate of heart beat
Lungs	Dilates bronchi and bronchioles Increases ventilation rate	Constricts bronchi and bronchioles Decreases ventilation rate
Gut	Inhibits peristalsis Inhibits secretion of alimentary juices Contracts anal sphincter muscle	Stimulates peristalsis Stimulates secretion of alimentary juices Inhibits contraction of anal sphincter muscle
Blood	Constricts arterioles to gut and smooth muscle Dilates arterioles to brain and skeletal muscle Increases blood pressure Increases blood volume by contraction of spleen	Maintains steady muscle tone in arterioles to gut, smooth muscle, brain and skeletal muscle Reduces blood pressure None
Skin	Contracts erector pili muscles of hair Constricts arterioles in skin of limbs Increases secretion of sweat	None Dilates arterioles in skin of face None
Kidney	Decreases output of urine	None
Bladder	Contracts bladder sphincter muscle	Inhibits contraction of bladder sphincter muscles
Penis	Induces ejaculation	Stimulates erection
Glands	Releases adrenaline from adrenal medulla	None

Source: Biological Science, Stout, Green and Taylor (ed. Soper), Cambridge University Press, 1985.

body to make rapid and precise adjustments to activities in order to maintain a steady state. (This can be compared to driving a car with an accelerator *and* a brake rather than just an accelerator!) Table 5.7 summarises the effect of the sympathetic and parasympathetic nervous systems in the body.

ACTIVITY 39

1 The sympathetic nervous system:
- contracts *erector pili* muscles of hair
- constricts the arterioles of skin in the limbs
- increases the secretion of sweat
- releases adrenaline from the adrenal glands

The parasympathetic nervous system:
- dilates arterioles in the skin of the face

Look at the list above of some of the effects of the autonomic nervous system on the body. What effect will each of these have on body temperature?

2 Figure 5.29 is a diagram of a reflex arc of the somatic nervous system. Find out how the neurones are arranged in the autonomic nervous system and how the arrangement differs between the sympathetic system and the parasympathetic system.

3 Looking at Table 5.7, which system is dominant during danger, stress and activity, and which is dominant during rest? Which increases metabolic levels and which decreases metabolic levels?

ACTIVITY 40

1 Draw a table to show the main differences between the nervous system and the hormonal system. To help you to do this, consider the following questions:
   • What is the nature of the 'message' passed through the system?
   • How quickly does the 'message' pass through the system?
   • What carries the 'message' through the body?
   • Are responses localised or widespread in the body?
   • Is the response short-lived, or does it continue over a long time?

2 The nervous system has been compared to a telephone system, and the hormonal system to a postal system. Why do you think this is?

THE PROCESS OF SEEING

The eyes are responsible for receiving the stimulus of light, and for converting this into nerve impulses.

The structure of the eye

The structure of the eye is shown in Figure 5.34.

ACTIVITY 41

1 Look into a mirror and draw a diagram of the front view of your eye. Use Figure 5.34 to help you label your diagram.

2 Cut a vertical section through a sheep's eye with a scalpel or sharp knife. Try to find all the labelled features. (It is currently recommended that bulls' eyes are not used because of the very small risk of infection by BSE.)

3 What are the functions of the eyelid and eyelashes, and lachrymal glands?

4 Explain why we need sight.

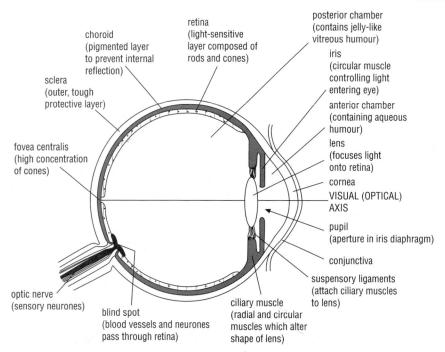

Figure 5.34 A diagram of a vertical section through the eye

Source: Stanley Thornes (Publishers) Ltd, *Understanding Biology for Advanced Level*, 2nd edition.

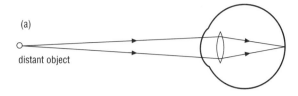

The wall of the eye consists of three layers: the *sclera*, the *choroid* and the *retina*.

The sclera is tough and fibrous, and protects the inner layers. At the front, it has a transparent area, the *cornea*, to allow light into the eye.

The choroid layer contains many blood vessels and is heavily pigmented to prevent light being reflected within the eye. At the front of the eye, the choroid is modified to form the *iris* which surrounds an aperture, the *pupil*.

ACTIVITY 42

Use a mirror to examine the effect on the diameter of the pupil of
(a)   a bright light
(b)   a very dim light

In the activity above, you will have found that the size of the pupil decreases in bright light (to protect the retina by preventing an excessive amount of light into the eye) and increases in dim light (to allow the maximum amount of light to fall on the retina). The size of the aperture is controlled by the iris which has two sets of muscles, *circular* and *radial*. These muscles are controlled by the autonomic nervous system (see p. 272 above).

ACTIVITY 43

Examine a camera and compare the mechanism for controlling the amount of light entering it with the mechanism described above.

Just behind the pupil is the *lens*. This is held in position by *suspensory ligaments* attached to a small ring of muscle called the *ciliary body*. The lens allows light to be focused onto the retina (see Figure 5.35). When looking at distant objects, the lens becomes flattened, and when looking at near objects, it becomes rounded.

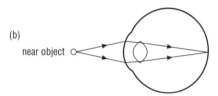

Figure 5.35   Focusing: (a) light from a distant object is focused on the retina by a flattened lens; (b) light from a near object is focused on the retina by a near-spherical lens
Source: Advanced Human Biology, Simpkins and Williams, Chapman and Hall, 1987.

ACTIVITY 44

Find out about the following abnormalities of the eye, and how they may be corrected:
• myopia (short-sightedness
• hypermetropia (long-sightedness)
• astigmatism

The retina contains the light-sensitive cells (*photoreceptors*) which convert the light waves they receive into nerve impulses which pass along neurones to the *optic nerve*, and hence to the brain. There are two types of light-sensitive cell: *rods* and *cones*. The basic structure of rods and cones is similar, but there are important differences which are shown in Table 5.8.

ACTIVITY 45

1   Because there are no photoreceptor cells in the region where the nerves converge to form the optic nerve, this region is known as the *blind spot*. To demonstrate these blind spots, close your right eye and hold Figure 5.37 about 30 cm away from your open left eye. Keep your left eye focused on the circle. Now move the

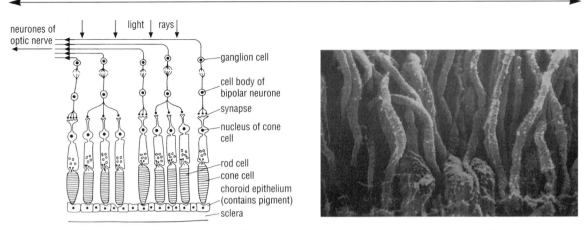

Figure 5.36   The retina and light-sensitive cells: (a) the microscopic structure of the retina; (b) a scanning electronmicrograph of rods and cones
Source: Stanley Thornes (Publishers) Ltd, *Understanding Biology for Advanced Level*, 2nd edition.

page slowly towards you, and notice that at a distance of about 15 cm from your left eye, the cross disappears. At this point, light from the cross falls on the blind spot of your left eye.

$+$ $\bigcirc$

Figure 5.37   The blind-spot demonstration

When you focus on the circle, it appears clearer than anything around it in the field of vision. This is because the light is focused onto the region of the retina known as the *fovea*. Only cones are found in this region (see Table 5.8). Figure 5.36(a) shows that many rods synapse with a sensory neurone. Because of this, cones can distinguish two dots which are very close together as separate entities, whereas rods cannot (see Figure 5.38).

Table 5.8   Differences between rods and cones

	Rods	Cones
Function	Sensitive to different intensities of light	Sensitive to different wavelengths of light (colour vision)
Distribution	Found throughout retina except in central region (fovea.) Rods 20 times more common than cones	Found in fovea
	Many rods synapse with each sensory neurone, therefore poor visual activity	In fovea, each cone synapses with one sensory neurone, therefore high visual activity
Photosensitive pigment	Rhodopsin: sensitive to low light intensity, therefore mostly used for night vision	Iodopsin (occurs in three forms): sensitive to high light intensity, therefore mostly used for day vision
Structure	Outer segment rod-shaped	Outer segment cone-shaped

2 Two simultaneously applied stimuli can only be distinguished if they activate two sensory neurones separated by one in between. Only in diagram (a) of Figure 5.38, therefore, are the two stimuli distinguished as two separate stimuli. Draw a diagram to show how rods can distinguish two separate stimuli.

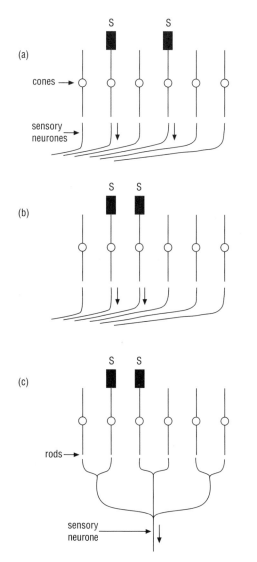

Figure 5.38 Rod and cone stimulus discrimination

THE FUNCTIONING OF RODS AND CONES

The functioning of rods and cones depends on *photosensitive pigments*. Rods contain *rhodopsin* or *visual purple*. This is made up of the protein *opsin* and a derivative of vitamin A, *retinal*. Light causes rhodopsin to split into opsin and retinal. This process is known as *bleaching*. This leads, in turn, to the creation of a *generator potential* in the rod cell which, if sufficiently large, generates an *action potential* along the sensory nerves leading to the brain. Once rhodopsin has been split, it has to be resynthesised to maintain the rods' ability to respond to light. This takes time, which is why your vision may be poor when going from a well-lit room or sunshine into a dimly lit room.

Cones, on their part, contain *iodopsin* which is less sensitive than rhodopsin to changes in light intensity. This is why cones are of little value in helping us to see in dim light. It is thought that there are three forms of iodopsin, each responding to a different wavelength corresponding to blue, green and red light. Each form is found in a separate cone, and the relative stimulation of each type is interpreted by the brain as a particular colour.

clear and sharp whereas the surrounding words are blurred?

(c) If you are trying to make out a faint star in the sky, why is it better not to look directly at it but slightly to one side of it?

(d) Why can the flicker on a cinema screen be seen when you look out of the corner of your eye, but not when you look directly at the screen?

4 From the information given above on the structure and functioning of the eye, decide which of the features in Fig. 5.34 are concerned with light detection in the eye, and which are concerned with allowing the light sensitive cells of the retina to operate to their maximum efficiency.

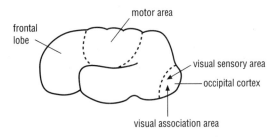

Figure 5.39   The position of the occipital cortex on the cerebral hemisphere

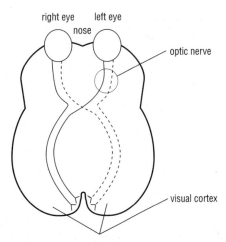

Figure 5.40   The pathway for impulses from the eyes to the visual cortex in the brain

THE MECHANISM OF HEARING

The ear is responsible for receiving the stimulus of sound waves, and for converting these sound waves into nerve impulses. Sound travels as waves consisting of alternating regions of high and low pressure. The *wavelength* is the time interval between each wave, and is measured in *hertz* (Hz). The shorter the wavelength, the higher the *pitch* of a sound. Our ears are sensitive to sounds between approximately 20 and 23,000 Hz.

The *loudness* or intensity of sound is determined by the amplitude of each wave. This is measured in decibels (dB). (See Figure 3.23 on p. 151 of Chapter 3.)

ACTIVITY 47

1 Look at Figure 5.41. Compare sound waves (a) and (b). Which gives the higher pitch? Compare sound waves (c) and (d). Which gives the loudest noise?

2 Hearing deteriorates with age, and it is usually the high frequencies which are lost first. If you have access to an oscillator, amplifier and loudspeaker, compare the range of frequencies different people can hear. Start with a

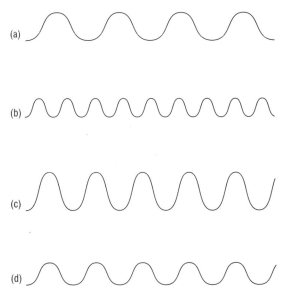

Figure 5.41   Examples of sound waves

high frequency of about 25 kHz, and gradually lower it until your subject indicates that they can hear a sound. Test people of various ages, and see if you find a correlation between age and highest frequency heard.

3 If a sound meter is available to you, investigate the level of sound as you move away from a busy main road. Find out about the legislation specifying the limits of exposure to sound in the workplace.

The structure of the ear is shown in Figure 5.42. It consists of the *outer*, *middle* and *inner* ear.

The outer ear consists of the *pinna* which funnels sound waves into the ear tube. The sound waves cause the *eardrum (tympanic membrane)* to vibrate.

In the middle ear, these vibrations cause the movement of the *middle ear ossicles*, the hammer, the anvil and the stirrup. The stirrup is connected to the *oval window* which thus vibrates (since the area of the oval window is about one-twentieth of that of the eardrum, the vibrations are amplified). The middle ear is air-filled, and it is therefore essential that the pressure within it be kept equal to that of the atmosphere. This is achieved by the *eustachian tube* which connects the middle ear to the pharynx.

The inner ear consists of an elaborate set of fluid-filled tubes embedded in the hardest

bone of the body. The part of this system concerned with hearing is the coiled *cochlea* (from the Latin for 'snail') (see Figure 5.43a). This is subdivided longitudinally into three canals (see Figure 5.43b). The upper and lower canals, which are filled with a liquid known as *perilymph*, are connected to form the upper and lower portions of a long hairpin bend (see Figure 5.43c). As the oval window vibrates, it pushes the perilymph in the upper canal. This pressure wave continues into the lower canal and causes similar displacements of the *round window*. It is thought that these pressure waves lead to movements of the membrane between the upper and lower chambers (*Reissner's membrane*), which in turn leads to movements of the *endolymph* in the central canal (see Figure 5.43b). This causes movements of the *basilar membrane* which is quite elastic. The *tectonial membrane*, by contrast, is more rigid, and so remains relatively fixed. Between these two membranes are sensory hair cells which become distorted. This sets up an action potential which is conveyed to the brain along a branch of the *auditory nerve*.

It appears that different pitches stimulate hairs in different regions of the cochlea. A low pitch stimulates hairs near the apex, and a high pitch stimulates hairs nearer to the round window. The number of hairs stimulated depends on the intensity of the sound. A loud sound stimulates more hairs than a quiet one.

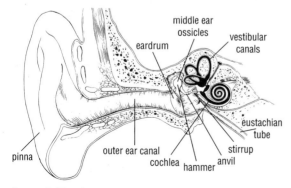

Figure 5.42 A cross-section of the outer, middle and inner ear

ACTIVITY 48

1 Investigate the range of hearing aids available. How do they work? What can you find out about *cochlea implants*?

2 Read the following article (by Dr Tony Smith):

COMMON COMPLAINTS

Earache
Earache mostly affects small children, swimmers and air travellers, but no one is

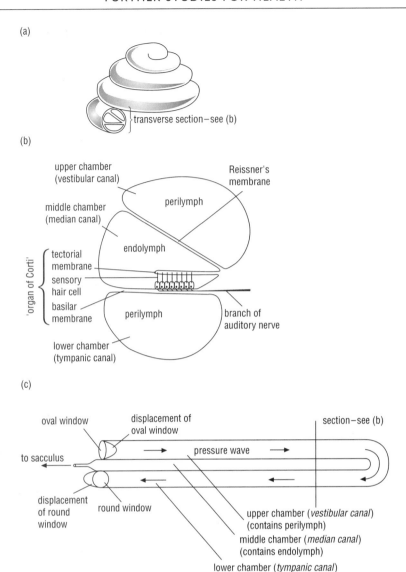

Figure 5.43 The structure of the cochlea: (a) the spiral shape of the cochlea; (b) a transverse section through the cochlea; (c) a diagrammatic section through an 'unwound' cochlea
Source: Stanley Thornes (Publishers) Ltd, *Understanding Biology for Advanced Level*, 2nd edition.

immune. Pain in the ear is peculiarly frustrating since ears are one of the least accessible parts of the body. We cannot peer at them in the mirror to see if they look odd or (fortunately) poke at any discomfort. Even the doctor who looks down the canal through a lighted funnel, the otoscope, can only inspect the outer surface of the eardrum; the working parts of the ears are internal organs . . .

Children get a lot of earache because they get a lot of throat infections, and the bacteria can easily find their way along the Eustachian tube and into the middle ear. Otitis media (inflammation of the middle ear) causes severe pain and a fever: if the child is too young to be able to say that his ear hurts, he will pull and rub at it. If no treatment is given the eardrum ruptures, releasing pus and easing the pain. This may be prevented by prompt administration of antibiotics.

A lot of children get repeated attacks and

some become deaf for months or years because the ear becomes filled with a sticky fluid – glue ear. Tiny drainage tubes called grommets are often inserted into the eardrum with variable results. In time, however, children have fewer throat infections, and as their heads get bigger the Eustachian tube gets longer and seems to provide better protection.

A painful ear in an adult is most likely to be due to inflammation of the external passage way, otitis externa; this is common in swimmers, since water softens the skin and makes it more vulnerable to infection. Swimming in polluted water and then pushing a dirty towel into the ear canal is almost guaranteed to cause an attack. A boil in the ear canal is very painful, because the skin cannot easily stretch. External ear infections are usually straightforward to treat.

Air travellers get pain if their ears cannot adjust to the air pressure in the middle ear cavity as the cabin pressure falls after take-off and then rises again as the aircraft comes in to land. This adjustment should happen automatically via the Eustachian tube; but if the tube is blocked or narrowed by a cold or by hay fever, repeated swallowing may be needed to encourage air to flow along the tube. If this doesn't work the stuffed-up passenger should pinch his nose between finger and thumb and then blow hard down the nose. This trick – Valsalva's manoeuvre – is a useful one. If you know you get ear problems when you fly, you should do it repeatedly as soon as you feel any fullness in the ears; if it is left too late the ear may stay blocked for hours.

(The Independent on Sunday, 14 April 1991)

If possible, interview an audiologist from your local clinic to find out more about how they diagnose and treat hearing disorders.

The mechanism of balance

Within the inner ear, just above the cochlea, is the *vestibular apparatus* (see Figure 5.44). This consists of two fluid-filled sacs called the *utricle* and the *saccule*. Connected to the top of the utricle are three semi-circular canals. Each of the three canals are arranged in a plane at right angles to the other two. When the head moves, this results in the movement of the semi-circular canals. However, the movement of the liquid within the canals lags behind, resulting in a relative movement between the canals and the liquid within them. The end of each of the canals is enlarged to form an *ampulla*. Within this is a flat gelatinous plate, the *cupula* (see Figure 5.45). The movement of the liquid displaces the cupula which is attached to sensory hairs. These detect the displacement and send impulses to the brain via the *vestibular nerve*.

The vestibular apparatus also aids balance by providing information about the position of the body relative to gravity. Within the utricle and saccule are chalk granules known as *otoliths*. These are embedded in a jelly-like material, and are attached to sensory hairs. Gravity causes the otoliths to pull on the sensory hairs, and this produces nerve impulses which pass along the vestibular nerve. If the head is moved to a different position, the otoliths pull the sensory hairs in a different direction, and the information from this can be interpreted in the brain.

Although the ear plays a vital part in balance, it should also be appreciated that there are receptors in the joints and muscles which provide the brain with essential information, and that visual information from the eyes also contributes information used to coordinate the movement and posture of the body.

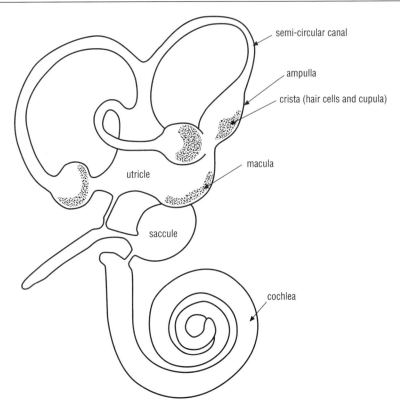

Figure 5.44   The vestibular apparatus
Source: Advanced Human Biology, Simpkins and Williams, Chapman and Hall, 1987.

ASSESSMENT OPPORTUNITY

Produce a report on an investigation into sensory and communication systems within the body, which includes:

- an explanation of the role of the endocrine system in communication
- an explanation of how hormones cause responses in cells
- a description of the nerve cell and its impulse
- an explanation of how the nervous system brings about communication
- a description, with annotated diagrams, of the structure and function of the eye
- a description, with annotated diagrams, of the structure and function of the ear

NB: you could work in pairs for this investigation and feed back information to one another to produce a joint project. (For example, one of the pair could investigate the eye, and the other the ear.) You should then produce an individual report on the investigation.

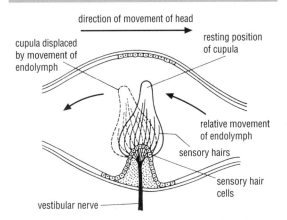

Figure 5.45   A section through the ampulla of a semi-circular canal
Source: Stanley Thornes (Publishers) Ltd,
Understanding Biology for Advanced Level, 2nd edition.

REFERENCES AND RESOURCES

It is assumed that the mandatory unit 'Health and social well-being' will have been completed prior to this unit. Information covering this mandatory unit can be found in Thomson et al. (1995) *Health and Social Care* (2nd edition), Chapter 3.

Any standard A-level biology or human-biology texts will be useful for further reading and research. Some of these are listed below:

Green, N. P. O., Stout, G. W. and Taylor, D. J. (1985); more recent editions available, *Biological Science*, Cambridge: Cambridge University Press.

Simpkins, J. and Williams, J. I. (1987), *Advanced Human Biology*, London: Chapman and Hall.

Toole, G. and Toole, S. (1991), *Understanding Biology for Advanced Level*, Cheltenham: Stanley Thornes Ltd.

There are also more specialised books available which, although they are aimed at students on higher-education courses, may be useful sources of reference. For example:

Tortora, G. and Anagnostakos, N. (1987), *Principles of Anatomy and Physiology*, New York: Harper and Row.

INDEX

α particles 230
acceleration 192–3
accidents 67, 72–3, 93
acetylcholine 271
acid rain 76, 104–5
acid/base balance 20–1
acids 17–18
    excretion by kidneys 22–3
action potential 270
active transport 251
adenine 49, 52
adenosine triphosphate (ATP) 15, 16, 32, 49, 264
adipose tissue 37, 264
adrenal glands 39, 253, 268
adrenalin 81, 268
ageing, diseases of 148, 150
agriculture
    intensive 90–1
    pollution 82, 83, 84
AIDS/HIV 69, 70, 71, 116, 131–33, 135
air 76
    pollution 103–4, 118–19
airborne diseases 159
alcohol 116
alcohol abuse 158
aldosterone 253, 268–9
algae 83
alimentary canal 29, 256–65
    regional structure 258
alkalis (bases) 18
allergies 65, 156, 175
alternating currents (AC) 214–15
aluminium 102, 150
    poisoning 83, 101
Alzheimer's disease 83, 150
amino acids 21, 40, 41, 254, 260
    absorption by gut 261
    breakdown of 250
    genetic code for 52, 53
ammonia 18, 20, 23, 83, 91
amniotic fluid 201
amphoteric substances 40
ampulla 281, 282
amylase 46, 48, 260
amylopectin 34–5
amylose 34–5
anabolism 10, 16
anaerobic respiration 14, 15
angiotensin 253
animal fats 36, 37–8, 39
anions 7
anorexia nervosa 155–6

antibiotics 44, 168
    resistance 69
antibodies 156, 164–5
antidiuretic hormone (ADH) 252, 253, 268
antigens 164–6
Archimedes' principle 206
arteries 39, 242, 244, 245
arthritis 116, 150
asbestos 97, 101, 154
asthma 54, 97, 156
atheroma 148
atherosclerosis 39, 148, 150, 156, 207
atmosphere 76
atomic forces 7–10
atomic number 5–6
atoms/atomic structure 2–3, 5, 229
atrioventricular (AV) node 239, 240
auditory nerve 279, 280
autonomic nervous system 272
Avogadro's constant 2

β particles 6–7, 230
back injuries 62, 67, 151
bacteria 70, 82, 107, 139, 140–1
    in eutrophication 83
    main types of 141
    see also food poisoning
balance and the ear 281–2
base pairing 49, 52
bases (alkalis) 18
basophils 241
Benedict's solution 32–3
beri-beri 256
bile 39, 259, 260
bilharzia 147
binary fission 141
biological control 109
biological oxygen demand (BOD) 83
birth defects 91, 124–5, 152
blood
    carbon dioxide transport 4, 22, 30–1, 246–7
    circulation of 242–3
    clotting 161, 163
    components 241
    control of sugar in 266–7, 268
    measurement of flow 206–9
    oxygen transport 4, 30–1, 243–6
blood pressure 150, 156, 181, 242
body mass index (BMI) 154–5
body scanning 223, 225
boiling 13
bowel disorders 255
Bowman's capsule 248–9, 250

Boyle's law 202–3
brain 269, 271–2, 277, 278
breast cancer 116, 137, 223
breathing mechanism 203–4
British Medical Association 72
Brownian motion 12
buffers
    chemical 20–2
    thermal 28–9
building legislation 109, 111–12
bundle of His 239, 240
buoyancy 205–6

caesium, radioactive 98
Camelford water incident 101
canaliculi 259
cancer 116
    detection of 26, 223, 224
    environmental causes 91, 97, 99–100, 101, 153, 154
    epidemiology of 128–9
    and lifestyle 116, 157, 265
    world distribution 137
capacitors 214
capillaries 242, 244, 245
car-exhausts see vehicle pollution
carbaminohaemoglobin 246
carbohydrates 29, 264
    breakdown of 260
    in diet 254, 255
    structure 28, 32–6
carbon 5, 6, 7–8, 9
carbon dioxide 8, 15, 16, 76
    in acid formation 4, 17, 20, 22–3, 247
    and combustion 29
    excretion 22
    pollution 78–9, 118–19
    solubility of 28, 30
    transport in blood 4, 22, 30–1, 246–7
carbon monoxide 76, 80, 97, 150
carbonic acid 4, 17, 20, 22–3, 247
carbonic anhydrase 22, 247
carcinogens 153
cardiac cycle 237–9
cardio-inhibitory centre 240
cardiovascular system 237–47
    diseases of 116, 129–31, 135, 156, 182, 254
CAT scanning 223, 225
catabolism 10, 16
catalase 43, 45
catalysis 16, 42
catalytic converters 104
catheters 190, 207
cathode ray tube 215, 216
cations 7
cell membranes 38, 39
cellular repair/growth 264
cellulose 32, 35–6, 255, 265
censuses 127
central nervous system (CNS) 269, 271–2
Centre of Communicable Diseases 72
cerebrospinal fluid (CSF) 201
cervical cancer 116, 137
charge
    atomic 5, 9
    electrostatic 209–10
    ionic 7
Charles's law 203
chemical science 1–57
    chemical basis for life 27–52
    chemical structures 1–10

physical chemistry 12–14
physiological chemical reactions 10–12, 14–17
chemicals
    in disease treatment 168–9
    working with 53–4, 63, 65
Chernobyl disaster 98–9
chitin 36
chloride ions 251
chloride shift 22, 247
chlorine 6, 7, 9–10
chlorofluorocarbons (CFCs) 79
cholera 82, 134–5, 141, 142, 159
cholesterol 39, 130, 148, 150, 156
chromatography 23–4, 25
chromosomes 49–50
    abnormalities 151
cigarettes see smoking
circulatory system 242–7
Clean Air Acts 103, 104
climate, and disease 135–6, 137
Clostridium 69, 71, 143, 144, 145
coal mining 101
cochlea 279, 280
collagen 41
collecting ducts 249, 252
colloids 29
colour blindness 277
combustion 10, 29–30
communication/sensory systems 265–73
compounds 1–2
condensation (of water) 13, 14, 16–17
condensation reactions 11, 33, 37
conduction (heat) 234
conductors, electrical 210
cones 275, 276–7
congenital disorders 91, 124–5, 152
contact tracing 170
contagious diseases 158–9
contrast media techniques 223, 224
Control of Substances Hazardous to Health (COSHH) Regulation
    52, 65
convection (heat) 234, 235
convoluted tubules 22–3, 248, 249, 251
Coulomb's law 209–10
council housing 109–10
counter-current multiplier 251, 252
covalent bonding 7–8
crop rotation 108
Crypts of Lieberkühn 258, 261
culture and health 178–9
cupula 281, 282
cysteine 52
cytochromes 15
cytoplasm 28, 29, 49
cytosine 49, 52

DDT 84, 91
defibrillation 214, 215
deficiency diseases 176–7, 256
deforestation 90
degenerative diseases 116, 148, 149–50
demographic trends 91–2
denaturation 44, 47, 48
density 205
deoxyribonucleic acid see DNA
dermatitis 151
detergent pollution 84
development of countries and disease 135, 136, 137
diarrhoeal diseases 124, 134, 135, 142
diastole 237, 238–9

diathermy 223
diet 38, 116, 130, 175–7
  healthy 254–6
dietary diseases 154–6
digestion 11, 259–64
  enzymes of 11, 43, 48
  use of products of 264–5
dioxan 91
dipeptides 40
diphtheria 71, 166
direct currents (DC) 214
disaccharides 32, 33, 254
disease
  bodily responses to 179–85
  causes and controlling factors 138–58
  control and prevention of 69–73, 160–71
  modes of transmission 70–2, 125, 158–60
  patterns of 123–38
    influences on 135–8
    national/worldwide distribution 128–35
    sources of information in 127–8
  socioeconomic factors affecting 171–9
diuretics 253
DNA (deoxyribonucleic acid) 49–52, 53
  fingerprinting 25–6
Doppler ultrasound 207–9
double bonds 11
droplet infection 158
drug abuse 158
duodenum 258, 260, 261
dysentery 94, 142, 159

ear 278–82
egestion 264–5
eggs 49–50
ego defence mechanisms 183, 184
electricity 209–15
  formula triangles 216
electrocardiograph 215, 217
electroencephalograph 215
electrolytes 18
electromagnetic fields/waves 218–31
  medical applications 221–31
  safety procedures 226
  spectrum 221
electron gun 228–9
electron microscopes 228–9
electron transfer system 15
electrons 5, 6, 7, 8, 14, 209
electrophoresis 24–6
electrostatic forces 209–10
elements 1
employers, safety at work 52, 61–73
endemics 142
endocrine system 265–9
energy 194–5
Entamoeba histolytica 82
environment and health
  and disease patterns 136–8
  environmental health provision 58–73
  harmful effects on 75–102
  reducing harm to 103–20
  socioeconomic influences on 74–5
environmental diseases 153–4
environmental poverty 74, 93–4
environmental pressure groups 74, 120
Environmental Protection Act (1990) 103–4, 105, 112
enzymes 10, 16–17, 41, 42
  classes of 48–9
  of digestion 260–1

factors affecting activity 45–8
  inhibitors 43–5
eosinophils 241
epidemics 139, 142
epidemiology 123–38
equilibria, chemical 17
equilibrium (of physical forces) 189–90
ergonomics 67
essential fatty acids 38
ethnic minorities 172–3, 178
European Commission 67, 119
European Community (EC) 59, 61, 67, 75, 117
eutrophication 83, 84
evaporation 13–14
excretion 249–51, 264–5
exercise 116
expenditure and health 171–2
eye 274–8
  functioning of rods and cones 277

Factories Act (1961) 61
farming, organic 108–9
fats see lipids
fatty acids 16, 36, 37, 38, 260
  absorption by gut 262
feedback mechanisms 266–7
fertilisers 79, 83–4, 91, 108, 138
fibre 36, 255, 265
fibroin 41
Fire Precautions Act (1971) 60–1
flies 72
flow, liquid 206
fluid mechanics 200–9
fluoride 106, 177
foetal abnormalities 91, 124–5
food
  allergies 156
  composition of 255
  contamination of 82, 83, 159
  energy in 195
  hygiene/safety 58–60, 71
food poisoning 58, 70, 71, 116, 133, 142–6
Food Safety Act (1990) 58–9
forces
  atomic 7–10
  in physics 189
formulas 2
fossil fuels 29, 76–8, 97, 104
freezing 13
friction 189–90
Friends of the Earth 74, 75, 95, 120
fructose 9, 33, 36
fungi 70, 139, 146
fuses 214
fusion 233

galactose 33, 36
gamma rays 6–7, 221, 226, 230, 231
gas gangrene 143
gases 4, 12–14, 200, 233
  gas laws 202–3
gastric juice 20, 260
gene therapy 169
genes 50
genetic code 52
genetic diseases 151–2, 160, 169
  screening for 24–6
glaucoma 201
global warming 79–80, 118–19
globular proteins 41–2

glomerulus 248, 250, 251, 252
glucose 9, 33–5, 254, 260, 264
    absorption by gut 261
    condensation/hydrolysis reactions 11, 16, 33
    control of blood level 266–7, 268
    oxidation 10–11, 14, 15
glycerol 16, 37, 38, 260, 262
glycogen 34, 254, 264
    in blood sugar control 266–7, 268
glycolysis 15
glycosidic bonds 16, 34, 35–6
gravity 189
greenhouse effect 79–80, 118–19
Greenpeace 74, 119, 120
growth, cellular 264
guanine 49

habitat destruction 90–1
haemoglobin 21–2, 40, 42
    abnormal forms of 24–5
    and carbon monoxide 80
    oxygen transport 30–1, 243–6
health
    defined 138–9
    reducing harm from pollution 103–20
    socioeconomic factors affecting 171–9
    see also diseases; environment
Health, Department of 58, 73, 127
health education 116, 125, 170–1, 177
health promotion 126, 171
health and safety at work 119
    Health and Safety at Work Act (1974) 52, 61–4, 68, 103,
        114
    Health and Safety Commission 61, 63, 65
    Health and Safety Executive 66, 67, 72, 100
    Health and Safety (First Aid) Regulations (1981) 66
hearing 88, 278–82
    damage to 151
heart
    defibrillation 214, 215
    structure and action of 237–40
heart disease 116, 129–31, 135, 156, 182
heat
    loss 234–5
    pollution 84
    transfer 234–5
Heat of Combustion 195
heavy metals 44, 58, 82–3, 91, 101
hemicelluloses 35–6
hepatic arteries/veins 257–8, 261
hepatitis viruses 69, 70, 72, 94, 123
Hiroshima nuclear explosion 99
homelessness 110
homeostasis 266
hormone replacement therapies 168–9
hormones 42, 265–9
housing 93–4, 116, 174–5
    legislation 109–11
human immunodeficiency virus (HIV) see AIDS
hydraulic press 199, 200
hydrochloric acid 17, 160, 260
hydrogen 1–3
    atom 5, 7–8, 28
    in electron transport 15
    ions 17, 18, 21
hydrogen bonds 9, 28, 41, 46–8, 49
hydrogen carbonate 21, 22, 246–7
hydrolysis 11, 48
hydrophilic/hydrophobic molecules 38
hydroxides 18

hygiene 69–73, 169
hypothalamus 181, 252, 265, 268

ileum 261
immune system/immunity 164–6
immunization 165–7
inclined plane 198, 199
income and health 171–4
industry
    safety in 61–3
    waste pollution 76, 82–3, 100–2, 153
infection and control 69–73
infectious diseases 139–48
inflammatory response 163, 164
influenza virus 139–40, 165
infrared radiation 76, 221, 223, 235
inherited diseases see genetic diseases
inorganic salts 256, 262
insecticides 45, 84, 91
insulators 210
insulin 2, 40, 41, 268
intermediate neurones 269, 270
intermolecular forces 9, 13–14
intravenous fluid administration 191, 192
inulin 36
iodine 176–7
    radioactive 98–9
iodopsin 276, 277
ionic bonding 7, 41
ionic molecules 28
ionisation 7, 17–18
iron 10, 30, 40
    deficiency in diet 177
isomers 9
isotopes 6–7

keratin 41, 160
kidneys 264
    and pH regulation 22–3
    structure of 247–53
kinetic energy 194
kinetic theory 12–13, 200
Krebs cycle 15, 20

laboratory safety 52–6
lactic acid 14, 15, 16
lactose 33
landfill sites 83, 101, 112, 113
large intestine 258, 262
lasers 226–7
latent heat 14, 233
lead 58, 80–1, 83, 97, 104, 154
lean burn engines 104
leukaemia 99, 100, 138, 153, 157
lever systems 196–8
lifestyle, and health/disease 116, 170
lifting 189, 190
light, visible 221
lignin 36
lipids 32, 36–9, 254–5, 260, 264
liquids 4, 10, 12–14, 200, 233
liver 18, 20, 34, 266–7
    structure 257, 259
Local Authority Plans 120
Local Government and Housing Act (1989) 109, 111
loop of Henlé 249, 251, 252
low density lipoproteins (LDLs) 39, 148
lung cancer 101, 128–9, 137, 138, 154, 157
lungs 21
    breathing mechanism 203–4

oxygen partial pressure 30–1
luteinizing hormone 267
lymphatic vessels 261
lymphocytes 164–5, 241

machines 196–9
magnetic resonance imaging (MRI) 231
magnets/magnetic fields 217–18
malaria 71, 72, 133, 134, 138, 146
maltose 11, 16, 33, 34, 254
mammography 223
mannose 9
manometers 201, 202
manual handling 189, 190
Manual Operations Handling Regulations (1992) 67–8
marine pollution 82, 83, 84, 87
mass 188
mass number 6
mass spectrometer 219, 220
measles 135, 165, 166, 167, 174
mechanics in care context 188–209
medical imaging techniques 221–3, 224–5
meiosis 49–50
melanoma 128
melting 13, 233
mental disorders 152–3
mercury 58, 83, 91, 101
metabolism 10
methane 7–8, 79, 83, 84, 101
methicillin-resistant *Staphylococcus aureus* (MRSA) 69, 70
microscopy 227–9
microwaves 221
minerals in diet 256, 262
Ministry of Agriculture, Fisheries and Food 58
mitosis 49
MMR vaccine 167
molar solutions 4–5
molecules 2
moles 2
monocytes 241
monosaccharides 32, 49, 254
mosquitoes 72, 138, 146
motor neurones 269, 270
motors 219
mucous membranes 160
mucus 29, 32, 36
mumps vaccine 165, 167
myalgic encephalitis (ME) 182–3

National Rivers Authority (NRA) 105
negative feedback 266–7
nematodes 139, 147–8, 149
nephrons 22–3, 247–53
nervous system 265
    impulses 270–1
    neurones 269, 270, 271
    organisation of 271–3
neurotransmitters 271
neutrons 5, 6
neutrophils 164, 241
Newton's Laws of Motion 193
nicotinamide adenine dinucleotide (NAD) 15
nitrates 83, 91, 105
nitrogen 30, 39, 76
nitrogen oxides 76, 79, 80, 95–7
noise 114, 115, 150–1
    pollution 88–9
nosocomial infections 70
notifiable diseases 73, 170
nuclear installations 63, 98–101, 138, 153

nucleic acids 24, 25–6, 49–52, 53
nucleotides 49
nucleus, atomic 5
nucleus, cellular 10, 49
nutrients, processing/transport 254–65

obesity 154–5, 156
occupational diseases 150–1
oesophagus 258, 260
Office of Population Censuses and Surveys (OPCS) 127
Offices, Shops and Railway Premises Act (1963) 61
Ohm's law 212
oil pollution 84
onchocerciasis 147–9
opsin 277
optic nerve 274, 275, 278
oral rehydration salts (ORS) 142, 143
organic farming 108–9
organic molecules 7
oscilloscope 215–17
osmoregulation 252–3
osteoporosis 150
overcrowding 110
oxidation 10–11, 14
oxides 10, 29
oxygen 14, 29, 76
    atomic structure 5, 7
    solubility of 28, 30
    transport in blood 4, 30–1, 243–6
oxyhaemoglobin 30–1, 244
oxytocin 267
ozone layer 76, 79–80
ozone pollution 79, 96, 97

pancreas 259–60, 267, 268
pandemics 139
parasites 139
parasympathetic nervous system 272–3
partial pressure 30–1, 244
particles, properties of 220–31
particulate pollution 97
pathogens 63, 139
pectin 36
pepsin 43, 48, 261
peptide bonds 21, 40, 254
peristalsis 36, 260
pernicious anaemia 256
pesticides 45, 84, 91, 108, 138
pH 17, 18–19
    biological importance of 20–3
    effect on enzyme catalysis 47–8
phagocytosis 163–4, 165
pharmaceuticals 168–9
phobias 152–3
phosphatase 43, 48
phosphates 83, 84, 91
phospholipids 36, 38, 39
photoreceptors 275
photosensitive pigments 277
photosynthesis 32, 254
    and pollution 76, 79
physical chemistry 12–14
physical science 188–236
physiology 237–83
    chemical reactions in 10–11
    physical chemistry and 12–14
physiotherapy 221, 223
pituitary gland 252, 265, 268
plant oils 36, 37–8, 254
plasma 21, 22, 29, 241

Plasmodium 146
platelets 148, 161, 162, 241
platyhelminthes 139, 147
pleural effusion 203
pneumonia 140, 141
polar molecules 9, 28
poliomyelitis 82, 135, 165, 166
pollution 74, 75–89, 93
   and disease 137–8
   reducing harm from 103–20
polychlorinated biphenyls (PCBs) 102
polymers 34, 49
polypeptides 9, 40, 41, 54, 254
polysaccharides 29, 32, 34–6, 254
population density 91–2
populations, disease patterns in 123–38
porphyrin molecules 30
positive feedback 267
potential difference 211
potential energy 194
poverty 172–3, 174
power
   electrical 213
   mechanical 196
pressure 200
   gas law 203
   measurement of 201–2
Project MONICA 129–30
proteins
   breakdown of 260
   in diet 254, 255
   separation of 24–5
   structure and functions 9, 21, 29, 39–42
   synthesis of 16, 51–2, 53
proteoglycans 29, 32, 36
protons 5–6, 15, 209
protozoa 82, 107, 139, 146
Pseudomonas aeruginosa 70
psychosomatic disorders 182
public health 125–6
pulse 206–7, 208
purines 49
Purkinje tissue 239, 240
pyrimadines 49
pyruvic acid 14, 15, 16

radiation (heat) 234, 235
radio waves 220–1
radioactive waste 76, 98–101, 153
radioactivity
   medical uses of 231
   types of 229–31
radiography 221–3
radioisotopes 6–7, 230–1
radiotherapy 153, 231
radon 138
rail companies 112–13
rain forests 90
rats 94
recycling 74, 108
red blood cells (erythrocytes) 22, 241, 244
redox reactions 11, 14, 15
reducing sugars 32–3
reduction 11, 14, 15
reflex arc 269, 270
relative atomic mass (RAM) 2, 6
renin 253
repair, cellular 264
repair mechanisms 160–4
repetitive strain injury (RSI) 150

replacement therapies 168–9
Reporting of Injuries, Diseases and Dangerous Occurrences
   Regulations (1985) 67, 72
resistance, electrical 213
respiration, cellular 11, 14–16, 32, 48, 264
respirators 203, 205
respiratory diseases 29, 76–7, 95, 97
retina 274, 275, 276–7
rheumatism 150
rhodopsin 274, 276
ribonucleic acid *see* RNA
rickets 256
river blindness 147–9
RNA (ribonucleic acid) 49, 51–3
rods 275, 276–7
roughage 36, 255, 265
rubella 140, 165, 167
rusting 10

safety at work *see* health and safety
safety in the laboratory 52–6
salmonella 70, 71, 72, 133, 144, 145
salts 17, 18, 28
sanitation 116, 159
saturated fatty acids 36, 39, 254–5
scalar quantities 191
schistosoma 147, 148
scurvy 256
sea, pollution of 82, 83, 84, 87
sebum 38, 160
Sellafield nuclear plant 98, 100
semi-circular canals 281, 282
sensory neurones 269, 270
sensory/communication systems 265–73
separation techniques 23–7
sewage 82, 83–4, 85, 106–8, 169
sexually transmitted diseases 71, 158
sharps 71, 72
sickle-cell anaemia 24–5
sino-atrial (SA) node 239, 240
skin
   as barrier to disease 160, 161
   disorders 182
   repair mechanisms 160–4
skin cancer 116, 124, 128
small intestine 258, 260–1
smog 77–8, 80, 104
smoke pollution 76
smoking 80, 116, 138, 150, 153, 157–8
social class 173, 177
Social Security, Department of 58
sodium 6, 7, 9–10, 23
   ions 251
   regulation in blood 253
sodium chloride 7, 18, 28, 247, 256
   absorption by gut 262
sodium-potassium exchange pump 270
soil erosion 90–1
solids 10, 12–13, 200, 233
solutes/solutions 4
solvent abuse 158
solvents 4
sound waves 278
specific gravity 206
specific heat capacity 28, 232
specific latent heat 233
speed 191
sperm 49–50
sphygmomanometer 202
spina bifida 124–5

spinal cord 269, 270, 271–2
Staphylococcus 69, 70, 141, 144
starch 16, 34–5, 46, 254
states of matter 12–14, 233
static electricity 209–10
sterilisation (of instruments) 225
steroids 36, 38–9
stomach 258, 260, 261, 262, 265
storage in body 264
stress 116, 180–5
strokes 157
strontium-90 98
structural formulas 8, 9
sucrase 45, 48
sucrose 33, 34, 45, 254
sugars *see* carbohydrates
sulphur dioxide pollution 96, 97, 104
surveys 127
sympathetic nervous system 272–3
synapses 271
synovial fluid 29
Systeme International (SI) units 188
systole 237

tapeworms 147
tears 29, 160
temperature 232
    and enzyme activity 43, 46–7
    and kinetic theory 12–13
    stabilisation of body 28
testicular cancer 116
tetanus 135, 166, 174
thermal buffering 28–9
thermal pollution 84
thermionic emission 215
thermodynamics 232–5
thermography 224, 225
thymine 49
thyroid gland and thyroxine 268
toxic substances 63, 65, 82
toxic waste *see* health and safety; pollution
toxins, bacterial 143
toxoids 166
tracers, radioactive 7, 231
traction 193
transcription 51
transport legislation 112–14
tri-carboxylic acid cycle 15
triglycerides 37, 39
tripeptides 40
tropical diseases 159
tuberculosis (TB) 131–2, 135, 175
    transmission 71, 72
    vaccine 165, 166
typhoid 70, 141
    case study 145–6
    in food/water 58, 71, 82, 159
    vaccine 165, 167

ulcers 116, 174, 182
ultrasound 207–9
ultraviolet radiation 221

and skin cancer 116, 128, 153
and vitamin D production 223, 225
unemployment 172, 174
unsaturated fatty acids 36, 39, 254–5
uracil 49, 52
uranium 5, 99
urbanisation 92–3, 94, 109–15
urea 250, 251, 264
urinary system 20, 23, 247, 249–51

vaccination 72, 125, 165–7
valency 9–10
vaporisation 14, 233
vasodilation/vasoconstriction 243
VDU screens 119–20
vector quantities 191
vectorborne disease 70, 72, 136, 159
vehicle pollution 76, 79, 80, 104, 118
    and health 95–7
veins 242, 244, 245
velocity 191, 192, 193
ventilators 203, 205
vestibular apparatus 281–2
villi 257, 259, 262
viruses 58, 70, 139–40
viscosity 29, 190
vitamins 262
    deficiencies 177, 223, 225, 256
    storage of 38, 264
voltage 211

waste 98–102
    collection/disposal 112
    see also industry; pollution
water
    absorption by gut 262
    biological importance of 27–9
    chemistry of 2, 3, 4, 10, 18
        bonding 7, 9
        evaporation/condensation 13–14
    as heat buffer 232–3
    need for clean 82–3, 94, 169
    pollution of 82–7, 105–8
    reabsorption by kidney 251, 252, 253
    and spread of disease 142, 145, 159
    treatment of 105–6
water legislation 105, 106
wavelength 278
waves, properties of 220–31
waxes 36, 38
weight 189
white blood cells (leucocytes) 164, 241
work (in physics) 193
World Health Organization (WHO) 74, 117, 174
    definition of health 138
    epidemiological information 127–8, 129
worms 82, 139, 147–9

X-rays 153, 221, 226, 230–1
    in diagnosis/screening 207, 222–3, 224